Applied Behavior Analysis

Kimberly Maich
Darren Levine
Carmen Hall

Applied Behavior Analysis

Fifty Case Studies in Home, School,
and Community Settings

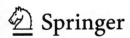 Springer

Kimberly Maich
Department of Teacher Education
Brock University
St. Catharines, ON
Canada

Darren Levine
Brock University
St. Catharines, ON
Canada

Carmen Hall
Fanshawe College
London, ON
Canada

ISBN 978-3-319-44792-6   ISBN 978-3-319-44794-0   (eBook)
DOI 10.1007/978-3-319-44794-0

Library of Congress Control Number: 2016949108

Printed on acid-free paper

This Springer imprint is published by Springer Nature
The registered company is Springer International Publishing AG
The registered company address is: Gewerbestrasse 11, 6330 Cham, Switzerland

Preface

Applying the Science of Behavior Across the Life span

The purpose of this publication is to provide ready-to-use case studies to accompany current academic textbooks and field training materials used by students and professionals studying, teaching, and working in the field of Applied Behavior Analysis (ABA). Through 50 case studies, learners are provided opportunities to apply ABA principles, processes, and practices to a range of scenarios across the life span. These scenarios offer a simulated platform for learners to design, implement, and evaluate behavior-change programs for children, adolescents, adults, and seniors across a range of home, school, and community settings.

The case studies within this work reflect the field experience of the authors as well as that of the academic faculty, field-based professionals, and students that contributed to the development of this valuable resource. Each case encourages users to reflect on, and think critically about, selected concepts and principles of ABA. When combined, the 50 cases within this text guide learners through the phases of behavior-analytic practice—from assessment and planning through implementation and evaluation—while offering a range of research and ethical considerations central to the science and practice of behavior analysis.

Supporting a Multidisciplinary Scientist-Practitioner Perspective

The cases offered challenge users to consider how to address complex behavior difficulties from the perspective of a scientist-practitioner (Hayes et al. 1999), giving consideration to evidence-informed practice, measurement and evaluation, and the production of new knowledge and understanding obtained through the delivery of services. Learners are guided, as well, to consider the interplay of biological, psychological, and social variables, while developing prevention, skill building, and intervention components of behavior-change programs. The case studies presented in this text further encourage learners to reflect on technical, interpersonal, and leadership challenges and opportunities associated with the translation of scientific principles into effective behavior-change programs.

Emphasizing Each Phase of Behavior-Analytic Practice

This publication is comprised of five parts: assessment, planning, implementation, evaluation, and research and ethics. Each part is subdivided into chapters focusing on either preschool to school-age or adolescence to adulthood. Each chapter is then made up of five cases, each with a unique focus and setting, supported by a guiding learning objective, Behavior Analyst Certification Board (BACB) task list links and Professional and Ethical Compliance Code, key terms, application and reflection questions, and links to Web-based resources.

A Valuable Resource for Both Academic- and Field-Based Professionals

This text offers a valuable ready-to-use resource for academic- and field-based professionals. The wide range of cases provided across the life span offer applied learning and professional development opportunities for students and practitioners in a multitude of disciplines. Examples include ABA, special education, disability studies, early childhood education, primary and secondary education, gerontology, and organizational behavior management.

Within academic contexts, these case studies offer students in college and university programs at the diploma, undergraduate, and graduate degree levels, a process to support the fusion of theoretical and practical components of ABA. Within service delivery contexts, this text offers a practical professional development resource for individuals or teams new to behavior analysis-based services, as well as a valuable refresher for more seasoned professionals. Case studies can be completed by individual practitioners as part of individualized professional development or supervision programs, or alternatively completed simultaneously by whole teams to support group learning and development.

Included in each chapter are sample figures, graphs, and templates. Exercises in each chapter offer hands-on activities to apply skills and complete exercises based on the case study and in online environments. Examples include visual displays of behavior data, behavior data sheet templates, and behavior assessment forms. These resources offer learners the opportunity to conduct simulated behavior assessment, data collection, data graphing, and data analysis activities: key components and hallmarks of ABA practice.

Highlighting the Standards of the Behavior Analyst Certification Board

Each case presented in this text includes links to the BACB Fourth Edition Task List (BACB 2012) including foundational knowledge, basic skills, and client-centered responsibilities. This feature makes this text a valuable resource for those preparing for future certification as Board Certified Behavior Analysts (BCBA) and Board Certified Assistant Behavior Analysts (BCaBA). Both the BCBA and BCaBA examinations are linked to the task list, and the structure, format, and content of each case offer learners opportunities to review definitions and applications of key terms, concepts, principles, and processes across the life span. In addition, embedded throughout the text and emphasized in Part V (Research and Ethics) are components of the BACB's Professional and Ethical Compliance Code for Behavior Analysts (Behavior Analyst Certification Board 2014). Complex ethical dilemmas arise frequently in ABA practice and research. The opportunity for students and practitioners to reflect on ethical standards and consider professional conduct through the simulated platform offered by this text is critical to ensuring high-quality services and the well-being of those supported by ABA practitioners.

Enhancing Student Engagement and Learning

Case-based pedagogy has been used across a range of disciplines (e.g., preservice teacher education, law, business, medicine, and engineering) to support the practical application of knowledge acquired in classroom settings (Neuhardt-Pritchett et al. 2004). Supplementing traditional teaching practices with case-based learning experiences has been shown to increase student exposure to real-world clinical cases (e.g., Wilson et al. 2015), and enhance students' problem solving and application skills (e.g., Hoag et al. 2001; Lee et al. 2009). Case-based approaches have further been found to result in more active learning, greater critical thinking, comprehension, and higher-order thinking skills, when compared to more traditional lecture-based approaches (e.g., Rybarczyk et al. 2007; Yadav et al. 2010). Further, they offer a mechanism by which to increase student interest and engagement (e.g., Lee et al. 2009; Tarnvik 2007), stimulate group learning and discussion, and have been well received by academic students and faculty (e.g., Flynn and Klein 2001; Srinivasan et al. 2007).

Supporting Tomorrow's Leaders

Applied Behavior Analysis: Fifty Case Studies in Home, School, and Community Settings is a valuable companion resource for those studying, teaching, and working in the field of ABA. Leading and guiding the implementation of ABA-based programs with, in many cases, vulnerable populations experiencing complex challenging behaviors, requires skills beyond an understanding of theoretical principles. Ongoing opportunities are needed to reflect on roles as part of multidisciplinary teams, the complex contextual considerations within home, school, and community settings, and the tact, diplomacy, and sensitivity needed to support individuals experiencing challenging behaviors and their families and caregivers. This text provides a springboard for this learning, and in doing so, is a critical resource for tomorrow's leaders in ABA.

St. Catharines, Canada   Kimberly Maich
St. Catharines, Canada   Darren Levine
London, Canada   Carmen Hall

References

Behavior Analyst Certification Board. (2012). *Fourth edition task list.* Retrieved from http://bacb.com/wp-content/uploads/2016/03/160101-BCBA-BCaBA-task-list-fourth-edition-english.pdf

Behavior Analyst Certification Board. (2014). *Professional and ethical compliance code for behavior analysts.* Retrieved from http://bacb.com/wp-content/uploads/2016/03/160321-compliance-code-english.pdf

Flynn, A., & Klein, J. (2001). The influence of discussion groups in a case-based learning environment. *Educational Technology Research and Development, 49*(3), 71–86.

Hayes, S., Barlow, D., & Nelson-Gray, R. (1999). *The scientist-practitioner: Research and accountability in the age of managed care* (2nd ed.). Boston: Allyn & Bacon.

Hoag, A., Brickley, D., & Cawley, J. (2001). Media management education and the case method. *Journalism and Mass Communication Educator, 55*(4), 49–59.

Lee, S., Lee, J., Liu, X., Bonk, C., & Magjuka, R. (2009). A review of case-based learning practices in an online MBA program: A program-level case study. *Educational Technology and Society, 12*(3), 178–190.

Neuhardt-Pritchett, S., Payne, B. D., & Reiff, J. C. (Eds.). (2004). *Diverse perspectives on elementary education: A casebook for critically analyzing issues of diversity.* Needham Heights, MA: Allyn & Bacon.

Rybarczyk, B., Baines, A., McVey, M., Thompson, J., & Wilkins, H. (2007). A case based approach increases student learning outcomes and comprehension of cellular respiration concepts. *Biochemistry and Molecular Biology Education, 35*(3), 181–186.

Srinivasan, M., Wilkes, M., Stevenson, F., Nguyen, T., & Slavin, S. (2007). Comparing problem-based learning with case-based learning: Effects of a major curricular shift at two institutions. *Academic Medicine, 82*(1), 74–82.

Tarnvik, A. (2007). Revival of the case method: a way to retain student-centred learning in a post-PBL era. *Medical Teacher, 29*(1), 32–36.

Wilson, A., Goodall, J., Ambrosini, G., Carruthers, D., Chan, H., Ong, S., et al. (2015). Development of an interactive learning tool for teaching rheumatology—A simulated clinical case studies program. *Rheumatology, 45*(9), 1158–1161.

Yadav, A., Shaver, G., & Meckl, P. (2010). Lessons learned: Implementing the case teaching method in a mechanical engineering course. *The Research Journal for Engineering Education, 99*(1), 55–69.

Acknowledgments

I would like to acknowledge my husband, John, and my children, Robert, Grace, and Hannah. for their collective tolerance for my long-term, time-consuming projects. They are my world, they have changed my world, and they are reflected in many small and significant ways in the narratives in this book—and others. Thank you to Brock University for my ABA training and to Carmen Hall for my ABA supervision which helped to support the direction of this book. All of the guest authors who contributed cases to this book also have my thanks for graciously contributing their creativity and time. My research assistants—Megan Henning, Susan Riecheld, and Sheri Mallabar—are also gratefully thanked for their time and energy in supporting its final steps toward submission. And, of course, to my co-authors Darren Levine and Carmen Hall: Thank you immensely for agreeing to be a huge, significant, unbeatable part of this journey. Let's do it again!

—Kimberly Maich

I would like to thank my wife Jen for her unwavering patience, support, encouragement, and belief in me. I would also like to express my gratitude to our three children, Maya, Noah, and Aiden. You are all a constant source of inspiration and a reminder never to take myself too seriously and that nothing is impossible. Thank you to my co-authors Kimberly Maich and Carmen Hall. This has been an exciting and rewarding journey!

—Darren Levine

I would like express my overwhelming gratitude to my husband, Tony, and son, Julian, in their patience, dedication, and commitment to this book, which took away from some of the time together as a family. Your belief in my career and me is unconditional and inspiring. Also, to all the friends and extended family who also contributed in many, many ways so that this book is possible—thank you! Special thanks to Erin Marshall for her dedication and commitment to helping bring some of our case studies to life and making them applicable to field settings. Lastly, I cannot thank the other authors on this team enough who pulled together time after time to make this project come to fruition!

—Carmen Hall

Contents

Part I Assessment

1 Assessment Case Studies for Preschool to School-Age Children ... 3
    CASE: i-A1... 4
    Why Won't Simon Listen to Me?........................... 5
    CASE: i-A2... 10
    Why Can't Erin Just Get Along? 12
    CASE: i-A3... 19
    What is Cyrus Trying To Tell Us? 20
    CASE: i-A4... 26
    Why Won't Serena Just Let Me Teach? 27
    CASE: i-A5 Guest Author: Monique Somma 35
    Where Did Siki Learn to Say That? 36
    References... 42

2 Assessment Case Studies from Adolescence to Adulthood 45
    CASE: i-A6... 46
    Emily's Worrying is Keeping Her Awake................... 47
    CASE: i-A7... 55
    Sam's Struggles with "Real-Life" Friends............... 56
    CASE: i-A8... 61
    Olivier's Challenges with Self-control................. 62
    CASE: i-A9... 67
    Miguel Used to Skip TO School, But Now He
    Is SKIPPING School!.................................... 68
    CASE: i-A10.. 77
    If Jaz Can't Get Here on Time, She Is Fired! 78
    References... 81

Part II Planning

3   Planning-Focused Case Studies for Preschool-Age to School-Age Children 85
   CASE: ii-P1 86
   We All Are Experts, But None of Us Alone Has All the Expertise . . . 87
   CASE: ii-P2 Guest Author: Adam Davies 91
   Change is Needed, But Who Is It That Has to Change? 93
   CASE: ii-P3 99
   You Mean You Want to Train My Student? 100
   CASE: ii-P4 105
   Zara's Ounce of Prevention 106
   CASE: ii-P5 110
   Let's Just Make Zara Stop 112
   References 117

4   Planning-Focused Case Studies from Adolescence to Adulthood 119
   CASE: ii-P6 119
   Why Does Jana Struggle in Some Places, And Not Others? 121
   CASE: ii-P7 126
   Changing Ilyas's Outcomes by Changing His Environment 127
   CASE: ii-P8 131
   Shape Up, Cris, Or Ship Out! 132
   CASE: ii-P9 Guest Author: Christina Belcher 140
   Is Garth's Experience Enough? 141
   CASE: ii-P10 146
   Is Daisy's Behavior a Message in Disguise? 148
   References 152

Part III Implementation

5   Implementation-Based Case Studies for Preschool-Age to School-Age Children 157
   CASE: iii-I1 158
   Important for ME, Or Important for YOU? 160
   CASE: iii-I2 163
   Robina's Data Are WRONG; My EXPERIENCES Are Right 165
   CASE: iii-I3 169
   Let's Just Get Moving Along! 171
   CASE: iii-I4 175
   When Is "ENOUGH"? 177
   CASE: iii-I5 182
   Big Changes for Bart, But Perhaps of Little Value? 184
   References 188

6   Implementation-Based Case Studies from Adolescence to
    Adulthood   191
    CASE: iii-I6   192
    Right, Wrong, or Different?   193
    CASE: iii-I7   198
    Jerry Just Needs to Learn a Lesson   199
    CASE: iii-I8 Guest Author: Drew MacNamara   204
    It's Just Too Time-consuming. I'm Pretty Sure That Things
    Are Getting Better. Is That Enough?   205
    CASE: iii-I9   210
    It Only Happens to Sophia When These People Are Here!   212
    CASE: iii-I10   216
    I Wish Hilde Could Just Tell Us!   218
    References   225

Part IV   Evaluation

7   Evaluation-Centered Case Studies for Preschool
    to School-Age Children   229
    CASE: iv-E1 Guest Author: Jocelyn Prosser   229
    My Teaching Strategies Are Working! Aren't They?   231
    CASE: iv-E2   237
    It's Working for Tito … Right?   239
    CASE: iv-E3   244
    It's Just Not Happening with Owen!   245
    CASE: iv-E4   252
    As Long as Molly's Improving, Nothing Else Matters   253
    CASE: iv-E5   258
    How Is It a Success for Ramsey, When WE Aren't Seeing
    Any Change?   259
    References   265

8   Evaluation-Centered Case Studies from Adolescence
    to Adulthood   267
    CASE: iv-E6   267
    I Think It Is Fair To Say That This Is Working!   269
    CASE: iv-E7   275
    Does It Matter WHAT Worked?   276
    CASE: iv-E8   284
    We Cannot Evaluate Our Program!   285
    CASE: iv-E9   287
    It Worked for Them; It Will Work for Us   288
    CASE: iv-E10 Guest Authors: Sharon Jimson and Renee Carriere   293
    Raja's Decreasing Disruptive Behavior   294
    References   306

Part V Research and Ethics

**9   Preschool-to-School-Age Case Studies Constructed Around
      Research and Ethics** 311
      CASE: v-R1 Guest Author: Tricia van Rhijn 312
      Stay, Play, and Talk with Me 312
      CASE: v-R2 319
      Show Me The Evidence 320
      CASE: v-R3 327
      Volunteered or Volun-*told*?................................ 328
      CASE: v-R4 331
      Settle In—Or Opt Out?...................................... 332
      CASE: v-R5 336
      Ask for Permission, or Ask for Forgiveness? 338
      References... 342

**10 Adolescence to Adulthood Case Studies Constructed Around
      Research and Ethics** 343
      CASE: v-R6 Guest Author: John LaPorta...................... 344
      Include or Exclude? 344
      CASE: v-R7 347
      Malcolm's in the Middle.................................... 348
      CASE: v-R8 353
      Skilled Practice or Practice Skills? 355
      CASE: v-R9 361
      What's Wrong with a Little Deception? 362
      CASE: v-R10 366
      Include or Exclude? 366
      References... 371

Ethics Index... 373

BACB 4th Edition Task List Index 377

Copyright Acknowledgements 383

Index 385

About the Authors

Kimberly Maich, Ph.D., OCT, is an associate professor in the Department of Teacher Education at Brock University and affiliated with the Center for Applied Disability Studies. She has studied and taught from coast-to-coast in Canada from Vancouver, BC, to St. Anthony, NL. She has spent most of her career as a resource teacher, supporting students with exceptionalities from Kindergarten to Grade 12, but has also worked as a guidance counselor, vice-principal, librarian, classroom teacher, and computer laboratory coordinator. Previously, she worked as an ASD Consultant and Program Coordinator with McMaster Children's Hospital. Before moving to Brock University, she was a professor in Fanshawe College's new Bachelor of Applied Arts in Early Childhood Leadership. Her primary interests lie in special education, primarily in autism spectrum disorders.

Darren Levine, Ed.D., is an adjunct faculty member in the Center for Applied Disability Studies at Brock University. He has taught graduate-level courses in Applied Behavior Analysis and supported student research and field-based learning and development. For more than fifteen years, Dr. Levine has held several progressively more senior positions implementing Applied Behavior Analysis intervention programs in home, school, and community settings, and conducting applied behavior-analytic measurement, evaluation, and research. Dr. Levine holds a doctorate in education from the Ontario Institute for Studies in Education at the University of Toronto (OISE/UT), specializing in adaptive instruction and special education.

Carmen Hall, MC, CCC, BCBA, has worked in the field of Autism Spectrum Disorders for more than 10 years, in both educational and clinical settings. She graduated from the University of Calgary (BA, Psychology), St. Lawrence College (Behavioural Science Technology Diploma), the University of Lethbridge (MC, Counseling Psychology), and is currently completing her Ph.D. in Clinical Psychology from Saybrook University. She is a Certified Canadian Counselor with the Canadian Counseling and Psychotherapy Association and is a Board Certified Behavior Analyst. Her primary focus has been on promoting and researching social skill development for children with disabilities in inclusive recreation, educational, and childcare settings, researching the use of the iPad to facilitate learning in K-Higher Education and the use of intensive ABA strategies for adults with developmental disabilities. Carmen has worked as an instructor therapist, educational assistant, and autism spectrum disorders consultant and is currently the Coordinator of the Autism and Behavioural Science Program at Fanshawe College. She regularly presents at provincial, national, and international conferences, and in 2013 was named an Apple Distinguished Educator, in 2014 received the College Sector Educator Award, and in 2015 received the President's Distinguished Achievement Award.

Part I
Assessment

Chapter 1
Assessment Case Studies for Preschool to School-Age Children

Abstract Behavior assessment is the first step in developing behavior support programs. Before attempts at changing behaviors can be made, information about target behaviors must be gathered, analyzed, synthesized, and translated into individualized support programs. This involves gathering information about the behaviors in question, the individuals, the specific environments, and individual histories of reinforcement and punishment in those contexts. More specifically, it is important to begin to gain insight into what the behavior in question looks like and what function it serves for the individual; when and where behaviors occur; why behaviors occur in some contexts, at certain times, and not in other contexts, at other times; and how the individuals and their skills, abilities, strengths, and limitations interact with the environment and his or her history of reinforcement and punishment to produce the observed behavior. The goal of behavior assessment is to develop a hypothesis as to why particular behaviors are occurring—their functions—and determine how the individuals might best be supported to be successful in the environments in which they are currently experiencing difficulties. The desired outcome is not only cessation of target problem behaviors, but also the learning of new skills that will provide access to reinforcement, make the problem behavior unnecessary, and contribute to improved quality of life for the individual involved. In this chapter, entitled "Assessment Case Studies for Preschool to School-age Children," behavior assessment principles, processes, and practices are explored through five case scenarios involving preschool and school-age children in home, school, clinical, and community settings.

Keywords Preschool · School-age children · Behavior assessment · Assessment · Behavior functions · Quality of life · Reinforcement · ABA

CASE: i-A1

Why Won't Simon Listen To Me?
Setting: Home   Age Group: Preschool

LEARNING OBJECTIVE:

- Design a behavior assessment plan.

TASK LIST LINKS:

- **Identification of the Problem**

  - (G-01) Review records and available data at the outset of the case.
  - (G-02) Consider biological/medical variables that may be affecting the client.
  - (G-03) Conduct a preliminary assessment of the client in order to identify the referral problem.

- **Assessment**

  - (I-01) Define behavior in observable and measurable terms.
  - (I-02) Define environmental variables in observable and measurable terms.
  - (I-03) Design and implement individualized behavioral assessment procedures.

KEY TERMS:

- **Behavior Consultation**

  - Behavior consultation typically has two purposes: (1) a behavior-change program for the individual displaying the target behavior; and (2) supporting the individual that will be implementing the intervention. It often utilizes a "mediator model" where someone other than the consultant (e.g., parent, teacher, and instructor therapist) implements ABA principles and processes. Behavior consultation requires both knowledge of the principles and processes of ABA (i.e., assessment procedures, program design, data collection, and evaluation), as well as skills in consultation (e.g., professional rapport and relationship building, collaborative problem solving, active learning techniques, training and support, and performance feedback) (Edmunds et al. 2013; Sanetti et al. 2013).

- **Behavioral Interview**

  - A behavioral interview is a discussion with those supporting the individual displaying the behavior identified for change such as a parent, teacher, or caregiver. In some cases, the individual that will be receiving the intervention may also be involved. These discussions attempt to identify problematic behaviors, determine the frequency at which they may be occurring, and identify associated antecedents and consequences (i.e., what seems to occur immediately before and after the behavior). Although these interviews focus on indirect accounts of the behavior, they can provide clues to the environmental variables that may be evoking and maintaining the target behavior. Behavioral interviews are often the first step in the functional behavior assessment process (O'Neill et al. 1997).

- **Developmentally Appropriate**

  – Behaviors that we expect from individuals of a particular chronological age or behaviors that most children of a particular age display, such as motor, language, cognitive, or social skills, are often referred to as developmentally appropriate behaviors. While children vary somewhat in terms of when they may achieve a particular skill, there are certain expectations, or sets of skills and behaviors, that are expected at certain ages. For example, by 4 or 5 years of age, children are expected to print letters, use a fork and spoon, and dress and undress independently (Health Canada 2013).

- **Social Significance**

  – Socially significant behaviors are those that are important to the individual that will be receiving an intervention. They are deemed socially significant when they help the individual function effectively, independently, and successfully in the environment. These may include social, language, academic, daily living, self-care, and/or recreational behaviors (Baer et al. 1968, 1987; Horner et al. 2005).

- **Target Behavior**

  – A target behavior is a behavior that is selected for change. It may be problematic behavior selected to decrease, or a new behavior or skill that is selected to increase. A target behavior is selected because its change would improve quality of life for the individual undergoing behavior change (Bosch and Fuqua 2001).

- **Typically Developing**

  – Children who are meeting developmental expectations and are displaying the behaviors and skills expected of a child of their age may be termed "typically developing" (Health Canada 2013).

Why Won't Simon Listen to Me?

Simon was a pretty perfect baby. His parents heard charming phrases thrown about when others discussed their little one: "Simon is just such a good baby!", "He will go to anyone!", "He laughs and smiles all the time!" They often made eye contact a little smugly over the brown curls on Simon's head, smiling together at the joy this feedback brought to their little family. Baby Simon met every single one of his typical milestones at just the right moments. Simon's parents knew this as they diligently transported him in his stroller to the local university medical center every few weeks, where medical doctors in training practiced their professional use of developmental assessment tools. Everyone—parents and professionals—agreed that Simon was a robustly healthy, **typically developing** child.

Simon grew—quickly, it seemed—into an equally delightful toddler. He was quite content to follow one of his parents, his six-year-old brother, or his eight-year-old sister around the house, the yard, or around the quiet suburban community. He was often found following one or the other of his siblings around, chortling while he joined in—or imitated—household chores, dramatic play, or his sister's wild dance moves! He was also quite happy to explore on his own, moving from room to room in their cozy bungalow. One day, he was only out of sight for a moment, when he was quickly discovered attempting to plunge the already-sparkling clean toilet. He was easily redirected, however, happily compliant in the continued attention of his family members, no matter what the context.

At the age of three, Simon transitioned part time into a childcare center—another service provided at the city's university center. It was the same time when his temperament seemed to shift. Although Simon appeared to transition without difficulty into the childcare setting, function extremely well in group play with other children his age, and bonded strongly with the educators at his center, his parents thought his behavior at home to be quite different. Simon seems to vary from **developmentally appropriate** behavior at school, to behavior at home that appears to be different than most children his age.

Late one night, after their three children were tucked in bed, either sleep or reading with bedside lamps glowing, Simon's parents—yet again—were talking about Simon's behavior far away from the listening ears of their three young children.

"He seems to listen more to me than he does to you," started Simon's mother. Simon's father nodded quickly, his eyebrows raised.

"Yes. Like today, when I ask him to clean up his fridge magnets from the table so that we could all have dinner," Simon's father recollected. "That was a bit of a disaster. I think maybe there were two things he didn't like: being asked to clean up, and he also likely figured out that coming to the table for dinner was on the horizon. These seem to be two of his hot buttons. When we press those—he's off!"

"I agree," nodded Simon's mother, emphatically. "I can hardly believe this is our little Simon. Where on earth did he learn that fighting and yelling with those little clenched fists of his was the right way to get along with everyone? I am really at a loss as to what we should do next. Let's see how tomorrow goes, and then maybe we are going to have to get some help. I am really at the point where I wonder if we should just not bother to ask him to do *anything*. It seems like it would be easier to give in than to figure out how to 'make' him do what we ask. Why doesn't he just listen?" Simon's father was well aware that this was a question that could not be answered—at least not right at the moment.

The next morning, however, was a breaking point for Simon's family. While trying to get a busy family of five ready for work, school, and childcare, Simon lay on his back in the midst of the narrow breezeway. His feet were propped up against the wall, and caught up in a fabric and belts of a number of spring coats. He thumped his heels rhythmically, causing the coats to fall in a messy pile, right into a boot tray filled with a wet puddle of melted slush. All of these were not happening in a void or without comment from those in Simon's family. Simon's father had asked him—quietly and kindly—to please get off the floor and put on his coat and boots, two or three times, with the frustration and volume level becoming more prominent with each repetition. Simon's siblings also "helped out" by stepping alongside their father and almost shouting, "Hurry up! Come on, Simon!" Their frustration and disgust was quite clear as they sighed and moaned while they picked up their soaked outdoor clothing. These interactions, however, seemed to get Simon's attention, and he started giggling about and rolling on the floor, while making no efforts to follow through with the direction he was given. Today, like many days, this ended in a physical altercation, Simon's siblings pulling and tugging at Simon, and Simon smacking wildly yet aimlessly until he came into contact with his brother and sister.

When everyone was finally lifted, seated, and belted into the backseat of the family sedan, Simon's parents again looked at one another, already exhausted. "Okay," said Simon's mother, knowing what she needed to do without any words exchanged, "I will call them again today." Previously, Simon's mother had been in contact with a behavior consultant—a Board Certified Behavior Analyst (BCBA)—recommended to her by the childcare center. At the time, though, she had not been willing to move ahead with **behavior consultation**. The BCBA had suggested beginning with a **behavioral interview**, as a starting point to pinpoint **socially significant target behaviors**. As she thought about what had been happening at home recently, she now felt prepared to move ahead. During her first break at work that morning, she took a deep breath, steadied herself, and took the first major step toward professional support for Simon—calling the BCBA.

The Response: Principles, Processes, Practices, and Reflections

Principles

(**Q1**) What is one behavior that you would identify for change for Simon? Why did you choose this behavior? Is this a socially significant target behavior? If so, please explain why. If not, please explain why not, and how you might ensure that a socially significant behavior is selected for change.

(**Q2**) The early stage of planning for behavioral intervention often involves developing a hypothesis about the function, or purpose, of a target behavior. An "Antecedent-Behavior-Consequence" (or ABC) chart can help to develop such a hypothesis. Extract information about one of Simon's challenging behaviors from the above case example and complete the attached ABC chart. Once completed, answer the following questions: What occurred immediately before the target behavior you selected? What occurred immediately following the behavior? Why is this important information (Table 1.1)?

Table 1.1 Sample ABC observation form

Individual:_____	Date:_____
Observer:_____	Setting:_____
Setting Events: _____	

Antecedent	Behavior	Consequence

Process

(Q3) Using the chart below as a guide, consider the following questions about the target behavior you selected: How might you measure the behavior? What type of data collection would you use? Who would be responsible for collecting these data? How often should data be collected? In what setting or settings should data collection happen? How do you think these data will help inform your assessment and guide your intervention planning (Fig. 1.1)?

(Q4) Consider the following ethical dilemma: Simon's parents decide that they would like you, as the behavior analyst, to focus on addressing a different target behavior than the one you have identified—a behavior that you believe to be of lesser social significance for Simon when compared to the behavior you selected for change. How might you approach this dilemma?

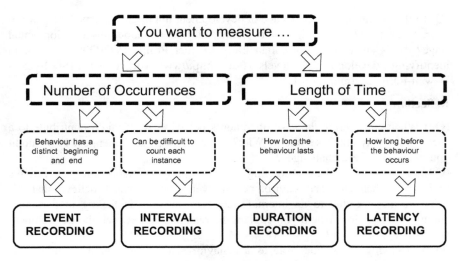

Fig. 1.1 Flowchart to help determine the type of data collection to use when selecting a data collection method to use (Bicard et al. 2012)

Practice

(Q5) Using the example below as a guide, write a behavioral objective for one of Simon's behaviors. There are four components that should be included: (1) reference to the individual, or who will conduct the behavior, (2) the target behavior, (3) conditions for the behavior to occur, and (4) criteria for acceptable performance (Fig. 1.2).

For example:
Navier will do up his zipper on his coat independently when asked to "put on his coat" by his teacher for 3 consecutive days in a row.

(Q6) Sometimes, when you are observing an individual to collect data about a behavior, your presence as an observer may influence the behaviors that you see (e.g., if someone knows they are being watched, they might change their behavior). Known as reactivity, this can be a concern because it might prevent you from collected data that accurately reflects the extent to which the target behavior is occurring. How might you observe occurrences of Simon's target behavior without your presence influencing the data being collected?

```
_____ will _____
        (Name)                          (Target Behavior)

when _____ for _____
                              (Conditions)

_____.
        (Criteria)
```

Fig. 1.2 A guide to assist in writing a behavioral objective

(Q7) Why is Simon's age and stage of development important to consider as part of your assessment? How might you gather information about his developmental stage? Tools such as the Hawaiian Early Learner Profile (VORT) can assist in identifying developmental levels (see http://www.vort.com/HELP-0-3-years-Hawaii-Early-Learning-Profile/).

Reflection

(Q8) When considering the case of Simon's behavior, what might contribute to a successful behavioral assessment? Why? What might pose challenges? How might you overcome these challenges?

(Q9) Simon's parents are struggling with accepting a relationship between his problematic behavior and environmental events, and instead believe that his behavior may be due to an internal state (i.e., how he is feeling in particular circumstances). How would you explain the relationship between the environment and Simon's behavior?

(Q10) *Thinking* about your role as a behavior analyst, how might you balance addressing the immediate behavior difficulty with focusing on longer-term behavioral, educational, and social goals for Simon?

Additional Web Links
Defining Behaviors:
http://iris.peabody.vanderbilt.edu/wp-content/uploads/2013/05/ICS-015.pdf
Seeking Outside Help:
http://csefel.vanderbilt.edu/documents/dmg_seek_outside_help.pdf
Developmental Milestones:
http://www.cdc.gov/ncbddd/actearly/milestones/index.html
Behavior Interviews:
http://challengingbehavior.fmhi.usf.edu/explore/pbs/step3_interviews.htm

CASE: i-A2

WHY CAN'T ERIN JUST GET ALONG?
Setting: School   Age Group: Preschool

LEARNING OBJECTIVE:

- Describe behavior using the three-term contingency of applied behavior analysis.

TASK LIST LINKS:

- **Measurement**

    - (A-01) Measure frequency (i.e., count).
    - (A-02) Measure rate (i.e., count per unit time).

- (A-04) Measure latency.
- (A-05) Measure inter-response time (IRT).
- (A-12) Design and implement continuous measurement procedures (e.g., event recording).

- **Fundamental Elements of Behavior Change**

  - (D-15) Identify punishers.

- **Behavior-Change Systems**

  - (F-07) Use functional communication training.

- **Identification of the Problem**

  - (G-03) Conduct a preliminary assessment of the client in order to identify the referral problem.
  - (G-04) Explain behavioral concepts using nontechnical language.
  - (G-06) Provide behavior-analytic services in collaboration with others who support and/or provide services to one's clients.

- **Measurement**

  - (H-01) Select a measurement system to obtain representative data given the dimensions of the behavior and the logistics of observing and recording.
  - (H-02) Select a schedule of observation and recording periods.
  - (H-03) Select a data display that effectively communicates relevant quantitative relations.

- **Assessment**

  - (I-01) Define behavior in observable and measurable terms.
  - (I-03) Design and implement individualized behavioral assessment procedures.

KEY TERMS:

- **Intensive Behavioral Intervention (IBI)**

  - IBI is an application of the principles and processes of applied behavior analysis, typically used with children with Autism Spectrum Disorder. It often involves an intense schedule of 20–40 hours of direct service each week. Programming includes a focus on reducing challenging behaviors and increasing a broad range of socially significant skills including communication, socialization, self-help, academics, and play (Howard et al. 2005).

- **Time-Out**

  - Also known as "time-out from positive reinforcement," this procedure involves the removal of access to reinforcement for a period of time as a consequence following displays of specific problematic behaviors (Cooper et al. 2007).

- **Functional Communication**
  - Functional communication is a form of behavior that conveys what we want, need, and/or are feeling, to others. This may involve verbal (e.g., words) or nonverbal behaviors (e.g., gestures). Communication is functional if it serves a particular purpose or results in a desired outcome (Dutton 2011).

Why Can't Erin Just Get Along?

"Home time!" exclaimed Erin's grandfather, who had just arrived at Erin's Kindergarten classroom at Tall Trees Therapy School, stomping snow from his boots near the inside doorway to Erin's classroom. Erin's teacher at the specialized setting, Ms. Grimes, looked up and smiled. Moving over to Erin's favorite place between the classroom's tablet computer table and the carefully stacked bins of math manipulatives, Ms. Grimes made sure she had Erin's attention. Then, she repeated the **verbal prompt** that Erin's grandfather had used and paired it with a color photograph of home taken from Erin's daily visual schedule. Without much difficulty—this time—Erin uncurled her legs, rose, and moved toward her grandfather, grasping her picture of home tightly in both hands. Ms. Grimes could hear Erin whisper quietly what she was sure was the word *home*. After Erin and her grandfather had departed from the Kindergarten classroom, Ms. Grimes had a few moments without lunch duty or yard duty where she had sometime to review Erin's Antecedent-Behavior-Consequence (ABC) chart, which she had been asked to complete by the school's behavior consultant. Ms. Grimes thought about Erin's afternoon program of individually designed home-based and privately funded **Intensive Behavior Intervention**. Erin's grandfather had been concerned about how expensive this intervention program has been, but recently has told her how pleased he is with Erin's progress.

Looking at the ABC chart, Ms. Grimes counted the number of so-called challenging behaviors (as she was learning to call them) which Erin had exhibited this morning alone. Across the top of the sheet was written "Target Behavior: Aggression" and a description of aggression which read: "Erin hits other children with her fist and pushes other children to the ground with the flat palms of both hands." Moving her eyes downward on the page, Ms. Grimes counted 1, 2, 3 … 8 ("Eight!" she exclaimed aloud) incidents of aggression with Erin and her classmates, just today. "I can't figure out why this isn't a problem at home for Erin and her grandfather," she murmured to herself, shaking her head with frustration, and *thinking* back through the day so far.

Today, Ms. Grimes had tried hard to uphold the social practices she was so proud of in her therapeutic classroom. When she saw that Erin's peers were not inviting Erin to play during child-directed center-based learning, she had helped out. She went to Erin and helped her to transition over to the squares of foam flooring in front of the math manipulatives—Erin's favorite—and poured out a pyramid of tiny rubber animals. She called one of Erin's peers over and suggested a patterning activity for them. She modeled a pattern on the floor and supported the children in developing their own patterns with these educational toys. But in her busy classroom, her attention was again inevitably drawn away from supporting Erin and her peer. After all, most of their students had extra-special needs! Out of the corner of her eye, Ms. Grimes almost immediately spotted a problem when she moved away from Erin. Erin reached out, put her hands roughly on the chest of her classmate, and pushed hard. In the flurry of tears that followed, Erin's peer landed hard on her bottom. Ms. Grimes had directed Erin to a time-out, telling her sternly, "No pushing!"

But it doesn't seem to work, thought Ms. Grimes. *No matter what I say to Erin, and no matter how many time outs I give her, nothing changes. At least, nothing changes for the better, except when she is doing intensive 1:1 work. It seems that whenever I encourage her peers to play with her, things get really bad really quickly. First thing this morning, I brought Ali over to the book center where Erin was flipping through a book, when they were both looking at a book I walked away. I turned back just in time to see Erin push Ali and Ali fall to the ground. As a result, I had to bring her to time out, and the morning wasn't even an hour in. No matter how much I try to supervise, I just can't be there all the time. When "play" happens, there always seems to be yelling and crying afterwards. After her time out from pushing Ali, she wondered over near a shelf containing a basket of textured squares. Pauline was nearby, so I encouraged the two to try to match the pairs of textures together. I stopped supporting their interactions and just watched, amazed at how well they were doing with one another, that is, until the class phone rang. While answering the phone I saw Erin hit Pauline. So it was back to time out, a great interaction turned bad again! I simply can't see the benefit to encouraging these peer interactions! I had all these excellent goals about friendship in Erin's Individual Education Plan, but we don't seem to get there—or even part of the way there! I really wonder if Erin is going to be able to stay in this social environment of ours. If the other parents keep complaining the way they are now, our principal might feel like she needs to move Erin across town to a more restrictive setting, or maybe do that expensive home program all day.* "Well," she said, interrupting her train of thought with her own words, "this is not solving anything." She put aside the ABC chart and her strong concerns about Erin and her behavior, and started to prepare for the second half of the instructional day. At the end of the day when all of her students had been bundled up and delivered to their parents, their buses, or their older siblings for a short walk home, she gathered her thoughts and her behavioral data, and headed off to the school's resource room for an after-school meeting with the behavior consultant, Erin's grandfather, and their IBI therapist. *I hope this is a short one*, she thought again to only herself. *I still need to get ready for our 100th day of school celebration tomorrow!*

When she arrived at the resource room after her long and busy after-school routine of assisting students who were still learning to be independent, she was greeted with smiles and thanks for the clipboard of information she brought with her to the meeting already in progress—quite the opposite of what she had expected. "This is really great," enthused the consultant. "You have already collected five full mornings of ABC data on that target behavior we had **prioritized**.

I am so pleased. This is really going to help us figure out Erin's patterns of challenging behavior. In fact, I think we should do the same thing at home, so we have information about all of Erin's environments where she spends a significant amount of time."

"But … just a minute," interrupted Erin's grandfather. "She doesn't do that at home. She doesn't hit me, or push me, and she certainly doesn't hit or push her older sister. What's the point? The only thing I really notice for sure is that she *seems* to be really frustrated when she is trying to tell me things. Usually I don't understand, and I think she finds that quite upsetting."

"Well," paused the consultant, "we need to have data on paper. And her therapy time is important too, which also happens at your house. Are you sure that she is never aggressive like this when the therapists are doing IBI at home?"

Erin's grandfather paused, thought for a few minutes, and eventually responded, "Maybe you are right. I don't really know what happens in terms of disruptions during the lessons that are going on. Usually I take that time for a bit of a break, and a lot of the time I am not even home: Erin's grandmother usually takes that shift around the house. Maybe you can walk me through what we need to do."

The positive tone of the meeting continued and ended much the same way, with consensus all around, a plan for data collection, and a goal set to figure out how to best support Erin in developing **functional communication** skills. Ms. Grimes only left with one thing on her to-do list: to talk with the Speech-Language Pathologist tomorrow when she will be in the Kindergarten classrooms doing screening for articulation issues with the whole class. *I think I can handle that!* She thought. *But can I handle Erin?*

The Response: Principles, Processes, Practices, and Reflections

Principles

(Q1) *Thinking* about Erin and the case outlined above, what might be one behavior that you would identify for change? Why did you choose this behavior? Is this a socially significant target behavior? If so, please explain why (Table 1.2).

(Q2) The early stage of planning for behavioral intervention often involves developing a hypothesis about the function, or purpose, of a target behavior. After completing the "Antecedent-Behavior-Consequence" (or A-B-C) chart with information provided in this case, what pattern(s) do you notice? How might this information help you in your assessment of this behavior (Table 1.3)?

Process

(Q3) What would be the intended outcome of the functional communication program for Erin? What might be your initial target? How might you proceed?

(Q4) *Thinking* further about the target behavior you selected, how might you measure this behavior? Who would be responsible for collecting these data? How often? In what setting or settings? Think about using different apps that are used for data collection, as listed on this Web site: http://www.positivelyautism.com/aba/mod4G.html

Table 1.2 A checklist to determine the social significance of program goals to consider when making goals for a learner (Carter, 2010)

Section 1 Client values	Yes	No	Comments
Is the goal of the program in line with the individuals' values and preferences?			
Does the individual and their caregiver agree with the outcomes that surround the program goal?			
Are there more goals the individual or their caregiver feel is important?			
Section 2 Normalization	Yes	No	Comments
Do the program outcomes increase chances for normalization?			
Are program goals age appropriate?			
Do program goals effect multiple areas of the individuals life?			
Do program goals generalize?			
Section 3 Choice	Yes	No	Comments
Do program goals encourage more occasions for the individual to make choices?			
Do program goals create opportunities for the individual to receive higher rates of reinforcement?			
Do program goals create opportunities for the individual to receive higher-quality reinforcement?			
Do program goals lessen the response effort required for the individual to meet reinforcement?			
Section 4 Habilitative potential	Yes	No	Comments
Will program goals teach new skills? • Skills necessary for long-term goals? • Social skills? • Life skills? • Vocational skills? • Leisure skills?			

(**Q5**) As a behavior consultant, your role is to synthesize information gathered surrounding observable behavior, construct an explanation as to why a challenging behavior may be occurring, and develop a behavior support program. In addition to the ABC data you have gathered, what additional types of information might important to gather? For each type of information you identify, explain why the information will be helpful, and how might you obtain it.

Table 1.3 Sample ABC chart with example behavior in each column that can work as a checklist for easier completion

Learner		Instructor:	
Date:		Time:	
Location/Setting:			
Antecedent	**Behavior**	**Consequence**	**Comments:**

☐ Demand
☐ Transition
☐ Peer
    interaction
☐ Tangible
    removed
☐ Attention
    removed
☐
☐
☐
☐
☐
	☐ Hit
	☐ Kick
	☐ Scratch
	☐ Pinch
	☐ Bite
	☐ Cry
	☐ Yell
	☐ Throw item
	☐ Run
	☐ Profanity
	☐
	☐
	☐
		☐ Demand removed
		☐ Demand reiterated
		☐ Demand remain
		☐ Verbal reprimand
		☐ Non-seclusion
		    timeout
		☐ Seclusion timeout
		☐ Blocking
		☐ Ignore behavior
		☐ Peer laugh,
		    commentary, or
		    other attention
		☐
		☐
		☐	

Duration of Behavior	(circle) :
	    <3 secs
	    5-15 sec
	    15-30 sec
	    30-60 sec
		1-2 min
		2 -5 min
		5 -10 min
		over 10 min
			over 30 min
			over 1 hour
			over 2 hours
			over 3 hours

Behavior Intensity:	low	medium	high

For each observation of a targeted behavior a new checklist would be completed

Practice

(Q6) In applied behavior analysis, the relationship between antecedents, behaviors, and consequences is referred to as "the three-term contingency." Educators and parents may rely on time-out as a consequence for behavior. However, time-out can sometimes be reinforcing given that the child is allowed to escape from the situation at hand. What is punishing about time-out? Looking at the ABC chart in Table 1.4, is the time-out reinforcing the behavior rather than punishing it as the teacher intended? How can you tell? Is the punishment working to reduce the behavior, as the time-out punishment procedure intended?

(Q7) It is not uncommon to observe different types of behaviors being displayed when Erin is with educators, parents, instructors, and peers. Looking once again at the ABC chart above in Table 1.4, what patterns do you notice? What might these patterns suggest about why certain behaviors are occurring with some people and not others?

Table 1.4 Analyze if the behavior below is being punished or reinforced by the time-out procedure the student's teachers are using

Antecedent	Behavior	Consequence
– Erin is driving car down car ramp at school – Peer joins in independently	– Erin grabs car out of peers hand and hits peer	– Teacher comes over – States "Erin, no hitting, go sit in time-out" – Teacher takes Erin by hand and brings her to the time-out chair, and gives her the car to play with
– Erin is playing the xylophone at school – Teacher brings peer over – Peer picks up tambourine and begins shaking it	– Erin places both hands on peer's chest and pushes	– Peer falls down – Teacher, "No, pushing!" – Takes Erin by hand and brings her to time out chair
– At home Erin is sitting on the couch making a stuffed elephant hop up and down – Her grandmother comes into the room, sits beside her, picks up a stuffed tiger and says, "watch this elephant! I can jump too!"	– Erin hits her grandmother on the knee with the elephant	– Grandmother says, "oh, if you hit me, then I do not want to play with you" – Erin stops and the grandmother leaves the room
– At school – Erin is coloring a picture at the table – Teacher walks over with peer – Peer sits down and begins coloring his own picture – Teacher walks away	– Erin gets up out of chair, walks over to peer, and pushes him out of his chair using both her hands	– Peer falls to the ground and shouts "Erin pushed me!" – Teacher walks over, says "Erin, there will be no pushing in this classroom. You need a time-out" – Takes Erin to time out chair and gives her a picture to color while she is there
– During morning circle time Erin is sitting next to peer – Class is singing, "ABC's" – Song ends and teacher hands each child a letter from the alphabet – Erin gets her letter ("E")	– Erin turns toward peer to her left, lifts her right hand up, and hits peer in the knee	– Peer says, "hey! that is mean!" – Teacher pauses circle time, takes Erin by the hand out of circle and to the time-out chair – Teacher resumes circle while Erin is in time-out

Reflection

(Q8) Have you been in a situation similar to the one above where an educator or parent was utilizing time-out?

- If so, did you find that it was working to punish the behavior (i.e., by reducing it) or to reinforce the behavior (i.e., by allowing the child to escape a situation or task)?

- If not, how would you respond to a situation if you believed that a parent or educator was unintentionally reinforcing a problematic behavior through the use of time-out, rather than reducing it?

(Q9) Considering that the behavior displayed by Erin involved physical injury and peers, how would you respond to the educators and other parents who want you to stop the behavior immediately, rather than take time to collect assessment data?

(Q10) When, if ever, is appropriate to begin an intervention before accumulating data? Explain your answer (Reference Ethics Box 1.1, Behavior Analyst Certification Board, 2014).

Ethics Box 1.1

Professional and Ethical Compliance Code for Behavior Analysts
- 1.04 Integrity.
   (d) The behavior analyst's behavior conforms to the legal and moral codes of the social and professional community of which the behavior analyst is a member.
- 2.09 Treatment/Intervention Efficacy.
   (d) Behavior analysts review and appraise the effects of any treatments about which they are aware that might impact the goals of the behavior-change program and their possible impact on the behavior-change program, to the extent possible.

Additional Web Links
Functional Assessment:
http://www.kipbs.org/new_kipbs/fsi/behavassess.html
Functional Communication Training:
http://csefel.vanderbilt.edu/briefs/wwb11.pdf
Early Intensive Intervention:
http://pediatrics.aappublications.org/content/early/2011/04/04/peds.2011-0426.full.pdf+html
ABC Analysis:
http://challengingbehavior.fmhi.usf.edu/explore/pbs/step3_antecedent_beh.htm
Time-Out:
http://csefel.vanderbilt.edu/briefs/wwb14.pdf

CASE: i-A3

"What is Cyrus trying to tell us?"
Setting: Clinic   Age Group: Preschool

LEARNING OBJECTIVE:

- Examine the role of a behavior analyst within a multidisciplinary behavior assessment process.

TASK LIST LINKS:

- Experimental Design

    - (B-01) Use the dimensions of applied behavior analysis (Baer et al. 1968) to evaluate whether interventions are behavior analytic in nature.

- **Identification of the Problem**

    - (G-01) Review records and available data at the outset of the case.
    - (G-02) Consider biological/medical variables that may be affecting the client.
    - (G-04) Explain behavioral concepts using nontechnical language.
    - (G-05) Describe and explain behavior, including private events, in behavior-analytic (nonmentalistic) terms.
    - (G-06) Provide behavior-analytic services in collaboration with others who support and/or provide services to one's clients.

- **Assessment**

    - (I-04) Design and implement the full range of functional assessment procedures.

KEY TERMS:

- **Occupational Therapists**

    - Occupational therapists engage in the study of human occupations to manage adaptive behavior to perform these occupations. They enable persons to achieve optimal functioning, prevent occupational dysfunction, and promote optimal performance (Reed and Sanderson 1999).

- **Speech and Language Pathologists**

    - Speech and Language Pathologists are professionals that specialize in the assessment and management of communication disorders. Services can be delivered to individuals, families, and groups and often focus on areas such as speech sound production, voice, fluency, language comprehension and expression, cognition, feeding, and swallowing. Clinical services also typically include prevention and screening, assessment and evaluation, diagnosis, and treatment (American Speech-Language-Hearing Association 2007).

- **Sign Language**
  - American Sign Language is a visual/gestural language used by deaf individuals in North America. "Signs" are the equivalent of letters and words used in spoken language. Using a combination of hand shapes, facial expressions, and body gestures, individuals express words and ideas (Kelly and Gobber 2011).

What is Cyrus Trying To Tell Us?

Five-year-old Cyrus sat in the middle of the clinic's waiting room, both of his legs splayed out in a v-shape. Within the "vee" of his legs, he had piled a mound of toys extracted from a plastic bucket, each with some type of musical sound or song. Both of his parents sat close to him, watching carefully from either side of his small play area, perched on the edges of their respective chairs, clearly waiting, wondering, and watching.

The clinic's name—Community Care Clinic—was prominently displayed above the reception area. Cyrus and his parents had been through its doors before, for a number of fairly brief visits with the developmental pediatrician recommended by their family doctor. His mother thought back to the journey that had brought them to the clinic today.

Both their family doctor and the developmental pediatrician had expressed concern about Cyrus when his mother and father first brought him in with reports that "something was just not right" with his development. During Cyrus's third and fourth years, his family waited—for a long while—then took Cyrus in for observations and interviews, while answering a full battery of questionnaires themselves. It was a confusing and stressful time, but they had held high hopes: Everyone told them that just knowing what was going on with Cyrus would help. So they waited for some words, a name, a diagnosis—and finally it came. Close to his fourth birthday, the developmental pediatrician told Cyrus's parents that Cyrus had an intellectual disability (American Psychiatric Association 2013). He explained that this used to be what was called "mental retardation," he patted their hands, "I know you will be fine," he emphasized. "Cyrus is a very lucky boy to have you." He suggested that, on their way out, they should make an appointment with the receptionist to meet with what he described as "everybody," waving his hands in a circular manner. He stood up, shook their hands, and walked them to the door of the office, and wished them good luck in the future. "Be good," he told Cyrus, and patted him on the head, gently closing his office door.

Since that date about six months ago, Cyrus's parents had cycled through episodes of shock, dismay, and fear. They had read everything they could find, they talked to everyone, and they continued to teach Cyrus at home, encouraging him to speak—which hadn't happened yet—and teaching him some signs from the baby sign language book they had borrowed from the library. So far, he had figured out "cookie" and "more." Mostly, though, he communicated by pointing, screaming, shaking his head, and jumping up and down on his tippy toes, almost vibrating in anger.

Today, hoped Cyrus's mother, *maybe we can get some answers and some help. I have heard so many good things about this team of professionals here. I sure hope we aren't disappointed after this second long wait.* She continued to watch Cyrus, fully engaged with playing the songs and sounds of his toys, one-by-one, and placing them back in his plastic bucket, signing "more" and "cookie" at regular intervals. *Well,* she considered, *I guess they are going to see one of his problems first-hand when they call us into the room for our appointment. And ... here we go!*

The door to the waiting room opened, and a smiling, professionally dressed woman emerged. She walked over to Cyrus, and greeted him softly, then greeted both of Cyrus's parents with a handshake and a welcome. "Let's head down to our family room," she suggested. "Cyrus can bring his things and we have some toys in the room for him to play with while we talk." Agreeing, Cyrus's mother and father looked at one another with concern, and looked down at Cyrus. Cyrus's mother spoke gently to him, and Cyrus's father began to pack up his plastic bucket of musical toys. Immediately, Cyrus leapt to his feet, began to scream in a high-pitched tone, signed "more" and "cookie" and rose up and down on his toes, clearly very agitated. Fifteen long and tiring minutes later, Cyrus's parents were seated around a large, oval table in the family room, Cyrus was seated happily again with his toys, and three other adults who appeared to have a kind, friendly, and welcoming manner, were also seated at the table.

"So let's begin," said the woman who had helped them transition to the family room from the reception area. "I am Dr. Ovid Smith, a Board-Certified Behavior Analyst, and I am here today to see what we can do to support you and Cyrus. I thought we could start with introductions, explaining our roles, why we are here, and how we can help. Then together, we can set some goals and next steps for Cyrus. How does that sound?"

Visibly relaxing, Cyrus's father—quiet until now—responded, "That sounds great! I would love to hear what you have to say, first, before we add our ideas."

"Perfect! Well, as I said, I am Ovid, and my role as a behavior analyst is to figure out WHY Cyrus is having some challenging behaviors—like the ones we witnessed today—and to help decrease them using what we call a 'functional analysis'. I can help at home, daycare, and I can also help at school, when Cyrus moves on to a classroom environment."

"I am Raleigh DiCaprio, and I am what's called a **Speech-Language Pathologist**. I help to figure out how best to help Cyrus learn to communicate with everyone around him, teaching him what is called 'functional communication skills'. One example of this could be building on the **sign language** that he has already started to use."

"I am an **Occupational Therapist**, and—oh—my name is Emily Needham. I will look at Cyrus's skills of daily living, and I can also check out his fine and gross motor skills as well as any sensory issues he might have with the environment around him."

Dr. Smith continued the conversation: "As you can see, we all work together here in what we like to call an interdisciplinary team. We find that we can best help children

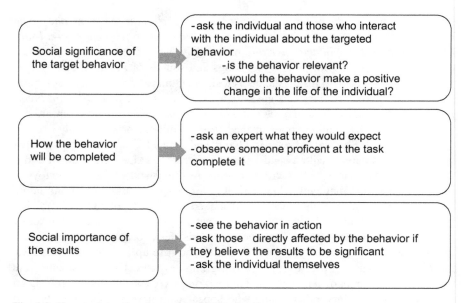

Fig. 1.3 How to determine the social validity of goals

and families when we all know what is going on with one another. And our ONLY reason for gathering together here is to support the three of you. So let's get started."

The Response: Principles, Processes, Practices, and Reflections

Principles

(Q1) How might you apply each of the defining characteristics of ABA outlined by Baer et al. (1968) to guide a behavior assessment process?

(Q2) Based on the information provided in this case, what might you identify as a priority target behavior? Please explain the social validity of your selected target behavior (Fig. 1.3).

Processes

(Q3) How might you operationally define your selected target behavior (Table 1.5)?

(Q4) Given the various disciplines involved in this case example, how might you, as the behavior analyst, lead and guide the development and implementation of a multidisciplinary assessment plan?

Here is a sample transition plan for a student with ASD from IBI to school and the inclusion of a multidisciplinary team (Fig. 1.4).

(Q5) Once the multidisciplinary assessment plan has been completed, how might you, as the behavior analyst, combine the outcomes attained from each professional involved into a single comprehensive formulation of why the problematic behavior may be occurring? What role might a functional behavior assessment play in this process?

Table 1.5 Considerations to include in an operational definition

The components of an operational definition	

1. Name the behavior (i.e., raising hand)
 2. Topography of the behavior
    (a) Inclusions (either left or right hand raised above shoulder)
    (b) Exclusions (hand resting on table and elbow lifted over the shoulder)
 3. What constitutes one incidence of the behavior
	4. Includes only one behavior (if more than 1 behavior is included, it will have its own definition)
	 5. Cannot be further broken down
	 6. Does not include explanation or hypothesis as to why behavior occurs
	 7. Clear, complete, concise, unambiguous, and objective

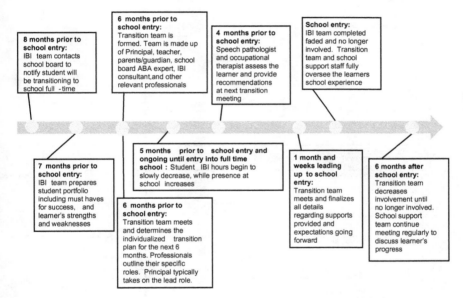

Fig. 1.4 Sample model and timeline for a multidisciplinary team when a child is transitioning from Intensive Behavior Intervention (IBI) to full-time school setting. *Source* Ontario Ministry of Children and Youth Services n.d.

Practices

(Q6) What are the benefits associated with a multidisciplinary assessment team? What are the limitations? What are some strategies you could use to overcome these limitations?

(Q7) How might you work together as part of a multidisciplinary team, despite possibly competing philosophical perspectives regarding why a behavior difficulty might be occurring?

Reflections

(Q8) How could you support Cyrus and his family to maintain an optimistic and hopeful view for the future, while recognizing the impact of Cyrus' intellectual disability? How could you incorporate strengths into her treatment plan?
Look at the following strengths checklist (Fig. 1.5).

	Never	Rarely	Some-times	Usually	Consis-tently
Learning					
The learner readily learns new skills in group teaching contexts					
The learner seeks help when s/he does not understand					
The learner can apply appropriate skills and knowledge even when situations are novel					
The learner will ask questions to clarify provided information					
The learner expresses interest by asking follow-up questions					
Self - Help					
The learner independently takes appropriate measures when s/he needs to go to the bathroom					
The learner cares for his or her belongings (e.g. remembers to bring backpack home from school, or brings pencil and notebook to class)					
The learner dresses and grooms his or herself appropriately (e.g. wears weather appropriate clothing)					
The learner expresses his or her feelings					
Does the learner prepare any meals for themselves? If so which ones:					
Is the learner able to navigate around their community? (i.e. can go to the corner store and get a snack)					
Problem Solving					
The learner shares relevant solutions to problems					
The learner identifies when a problem arises					
The learner asks for help when unable to solve a problem independently					
Can come up with creative solutions to unique problems /					
Creativity and Talents					
Learner expresses joy about activities from the past, or when currently engaged					
Plays sport(s). Which one(s):					
Artistic —circle: clay, paint, pencil, paper craft, construction, other:					
Interests and passions. List them:					
Learner recognizes when s/he has done something well					
Does the learner have any collections? If so what kind?					
Is the learner involved in any clubs or organizations? If so which one(s) and what is their role within it?					
Social Interactions					
The learner is able to carry a give and take conversation with a same aged peer					
The learner is able to join peers currently playing appropriately					
The learner can interrupt a conversation appropriately					
The learner is able to respond to WH questions					
The learner is able to ask WH questions					
The learner will approach peers during recess or lunch to instead of being alone					
Communication					
How does the learner primarily communicate? (circle) Verbally, sign language, PECS, augmented communication device, other:					
The learner responds to non-verbal communicative cues					
The learner uses non-verbal communication (e.g. s/he will point to an object s/he wants)					

Fig. 1.5 Excerpt of a strengths checklist that can be filled out by a parent or guardian and then used by professional when creating treatment goals for the learner (Able Differently, n.d.)

(Q9) What are the benefits and limitations of conducting an assessment in a clinical setting? How might you overcome these limitations?

(Q10) After the initial interdisciplinary meeting Cyrus' parents left feeling like a weight had been lifted. The team spoke to them using language they understood, while conveying professionalism and knowledge. The field of behavior analysis is filled with many terms, when speaking to families how can you ensure they comprehend what is being said and the plan going forward? In the case study above locate the behavioral jargon used and determine nonbehavioral replacement words that could be used in their place (Reference Ethics Box 1.2, Behavior Analyst Certification Board, 2014).

Ethics Box 1.2

Professional and Ethical Compliance Code for Behavior Analysts

- 1.05 Professional and Scientific Relationships.

  (a) Behavior analysts provide behavior-analytic services only in the context of a defined, professional, or scientific relationship or role.

  (b) When behavior analysts provide behavior-analytic services, they use language that is fully understandable to the recipient of those services while remaining conceptually systematic with the profession of behavior analysis. They provide appropriate information prior to service delivery about the nature of such services and appropriate information later about results and conclusions.

  (c) Where differences of age, gender, race, culture, ethnicity, national origin, religion, sexual orientation, disability, language, or socioeconomic status significantly affect behavior analysts' work concerning particular individuals or groups, behavior analysts obtain the training, experience, consultation, and/or supervision necessary to ensure the competence of their services, or they make appropriate referrals.

  (d) In their work-related activities, behavior analysts do not engage in discrimination against individuals or groups based on age, gender, race, culture, ethnicity, national origin, religion, sexual orientation, disability, language, socioeconomic status, or any basis proscribed by law.

  (e) Behavior analysts do not knowingly engage in behavior that is harassing or demeaning to persons with whom they interact in their work based on factors such as those persons' age, gender, race, culture, ethnicity, national origin, religion, sexual orientation, disability, language, or socioeconomic status, in accordance with law.

  (f) Behavior analysts recognize that their personal problems and conflicts may interfere with their effectiveness. Behavior analysts refrain from providing services when their personal circumstances may compromise delivering services to the best of their abilities.

Additional Web Links
Intellectual Disability:
http://aaidd.org/intellectual-disability/definition
Multidisciplinary Assessment:
http://www.selectivemutism.org/resources/library/Educational%20Planning%
20IEP%20IDEA%20%20and%20504/Multidisciplinary%20Assessment-%20A%
20Parents%20Guide.pdf/view?searchterm=assessment
Sign Language and ASD:
www.txautism.net/uploads/target/SignLanguage.pdf

CASE: i-A4

Why won't Serena just let me teach?
Setting: Classroom   Age Group: School-Age

LEARNING OBJECTIVE:

- Apply applied behavior analysis assessment processes within an inclusive classroom setting.

TASK LIST LINKS:

- **Identification of the Problem**

  - (G-03) Conduct a preliminary assessment of the client in order to identify the referral problem.
  - (G-06) Provide behavior-analytic services in collaboration with others who support and/or provide services to one's clients.
  - (G-08) Identify and make environmental changes that reduce the need for behavior analysis services.

- **Measurement**

  - (H-01) Select a measurement system to obtain representative data given the dimensions of the behavior and the logistics of observing and recording.

- **Assessment**

  - (I-06) Make recommendations regarding behaviors that must be established, maintained, increased, or decreased.

KEY TERMS:

- **Classroom Management**

  - Classroom management typically refers to the techniques a teacher uses within a classroom setting to keep students on-task and displaying expected behaviors, and to ensure academic activities are completed within the allotted time (Simonsen et al. 2008).

- **Habilitation**
  - Habilitation is the process of teaching new behaviors that increase access to shorter-term and longer-term reinforcers and reduce access to shorter-term and longer-term punishers (Cooper et al. 2007).

- **Paraprofessional**
  - A paraprofessional is an individual working in a classroom setting under the direction of a teacher to provide specialized support to students. Such individuals are not licensed to teach, but instead provide either individual or small group guidance to students within a classroom. Paraprofessionals will often work in partnership with teachers to support children with disabilities in inclusive classrooms (Giangreco 2003).

- **"Relevance of Behavior" Rule**
  - Many applied behavior Analysis (ABA)-based programs involve not only reducing problematic behavior, but also teaching new skills. The relevance of behavior rule is a guide when selecting a new skill to be taught. The rule is that only those behaviors that will continue to be reinforced after training in the natural setting should be selected because this will increase the likelihood that the new skill is maintained and generalized after the teaching program has ended (Ayllon and Azrin 1968; Alber and Heward 1996).

Why Won't Serena Just Let Me Teach?

Mr. Thiessen's grade one class is a soothing class. He takes great pains to continue the "natural look" that the Kindergarten class before him offered, that he learned about in depth in the months before graduation last year from his teacher education program. The lights are natural, and lamps are plugged in around the classroom but kept low. Brightly colored wall decorations cannot be found: The room follows the colors of the natural environment. Bulletin boards are covered with crinkly brown paper, floors are covered with snuggly area rugs soothing to the feet, and the door to the school's major hallway has a special mechanism that helps it to close slowly and softly. Transitions from activity to activity are signaled with familiar sounds, a gentle rain stick, or sometimes the unavoidable school buzzer amplified throughout the public address system. Although the school itself is mid-sized, with about 600 children filling its classes, the classroom itself is a joyously large, open rectangle with only 14 small students: a cause for celebration!

Even with the small numbers of children in the grade one class, Mr. Thiessen and his students are further supported by a **paraprofessional**—an experienced, energetic educator whom the students called "Mrs. Bee" for her favorite black-and-yellow-striped jacket she wears while on yard duty—who was assigned to the grade one class on a full-time basis this year due to the presence of many students with complex needs. In addition to students with social-emotional needs like frequent bouts of crying, physical needs like toilet training, and basic needs like healthy foods and weather-appropriate clothing, the grade one classroom included three students diagnosed with disabilities (quite unusual for the early years of school).

One particular student typically demands a high frequency and intensity of attention from both educators in the room: six-year-old Serena. *Her name*, Mr. Thiessen considered, *is quite the juxtaposition to her everyday behavior.* Serena had no "diagnosis" and wasn't considered to have a disability of any sort (yet), but she certainly is—in Mr. Thiessen's opinion—a high-needs child!

He thought back to yesterday ...

Yesterday, Mr. Thiessen and "Mrs. Bee" started the morning by transitioning the students into the well-planned day by spreading out bins of math manipulatives across the classroom. They laid them on desks, carpets, and the tops of low book-shelves—anywhere that was not an individual student's desk or table. Immediately upon entering the room from the crisp fall morning from the classroom's private exterior door, Serena threw up her hands and screeched excitedly. She thumped down her colorful knapsack onto the wet floor, stomped her boots repeatedly in the dressing and undressing alcove, then threw her knitted hat and matching mittens in the general direction of her three-pronged hook, leaving them in a shallow puddle of collective drippings from a classroom full of outdoor clothing. Despite repeated requests by both educators to please "put away her things properly," Serena did not. Instead, she bounced her way over to the closest math bin and stretched out on top of the classroom's largest beanbag chairs, scrunching and wiggling until she was comfortable. Then—in a well-experienced way—she grabbed an adjacent beanbag chair and slung it over her lower back and upper legs, calling for Mrs. Bee to "make it good." This was Mrs. Bee's prompt to "fluff up" the beanbag until it was "just right" (according to Serena's needs). Mrs. Bee knew to go right away, or Serena would call her and call her in an increasingly high-pitched, demanding voice until she "finally" appeared. *It isn't worth making her wait*, insisted Mrs. Bee.

Fast-forward to the present "carpet time" where the grade one students gathered together for 15 min to plan the day ahead, sing and talk together, and complete some literacy exercises in a fun, interactive way, Mr. Thiessen was leading the class in a familiar song—one without actions, this time. While all the other student were seated, legs crossed, around the edge of the carpet, Serena hopped up boldly and proceeded to wiggle her bottom to the beat of the song, eyes tightly closed, elbows out, and flapping. Naturally—like usual—the other students started giggling.

Even though we keep our carpet time to less than 15 min, reflected the teacher, *it's almost impossible to get through it without Serena getting everyone else off track. How frustrating! When she isn't disrupting EVERYONE, she is sure to be disrupting SOMEONE. Why won't she just let me teach? I may have to use* **habilitation** *as well as the curriculum itself to assist her to learn basic skills like sitting and attending, even for short periods of time to start. I remember from a presentation I attended that the* **relevance of behavior rule** *needed to be followed.* Although Mr. Thiessen would never voice these inner thoughts, it was difficult to keep them from recurring— especially when he was trying to drop off to sleep at night.

After what he felt was a debacle at carpet time, Mr. Thiessan had asked if "Mrs. Bee" would take Serena across the hall for some special attention time. Across the hall was an empty classroom that was not assigned to a specific class. Various staff members accessed it for a range of reasons, from a private area for parent–teacher interviews, to a meeting room, to reasons just like this one: for some flexible time and space on an as-needed basis.

"Mrs. Bee" and Serena worked together on the same lesson that was planned for the whole class. In this case, it was sorting out small items into labeled containers, placing them into the containers that represented the first letter of each item. Throughout the 15 minutes they were across the hall, Serena seemed completely immersed. For example, she put her tiny toy car in the "C" container, and her miniscule plastic ladybug into the "L" container.

Mr. Thiessan knew, however, that today's **classroom management** decisions were not going to please Serena's mother or father. While they lived in two separate households, they were solidly and collectively opposed to Serena being separated from her playmates in any way. In addition—like all parents—they want the best education for Serena and both repeatedly expressed that they felt the best education was the teacher and not the paraprofessional. Mr. Thiessen, "Mrs. Bee," their principal, and Serena's two parents had already had a few meetings about these issues. *But*, concluded Mr. Thiessen, *I still need to survive the day. Maybe we SHOULD think about calling in a behavior consultant, like the principal suggested. I know that they do more than dealing with problem behaviours, they do help with skill-building as well and there are definitely areas where Serena and a few others in the class could keep learning—like sitting at carpet time, like waiting for help, like putting their outdoor clothes on their indoor hooks. But I don't know if the parents would go for it. I think they believe that I am the problem, and not Serena. But maybe it's both.*

The Response: Principles, Processes, Practices, and Reflections

Principles

(Q1) How might the principle of habilitation and the relevance of behavior rule guide and inform your behavior assessment process? Please discuss each using examples from Serena's case.

(Q2) In Serena's situation, what type of data collection would you start with to understand the frequency of the behavior that is occurring throughout the day before you meet with the parents?

Processes

(Q3) Why is it important to include the professionals supporting the child experiencing the behavior difficulty in the assessment process? Considering Serena's case, how might you include the teacher in the assessment process? Please provide a rationale for your decision.

Students can also be involved in assessments and interventions. See the following website for additional information: http://www.parentcenterhub.org/repository/student-involvement/

(Q4) Please describe how you would approach both indirect and direct assessments of the problematic behavior and provide a rationale for your approach (Table 1.6).

(Q5) When meeting with Serena's parents, they will be looking to ensure that Serena is included with her peers, but she seems to do better and be more focused when she is one-on-one with the paraprofessional. What types of data and what support would you have prepared for the meeting with the parents to ensure a plan to support full inclusion? Would you start with full inclusion or partial inclusion?

Table 1.6 A guide to differentiating between and planning direct and indirect assessments with an individual

	• First operationally define the behavior • Take into consideration setting events (medication, sleep, interruptions in schedule, variations in staff or peers in the environment, sleep, etc.)	
Type of assessment	Indirect assessments	Direct assessments
What it looks like	• Based on parent, support staff, individuals personal description of events and pattern • More subjective	• Based on observations of the individual • Can be in vivo or video recordings • More objective
How it is done	• Written questionnaire paired with verbal interview	• Observer takes data (for example, ABC chart or frequency count) simultaneously with their observation

Practices

(Q6) Insert the carpet time scenario outlined in this case above documenting the antecedents, behaviors, and consequences into Fig. 1.6. What hypothesis might you draft based on this analysis? Please explain how you reached this hypothesis and how you might further test this hypothesis (Table 1.7).

Student Name: _____   _____ _____

Behavior of Interest: _____

Operational definition of the behavior: Operationally define the behavior of interest ensuring to include information regarding what it looks like, and examples of the behavior that will not be included (if applicable)

_____   _____ _____ _____

_____   _____ ___ ____

_____   ___ ___

Are there any situations, people, times of day, etc. when the behavior con sistently does not occur? If so list them here:

_____   ____ ___

Known setting events (i.e. hunger, change in routine, medication change, noise level):

_____   ____ ___

Antecedents & Consequences

Immediate Antecedent	Consequences
_ Seat task (non‑preferred)	_ Behavior unacknowledged
_ Demand/request	_ Verbal warning
_ Transition from: _____ to _____	_ Verbal redirection
_ Unprepared (missing material)	_ Non‑verbal redirection
_ Toy inaccessible	_ Physical redirection
_ Peer interaction	_ Time‑out (duration: _____ _____)
_ Alone	(non‑seclusion/seclusion)
_ Other _____	_ Privileges removed (type: _____ ____)
	_ Blocking
	_ Other _____

Hypothesis for the function (s) of the behavior:
_ Escape from: _____
_ Attention from : _____
_ Gain tangible : _____
_ Automatic Reinforcement (sensory stimulation): _____

Statement: When the learner _____
(antecedent)
and s/he engages in _____ it is in order to _____
(behavior of interest)
_____. The behavior is more likely to
(perceived function)
occur if _____.
(setting event)

Completed by: _____   _____

Date: _____

Revision date: _____

Fig. 1.6 Sample template for understanding the function of a behavior in a classroom (Barnhill 2005)

Table 1.7 An ABC chart for taking direct observational data

Antecedent	Behavior	Consequence

(Q7) Conducting a behavior assessment requires parental informed consent. What information needs to be included in an informed consent? Since Serena's parents are separated, do they both need to sign the informed consent or is one parent's consent satisfactory (Table 1.8) (Reference Ethics Box 1.3, Behavior Analyst Certification Board, 2014)?

Table 1.8 Informed consent checklist (Institute for applied behavior analysis, n.d.)

General topics
☐ Type of program and goals of the program
☐ Where intervention will take place
☐ Day and time of intervention
☐ Any different treatment methods that may be utilized
☐ Intrusiveness
☐ Estimate of how long the intervention will be necessary
☐ Levels of responsibility and roles of each individual involved
☐ Accessibility to records
☐ Phone numbers and contact information
☐ Freedom to participate and end the intervention
☐ Qualifications
Professional's obligations and responsibilities
☐ Confidentiality and limits of confidentiality
☐ Compliance with set appointments and session times
☐ Collection of data
☐ Writing reports
☐ Assessments—note assessments that may be used
☐ Development of intervention plan and necessary programs
☐ Train and model aspects of intervention and program
☐ Practice within area of competence
☐ Answer all questions regarding intervention, program, and interaction
☐ Obtain caregiver/guardian permission for all programs to be implemented
☐ Inform caregiver/guardian of all potential side effects
☐ Attend all meetings related to intervention, and program with other agencies
☐ Terminate upon request
☐ Upon request provide additional information and resources
Obligations of caregiver/guardian
☐ Provide input regarding program goals
☐ Be involved and participate in all aspects of program
☐ Comply with set appointments and sessions
☐ Active involvement in meetings
☐ Collect data
☐ Communicate openly regarding program, staff, and challenges

Ethics Box 1.3

> ## Professional and Ethical Compliance Code for Behavior Analysts
>
> - 2.04 Third-Party Involvement in Services.
>   (a) When behavior analysts agree to provide services to a person or entity at the request of a third party, behavior analysts clarify, to the extent feasible and at the outset of the service, the nature of the relationship with each party and any potential conflicts. This clarification includes the role of the behavior analyst (such as therapist, organizational consultant, or expert witness), the probable uses of the services provided or the information obtained, and the fact that there may be limits to confidentiality.
>   (b) If there is a foreseeable risk of behavior analysts being called upon to perform conflicting roles because of the involvement of a third party, behavior analysts clarify the nature and direction of their responsibilities, keep all parties appropriately informed as matters develop, and resolve the situation in accordance with the code.
>   (c) When providing services to a minor or individual who is a member of a protected population at the request of a third party, behavior analysts ensure that the parent or client surrogate of the ultimate recipient of services is informed of the nature and scope of services to be provided, as well as their right to all service records and data.
>   (d) Behavior analysts put the client's care above all others and, should the third party make requirements for services that are contradicted by the behavior analyst's recommendations, behavior analysts are obligated to resolve such conflicts in the best interest of the client. If said conflict cannot be resolved, that behavior analyst's services to the client may be discontinued following appropriate transition.

(Q8) If a behavior analyst were to come into the school to assess Serena's behavior, who would be able to access the records? Could the behavior analyst leave the records regarding Serena in the classroom filing cabinet? Explain your answers.

Reflections

(Q9) Conducting a behavior assessment requires parental informed consent. How might you respond if you were faced with a scenario where a child is experiencing behavior difficulties, the teacher is recommending a behavior assessment, but the parents are refusing to provide consent?
*see Ethics Box 1.3 above
(Q10) In addition to parental informed consent, it is important to include children in the consent process, and this is often called assent. Please explain how you would

involve Serena in aspects of the decision-making process? How could you verify that Serena understood the assent?

For a sample assent tutorial, see here:
http://www.irb.vt.edu/pages/assent.htm
Additional Web Links
Classroom Inclusion:
kc.vanderbilt.edu/kennedy_files/InclusioninClassroomTips.pdf
Inclusion and ASD:
http://www.asatonline.org/research-treatment/clinical-corner/inclusion/
A Resource Guide for Teachers:
https://www.bced.gov.bc.ca/specialed/sid/

CASE: i-A5 Guest Author: Monique Somma

Monique Somma: PhD Student, Brock University
Where did Siki learn to say that?
Setting: Community   Age Group: School Age

LEARNING OBJECTIVE:

- Construct a behavior assessment process in a community setting.

TASK LIST LINKS:

- **Fundamental Elements of Behavior Change**

    – (D-11) Use mand training.
    – (D-13) Use intraverbal training.
    – (D-15) Identify punishers.

- **Specific Behavior-Change Procedures**

    – (E-04) Use contingency contracting (i.e., behavioral contracts).

- **Identification of the Problem**

    – (G-01) Review records and available data at the outset of the case.

- **Measurement**

    – (H-01) Select a measurement system to obtain representative data given the dimensions of the behavior and the logistics of observing and recording.
    – (H-02) Select a schedule of observation and recording periods.

KEY TERMS:

- **Differentiated instruction**

  - Differentiated instruction is an approach to teaching in which different students in the same classroom are provided with different types of learning opportunities based on areas such as students' interests, readiness, and preferences (Levy 2008).

- **Full Inclusion**

  - Full inclusion is a variation of inclusion in which students with exceptionalities are placed full time in an inclusive classroom with their same-age peers. Within this context, emphasis is often placed on teaching social skills to children with exceptionalities in order to foster successful interactions and relationships with their nondisabled peers (Fuchs and Fuchs 1998).

- **Inclusive classroom**

  - An inclusive classroom is an approach to special education in which students with exceptionalities spend most of their time in the same classroom, and engaged in the same activities, as their same-age peers. This contrasts with a segregated classroom in which children with exceptionalities are placed in a classroom separate from their same-age peers without disabilities, and spend most of their time in this specialized classroom interacting with other children with exceptionalities (Florian 2008).

- **Intraverbal**

  - Intraverbals are "verbal operants characterized by the emission of a verbal response after the presentation of a verbal stimulus that shows no point-to-point correspondence with the response" (Belloso-Díazn and Pérez-González 2015, p. 749).

- **Mand**

  - A mand is "a verbal operant in which the response is reinforced by a characteristic consequence and is therefore under the functional control of relevant conditions of deprivation or aversive stimulation" (Skinner 1957, pp. 35–36).

Where Did Siki Learn to Say That?

"Hey butt-face!" The cry out is heard over the busy rustling and talking during the typical dinner rush at the local pizza joint.

"Siki! Stop that!" Mrs. Adams whispered with vehemence, and she felt her ears and neck growing hot, red, and blotchy.

"Butt-face! Butt-face!" Matteo and Teal piped in while giggling loudly. "That's it! No TV or video games, that includes your iPad, Siki, when we get home!" snapped Mrs. Adam who was barely holding it together and completely unable to swallow the food that was now stuck in the back of her throat. Her eyes welled up with tears and she gazed away from the table, noticing several patrons awkwardly look away to avoid her gaze. This was the final straw of the evening, for her, as Siki had cursed at least seven other times prior in the past 45 min. Mr. Adam knew without asking what his wife was feeling, and rubbed her back with sympathy, glancing at his three children as they munched their pizza as if their mother had not just taken away their favorite leisure activities. He felt fortunate to have three healthy, beautiful children, Matteo and Teal who were four and five years old, respectively, and Siki, the 9-year-old apple of his eye since the day she was born.

Mr. Adam, now lost in his thoughts, remembered that ever since Siki was a small child, he knew that she was not quite like the other kids around her. She had always preferred to play her own games, which she often perseverated on for long periods of time. These games had never made much sense to him, but Mrs. Adams had repeatedly assured him that she was "just being creative." Having two younger brothers, though, had allowed her to expand on her interactions with other children as they constantly seek her out to play with them, he thought. Life at home has been pretty good for his three young children and Siki has really grown socially as a result of having the boys around. At school, this year especially, she had been more successful in the **inclusive** grade 4 classroom. *There have been fewer calls home about Siki being frustrated and upset and most days she has received a happy face in her agenda*, he thought.

Although Siki sees Dr. Remanuski, her pediatrician, regularly, Mr. and Mrs. Adams have not wished to move forward with further testing as far as obtaining a diagnosis for Siki. But some things were definitely unusual: both past and present. At the age of four, for example, Siki had already started reading most children's books and had usually been able to exceed the academic expectations in class as long as she was interested in the topic. As far as Mr. and Mrs. Adam were concerned, Siki interacts better with adults as a result of her being an only child for four years and her not being in any structured, or social programs until she went to Junior Kindergarten. For the first two months of school, Siki cried off and on for much of the morning. When directed to play in the Discovery Centre, she would often throw toys and materials such as pencils, erasers, and small pebbles. At one point, the school personnel had encouraged the Adams to look into sending Siki to a specialized program, but Mrs. Adam was very persistent and she worked diligently with the teachers to keep Siki in an inclusive setting. Once the teachers had figured out that Siki was most content when in the classroom library reading stories out loud to herself or lining them up in a particular order on the carpet, Siki was permitted to choose this for a discovery time activity. The crying and throwing subsided tremendously and Siki seemed much happier in Kindergarten.

As Siki progressed through the early elementary grades, formal and informal meetings at the school urged the Adams to consider further testing in order for Siki to receive some additional supports and programs. Although the teachers, principal, and school psychologist had recommended further assessment more frequently as time passed, her parents continued to feel that although it takes Siki and the teacher a couple of months to get to know one other, and it is the school and classroom teacher's job to figure out what works. They have never believed that any diagnosis would ever help the teacher and Siki to get to know each other better. With a lot of strength and advocacy, they have been reasonably happy with the school, which has a strong focus on **full inclusion** and **differentiated instruction**.

Lately though, as Siki has been displaying more inappropriate behavior, especially cursing when out with her family, Mr. and Mrs. Adam have begun to reluctantly discuss revisiting the idea of further testing with Dr. Remanuski.

"It seems as though in the past year or so, we cannot go anywhere without at least one episode of Siki shouting out swear words. Whenever we are out, like the grocery store or a restaurant, she seems to just blurt out profanity for no apparent reason. Lately, the boys have been copying whatever Siki says, shouting it out and laughing because they know the words are making us angry. Have you noticed this?" Mrs. Adams continued to whisper at her spouse.

In general, the Adams were puzzled as to where Siki had learned the inappropriate language, and why she thinks it is okay to shout out in public. Neither of them uses profanity (at least when the children are around) and Mrs. Adam is very strict with the television programs that the children are permitted to watch. They even closely monitored Siki's use of the Internet, her online interactions, and the games she plays on the iPad. Siki had actually been grounded from the iPad a lot lately since this seemed to be the best **punishment** when she showed this type of disruptive behavior. Although recently, it seemed that Siki had little care for this **consequence**, as she continued to use profanity on a regular basis, often daily. Even when she was grounded from the iPad, she continued to swear in public.

At home the swearing had been more tolerable; however, the boys were really picking up a lot of inappropriate language because of it. Matteo's daycare teacher actually mentioned that the other day he had called another child "Butt-face!" when they were fighting over a toy truck.

When Mrs. Adam spoke to Siki's teacher, Miss Pri, last week, she asked if Siki had been using foul language at school. Miss Pri replied that she has not heard Siki use profanity of any kind in the classroom or when she has been outside on yard duty. She assured Mrs. Adam that she would let the other teachers who interact with Siki know so that they could be aware in case there was an incident at school. They had a behavior contract in place from the previous years that had broad expectations, but Mrs. Adams said she rarely had to reference it. Although Mrs. Adam was reassured by Siki's behavior at school, she still felt very discouraged as to the reason for her newest and ever-increasing behavior issues outside of school. She had also felt silly for asking Miss Pri because in hindsight of course the teacher would have contacted her or written in Siki's agenda if there was a problem at school.

"Let's go, ploppy turd-faces!" Siki shouted as she jumped up from the table and began to put her jacket on. Mr. Adam's thoughts were interrupted as he was reminded of the challenges they face as a family when doing simple things like going out shopping or to a restaurant which was something the Adams did as a way of spending "family time" together.

Mr. Adam piped in as he stood and gestured for her to sit down. "Just a minute Siki. We still have to pay the bill." At that moment the waiter appeared with the check and waited somewhat impatiently as Mr. Adam fumbled to retrieve the cash from his wallet. He felt relieved to finally be leaving the restaurant. "Bye, butt-face, poo-brain!" could be heard trailing out of the restaurant along with the echo and giggles of the two young boys on the way to the car.

Although the ride home was less than three minutes, it felt like an eternity. Mrs. Adam was nearly in tears, which she had been holding in for the latter half of the evening. The only words uttered were by Mr. Adams, who, upon arrival at home, directed all three children to go upstairs and prepare themselves for bed, and he would be up shortly to tuck them in. The boys whispered to each other and Siki expressed her discontentment with an "Ugh, it's not fair!" and crossed her arms with a pout.

A few hours later, as Mr. and Mrs. Adam settled into bed, they discussed the events of that evening, which seem to be the norm lately. "I feel as though people are judging us as parents. I know they are staring!" Mrs. Adam sobbed—even though she thought she was done with tears for the evening. "Now the boys are also giggling and repeating these swear words all the time as though it were a funny joke."

Mr. Adams dared not tell her about what the childcare educator had said to him the other day. It seemed as though he remembered less and less what it felt like to be relaxed going out in public, and more and more feeling stressed about the unknowns. What will Siki do? How will she act? What will she say this time?

Mrs. Adam commented that she felt like it was a circus whenever they go out, except they are the main act. Mr. Adam emphasized that ordering in and eating at home would be a better option from now on. Moving forward with an assessment for Siki seemed to be the only next logical step, to seek out some answers that would calm the roiling sea of emotional turbulence where they were precariously balanced.

The Response: Principles, Processes, Practices, and Reflections

Principles

(Q1) Based on the information provided in this case study, what consequences are increasing Siki's behavior and which are decreasing it?

(Q2) How might you describe Siki's behavior topographically? How might you describe it by function? What are the benefits and limitations associated with each of these methods of describing behavior?

Processes

(Q3) Based on the information provided in this case study, indicate the antecedents and consequences that might be surrounding Siki's problematic verbal behavior.

What patterns emerge? Based on these patterns, hypothesize why these problematic behaviors might be occurring (Fig. 1.6).

(Q4) What would be your first step to determine why the behavior may be occurring with Siki's family and not at school? Based on the information in the case, what is your initial hypothesis on why this is occurring?

Practices

(Q5) How could you approach the assessment of Siki's problematic behavior across multiple settings such as home, community, and school? Which parties would need to give consent? In what manner would you explain the results of the assessment to, and to whom (Reference Ethics Box 1.4, Behavior Analyst Certification Board, 2014)?

Ethics Box 1.4

Professional and Ethical Compliance Code for Behavior Analysts

- 2.03 Consultation.
  (a) Behavior analysts arrange for appropriate consultations and referrals based principally on the best interests of their clients, with appropriate consent, and subject to other relevant considerations, including applicable law and contractual obligations.
  (b) When indicated and professionally appropriate, behavior analysts cooperate with other professionals, in a manner that is consistent with the philosophical assumptions and principles of behavior analysis, in order to effectively and appropriately serve their clients.
- 3.04 Explaining Assessment Results.
  Behavior analysts explain assessment results using language and graphic displays of data that are reasonably understandable to the client.
- 3.05 Consent-Client Records.
  Behavior analysts obtain the written consent of the client before obtaining or disclosing client records from or to other sources, for assessment purposes.

(Q6) Which dimension would you use to collect behavior in the assessment observation (Fig. 1.7)?

(Q7) Mrs. Adams directly mentions that Siki may not use the iPad when they get home from dinner. What is a behavior contract and how could the Adams family potentially utilize this with Siki and her iPad?

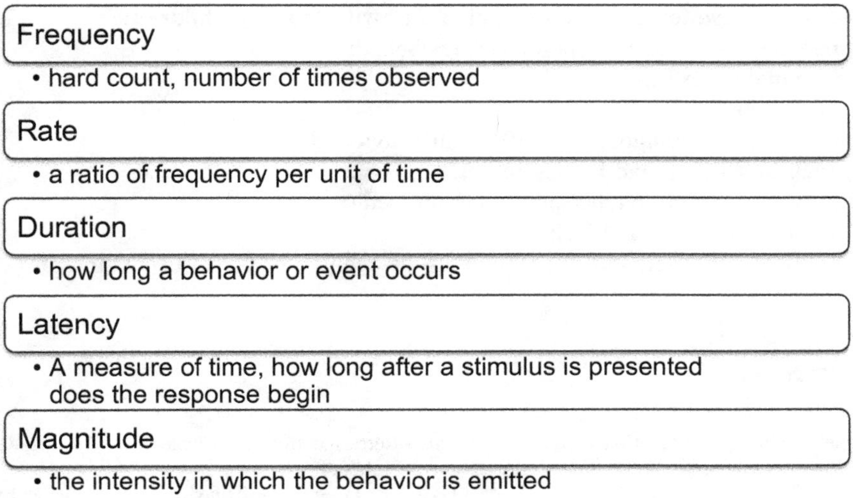

Frequency

• hard count, number of times observed

Rate

• a ratio of frequency per unit of time

Duration

• how long a behavior or event occurs

Latency

• A measure of time, how long after a stimulus is presented does the response begin

Magnitude

• the intensity in which the behavior is emitted

Fig. 1.7 Dimensions of behavior

Reflections

(**Q8**) *Thinking* not just about reducing the immediate frequency of Siki's problematic behaviors, but rather about longer-term behavioral improvements, how might you balance a focus on the specific presenting behavior difficulties and the quality of life for Siki's family?

(**Q9**) As a behavior analyst you are responsible to everyone who is affected by the services being offered. What implications could be present for Siki's siblings if you were brought into the home to assess Siki's behavior (Reference Ethics Box 1.5, Behavior Analyst Certification Board, 2014)?

Ethics Box 1.5

Professional and Ethical Compliance Code for Behavior Analysts

- 2.02 Responsibility.
  The behavior analyst's responsibility is to all parties affected by behavioral services. When multiple parties are involved and could be defined as a client, a hierarchy of parties must be established and communicated from the outset of the defined relationship. Behavior analysts identify and communicate who the primary ultimate beneficiary of services is in any given situation and advocates for his or her best interests.

(**Q10**) Consider the stigmas that can often come with labels and diagnoses, why may Siki's parents be reluctant to engage in an assessment with professionals?

See this article for examples of difficulties with labeling children:
http://smhp.psych.ucla.edu/pdfdocs/diaglabel.pdf
Additional Web Links
Verbal Behavior:
www.txautism.net/uploads/target/VerbalBehavior.pdf
Speech and Language Development:
http://www.asha.org/public/speech/development/
The Analysis of Verbal Behavior:
https://www.abainternational.org/journals/the-analysis-of-verbal-behavior.aspx

References

Able Differently. (n.d.). *Child strengths checklist*. Retrieved from http://able-differently.org/wp-content/uploads/2012/01/Strengths-Assessment-Child.pdf

Alber, S. R., & Heward, W. L. (1996). "GOTCHA!" Twenty-five behavior traps guaranteed to extend your students' academic and social skills. *Intervention in School and Clinic, 31,* 285–289.

American Psychiatric Association. (2013). *Intellectual disability fact sheet*. Retrieved from http://www.dsm5.org/documents/intellectual%20disability%20fact%20sheet.pdf

American Speech-Language-Hearing Association. (2007). *Scope of practice in speech-language pathology*. Retrieved from http://www.asha.org/policy/SP2007-00283.htm

Ayllon, T., & Azrin, N. H. (1968). *The token economy: A motivational system for therapy and rehabilitation*. New York: Appleton-Century-Crofts.

Baer, D. M., Wolf, M. M., & Risley, T. R. (1968). Some current dimensions of applied behavior analysis. *Journal of Applied Behavior Analysis, 1*(1), 91–97.

Baer, D. M., Wolf, M. M., & Risley, T. R. (1987). Some still current dimensions of applied behavior analysis. *Journal of Applied Behavior Analysis, 20*(4), 313–327.

Behavior Analyst Certification Board (2014). *Professional and ethical compliance code for behavior analysts*. Retrieved from http://bacb.com/wp-content/uploads/2016/01/160120-compliance-code-english.pdf

Barnhill, G. P. (2005). Functional behavioral assessment in schools. *Intervention in School and Clinic, 40*(3), 131–143.

Belloso-Díaz, C., & Pérez-González, L. (2015). Effect of learning tacts or tacts and intraverbals on the emergence of intraverbals about verbal categorization. *Psychological Record, 65*(4), 749–760. doi:10.1007/s40732-015-0145-0.

Bicard, S. C., Bicard, D. F., & the IRIS Center. (2012). *Measuring behavior*. Retrieved on from http://iris.peabody.vanderbilt.edu/wp-content/uploads/pdf_case_studies/ics_measbeh.pdf

Bosch, S., & Fuqua, R. (2001). Behavioral cusps: A model for selecting target behaviors. *Journal of Applied Behavior Analysis, 34*(1), 123–125.

Carter, S. (2010). *The social validity manual: A guide to subjective evaluation of behavior interventions*. London: Academic Press.

Cooper, J. O., Heron, T. E., & Heward, W. L. (2007). *Applied behavior analysis* (2nd ed.). Upper Saddle River, NJ: Pearson.

Dutton, L. (2011). Functional communication and special education: Giving a voice to those who can't speak. *Southeast Education Network, 16*(1). Retrieved from http://seenmagazine.us/articles/article-detail/articleid/1660/functional-communication-and-special-education.aspx

Edmunds, J., Kendal, P., Ringle, V., Read, K., Brodman, D., Pimentel, S., et al. (2013). An examination of behavioral rehearsal during consultation as a predictor of training outcomes. *Administration and Policy In Mental Health, 40*(6), 456–466.

Escambia County School District. (n.d.). *ABC checklist—version 2*. Retrieved from http://www. escambia.k12.fl.us/pbis/fbadata/

Florian, L. (2008). Inclusion: Special or inclusive education: Future trends. *British Journal of Special Education, 35*(4), 202–208.

Fuchs, D., & Fuchs, L. (1998). Competing visions for education students with disabilities: Inclusion versus full inclusion. *Childhood Education, 74*(5), 80–81.

Giangreco, M. (2003). Working with paraprofessionals. *Educational Leadership, 61*(2), 50–53.

Health Canada. (2013). *A young child's assessment and diagnosis*. Retrieved from http://www. gov.mb.ca/fs/imd/young_child_assess.html

Horner, R., Carr, E., Halle, J., McGee, G., Odom, S., & Wolery, M. (2005). The use of single-subject research to identify evidence-based practice in special education. *Exceptional Children, 71*(2), 165–179.

Howard, J., Sparkman, C., Cohen, H., Green, G., & Stanislaw, H. (2005). A comparison of intensive behavior analytic and eclectic treatments for young children with autism. *Research in Developmental Disabilities, 26*(4), 359–383.

Institute for Applied Behavior Analysis. (n.d.). *Informed consent checklist*. Retrieved from http:// iaba.com/downloads/Forms_and_Procedures_Manual/tab04.pdf

Kelly, R., & Gobber, B. (2011). *Toward a more flexible, believable model of the human hand for American Sign Language*. Retrieved from http://socrs.cdm.depaul.edu/2011/program/SOCRS-11.pdf#page=87

Levy, H. (2008). Meeting the needs of all students through differentiated instruction: Helping every child reach and exceed standards. *The Clearing House: A Journal of Educational Strategies, Issues, and Ideas, 81*(4), 161–164.

Ontario Ministry of Children and Youth Services. (n.d.). *Transition team model*. Retrieved from http://www.autismontario.com/client/aso/ao.nsf/0/15006C97042D3DDD8525756D00683967/ $FILE/Supporting%20Seamless%20Transitions%20Appendix%20A.%20Connections%20for %20Students.pdf?openelement

O'Neill, R., Horner, R., Albin, R., Sprague, J., Storey, K., & Newton, J. (1997). *Functional assessment for problem behavior: A practical handbook* (2nd ed.). Pacific Grove, CA: Brooks/Cole.

Reed, K. L., & Sanderson, S. N. (1999). *Concepts of occupational therapy*. Baltimore, MA: Lippincott Williams & Wilkins.

Simonsen, B., Fairbanks, S., Briesch, A., Myers, D., & Sugai, G. (2008). Evidence-based practices in classroom management: Considerations for research to practice. *Education and Treatment of Children, 31*(3), 351–380.

Skinner, B. F. (1957). *Verbal behavior*. New York, NY: Appleton- Century-Crofts.

Chapter 2
Assessment Case Studies from Adolescence to Adulthood

Abstract Applied Behavior Analysis (ABA) is the scientific study of human behavior. The principles and processes of ABA, including those involved in the assessment of behavior, can be used to gain insight and understanding into human behavior across the life span. In Chap. 1, behavior assessment principles, processes, and practices were explored through five case scenarios involving preschool- and school-age children in home, school, clinical, and community settings. In Chap. 2, the behavior assessment process is explored with adolescents and adults in a range of settings and contexts including high school and employment. In adolescence and adulthood, peer relationships, independence, empowerment, and self-sufficiency become increasingly important. The outcome of behavior assessment therefore is not only to design and implement a behavior-change program to reduce a specific problematic behavior, but also to create the conditions for the individual to be successfully independent in the context in which he or she is learning (e.g., high school, college, and university), living (e.g., apartment, house, and supportive living arrangement), or working (e.g., employment placement). For behavior analysts, this requires a dual focus on shorter-term outcomes such as the reduction of presenting problem behaviors and longer-term outcomes such as knowledge and skill acquisition. The environment–behavior relationship that is the hallmark of ABA allows behavior analysts to maintain an optimistic and hopeful view of the future for each individual they are supporting—recognizing that once environmental and experiential factors are identified through assessment, behavior change and improved outcomes are within reach for everyone, irrespective of age and stage of life.

Keywords Adolescence · Adulthood · Assessment · Behavior assessment · ABA · Life span · Peer relationships · Learning · Living · Environment–behavior relationship · Experiential factors

© Springer International Publishing AG 2016
K. Maich et al., *Applied Behavior Analysis*,
DOI 10.1007/978-3-319-44794-0_2

CASE: i-A6

"Emily's worrying is keeping her awake."
Setting: Home   Age Group: Adolescence

LEARNING OBJECTIVE:

- Analyze graphic displays of behavior.

TASK LIST LINKS

- **Measurement**

    - (A-06) Measure percent of occurrence.
    - (A-10) Design, plot, and interpret data using equal-interval graphs

- **Fundamental Elements of Behavior Change**

    - (D-02) Use appropriate parameters and schedules of reinforcement.

- **Measurement**

    - (H-04) Evaluate changes in level, trend, and variability.

- **Assessment**

    - (I-02) Define environmental variables in observable and measurable terms.
    - (I-03) Design and implement individualized behavioral assessment procedures.
    - (I-05) Organize, analyze, and interpret observed data.

KEY TERMS

- **Acceptance and Commitment Therapy**

    - A third-wave approach to behavior and cognitive therapy that is a type of psychotherapy that focuses on mindfulness, acceptance of problems rather than "fixing" them, and commitment and value-based living (Hayes and Smith 2005).

- **Equal-Interval Graphs**

    - Types of graphs where the x-axis and y-axis are equally spaced compared to graphs, like standard celeration charts that use logarithmic units. Line graphs, bar graphs, and cumulative graphs are usually classified as this type of graph (Mayer et al. 2014).

- **Graphic displays of behavioral data:**

    - In applied behavior analysis, behavior is documented and analyzed through repeated measurement over time. The data gathered are then displayed visually on a graph. A graph is made up of a horizontal axis (the x-axis) that typically represents the passage of time and a vertical axis (the y-axis) that typically represents a quantifiable dimension of the behavior under observation (Horner et al. 2005).

- **Skills Assessment**
  - An assessment that examines an individual's skills and deficits, allowing the creation of a program that will meet a person's needs. These can be published skills assessments (i.e., VB-MAPP or ABLLS-R) or unpublished and based on observation. Often skills assessments are done biannually to track progress and determine the next skills to teach (BCOTB 2012).

Emily's Worrying is Keeping Her Awake

Emily is an 11-year-old girl, treasured by her parents as what they often describe as a responsible, caring, and helpful daughter. She has always had many friends—the same core group since Kindergarten—and is always striving to be one of the near-the-top achievers in her grade six class at the local public school. She tends to spend her spare time either with friends in various athletic pursuits or just "hanging out," participating in local school and community initiatives such as gathering nonperishable goods for the food bank, helping to house-build in the downtown core, and, of course, helping with her two red-headed, much younger siblings: Michael, aged five, and Sarah, a three-year-old preschooler.

Her parents also laughingly call her a "mother hen." Since Emily's mom met her current partner—Emily's stepfather—she begged almost daily for what she called "babies." She hounded the happy pair constantly for a baby brother and a baby sister, practiced in her play stroller and her play high chair with her life-sized dolls, and seemed like quite the nurturing little character. This care for others, in Emily's preadolescence, seems to have broadened even beyond these two longed-for additions to the family, but also to issues around her: what she saw on television, encountered on the Internet, and overheard from others. She spoke with constant concern about medical epidemics, children without parents, and lack of access to food and water. As soon as she became old enough to volunteer—she did!

Emily's parents continued to watch her with pride—and amazement—as she was out almost every evening and at least one day of the weekend, with her parents, with her friends, with her community organizations, and even with her grandparents! *If Emily were a cheerleader,* her mother thought *she would be the head cheerleader, twisting and turning in the air before landing with perfect precision. I can envision it perfectly!* Everything continued smoothly but busily for months on end, with a few seemingly minor adjustments in the family, like more fast food, eating on the run, and less time for previously enjoyed family leisure activities such as reading together, watching movies together, and concocting fancy meals from newly acquired cookbooks together.

However, the smooth pathway became bumpy over time—and even contained a few jarring speed bumps. Over the past few weeks, just a few months into her grade six school year, Emily's parents began to notice some difficulties in Emily's day-to-day functioning that quickly became quite concerning. Often, Emily would not return home until 8:00 or sometimes 9:00 PM, often accompanied by a leader from one of the well-trusted community organizations, leaving her little time to complete her school assignments and help pack her lunch for tomorrow. After she quickly brushed her teeth, washed her face, and put on her pajamas, she would collapse into bed.

Emily's mother—who usually tucked her in at night on her way to her own bedroom—began to notice Emily repeatedly checking the digital clock glowing in the kitchen. At first, Emily's mother did not think much of it. However, after watching this happened night after night, she was becoming concerned. Clearly, she was *thinking* about the day's events and beginning to worry. At first, she would just ask her parents a few questions about an assignment that she completed at school. For example, several weeks ago, on a rare evening at home, as her parents were helping her two younger siblings get into their pajamas and into their beds, Emily interrupted the process and said, "Is it okay if I made a mistake in class today?", "I am worried I won't get a good mark when I write my test next week." After some reassurance from her parents, Emily outwardly appeared to calm down and eventually went off to complete her before-bed routine, walking with a book in her hand.

Since that day, however, at least two—and even three—evenings each week, Emily will express worries to her parents about mistakes she feels she may have made on her coursework. Over the last week, Emily's worries have ramped up, and her parents are becoming highly concerned, passing looks back and forth, and having private conversations about Emily late into the night. Emily began to perseverate on her daily activities, asking her parents repeatedly if she is going to get in trouble at school for a possible mistake on an assignment or activity, or test. She is also lying awake, which is additionally concerning, given that she has always been in the habit of falling asleep after about 10 min of reading in bed, with her light on, the book tossed aside or open on her sleeping face. Quick bedroom checks have indicated that she is taking upward of two hours to fall asleep, which is impacting her parents' sleep, as they are only sleeping consecutively for short periods of time so that they can check on Emily throughout the night. This has begun to impact both Emily and her parents' quality and quantity of sleep, resulting in everyone being irritable, tired, and short with one another.

Just yesterday, Emily's mother received a call at work from Emily's teacher, saying that Emily fell asleep in class: not just once, but twice. Emily's mother began to think about the impact on the entire family. Most nights, as her parents are helping Michael and Sara get ready for bed, or are trying to clean up from a busy day with a busy family, Emily frequently interrupts, wanting her parents to talk with her about the day's events. This has angered Michael and Sara and has resulted in raised voices and clenched fists, and Emily's parents were having to spend close to an hour each time working hard to de-escalate these situations—far beyond the bounds that they have parented within before.

Emily's parents are worried about Emily and have placed a call to Emily's teacher; however, her teacher did not report any concerns with Emily's behavior or academic achievement at school—other than the unexpected napping. Worried, confused, and unsure how to support Emily and restore the previous calm in their home, Emily's parents have received—and taken—the advice to contact a local behavior consultant. After an initial meeting with Emily's parents, who sat down at the agency, fraught with anxiety, the behavior consultant asked whether Emily would join a behavior-based anxiety group for adolescents that was running in the community. She explained that it is based on applied behavior analysis and **Acceptance and Commitment Therapy.** They enthusiastically agreed.

After the first number of sessions, the direct-support professionals observed and recorded Emily's specific behavior difficulties for a two-week period and then plotted the data collected on a graph. During a meeting, the behavior consultant explained the importance of **graphic displays of behavior data**, which she explained how to graph data, and why the level, trend, and variability of the data collected are important. In graphs like this, the values on the x-axis and y-axis are generally the same, she explained, and they are called **equal-interval graphs**.

Seeing the focus on the anxiety, the consultant also asked the direct-support professional what skills they felt Emily needed to learn and provided them a **skills assessment** to complete. They talked initially that the first skill they would start to collect data on was the number of times Emily responded to peers within 5 s. The direct-support professionals had stated that they had noticed that she often looked consumed in thought and thus took a while to answer or even notice when a peer asked a question. When asking what type of data collection should be used, they responded, "Percentage of occurrence" in unison. "That's right" said the consultant, "We need to ensure that we measure her responses based on the number of opportunities that her peers provide her." The consultant also spoke about schedules of reinforcement, and how daily events and responses together can influence the quantity and intensity in which certain behaviors occur. Together, they decided they would focus on increasing Emily's skills, hoping that everyone in her family might begin to get more rest and be better able to work as a team to resolve the challenges Emily and her family are facing.

The Response: Principles, Processes, Practices, and Reflections

Principles

(Q1) From the case above, identify two target behaviors. How would you define, in observable and measureable terms, the two behaviors you have selected? How would you rate each behavior on the following matrix (Table 2.1)?

(Q2) Explain why developing a hypothesis about the schedules of reinforcement surrounding the behaviors selected for observation is an important part of the assessment process (Fig. 2.1).

Table 2.1 Sample rating matrix (Pearson Education, 2007)

Behavior of interest	
Is the behavior dangerous to the individual or those around the individual?	☐ No ☐ Slightly ☐ Significantly
Has the behavior been occurring for a long time? Is it a recurring problem?	☐ No ☐ Somewhat ☐ Yes
Will changing the behavior effect the learners access to reinforcement in a beneficial manner (quantity, quality, access to, etc)?	☐ No ☐ Possibly/slightly ☐ Significantly
Has this behavior been targeted for change in the past by a behavior consultant and been unsuccessful?	☐ No ☐ Between 1 and 3 times ☐ More than 3 times

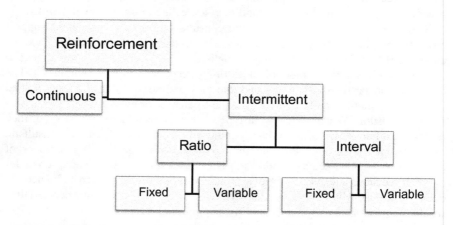

Fig. 2.1 Schedules of reinforcement (Pearson Education, 2007)

(Q3) Define how the three aspects of the visual analysis of a graph (level, trend, variability) are important to determine whether the behavior change is significant (Table 2.2).

Table 2.2 Graphs portraying the three aspects of visual analysis (Cooper et al. 2007)

Level	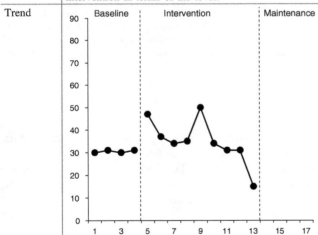
	Changes in the level of data are determined by comparing the phases and data vertically. In the above example, there is a jump in the data from baseline to intervention in terms of the level.
Trend	
	Trend is the direction or path the data are going in. There are three options, increasing, decreasing, or no trend. Data trends can also be stable or variable. The example above depicts no increasing trend in the baseline phase, followed by a decreasing trend in intervention phase, and no trend in the maintenance phase.

(continued)

Table 2.2 (continued)

Variability	
	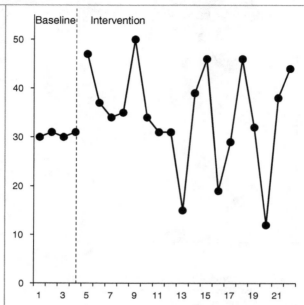

Variability refers to how different the data points are from one another. The graph depicted above shows little to no variability during the baseline phase, as a result predictability in future data points in the same phase is established. In contrast, the intervention phase has high variability and requires many more data points before a predictable pattern can emerge.

Processes

(Q4) Research published skills assessments that you could use with Emily. What other informal assessments could you use to assess her skills?

(Q5) Research Acceptance and Commitment Therapy—a popular treatment for anxiety, based on the third wave of behaviorism. How could this program be implemented with Emily? How is it similar/dissimilar to ABA?

Practices

(Q6) Using the attached graph in Fig. 2.2, what might you hypothesize regarding the behaviors depicted, per day? Please include a summary of the level, trend, and variability of the data.

(Q7) After the behavior consultant and Emily's parents implement an intervention, would they start a new graph, or could it be noted on the graph that a change has occurred? If so how could this be done?

For more information see http://www.kipbs.org/new_kipbs/fsi/files/graphingtips.pdf

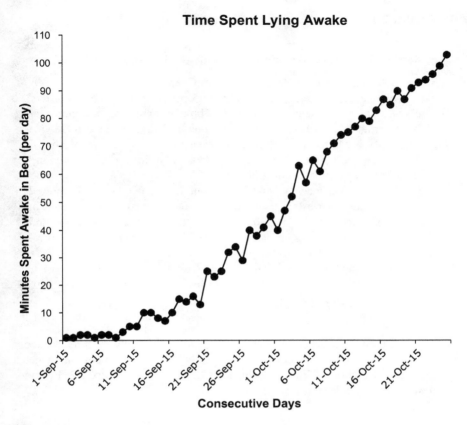

Fig. 2.2 The number of minutes Emily spent lying awake per day, in her bed, from September 1, 2015, to October 25, 2015

(**Q8**) Using Fig. 2.1 above, what current schedule of reinforcement is in place? Is this maintaining or decreasing the behavior? What would be your suggested schedules or reinforcement when you start the intervention and once the intervention is in place?

Reflections

(**Q9**) In addition to being the subject of the behavioral observations, how might you include Emily in the consent, decision-making, and data collection processes? Why is it important, from both an ethical and clinical perspective, for Emily to be included in the process (Reference Ethics Box 2.1, Behavior Analyst Certification Board, 2014)?

Ethics Box 2.1

Professional and Ethical Compliance Code for Behavior Analysts

- 2.0 Behavior Analysts' Responsibility to Clients.
  Behavior analyst has a responsibility to operate in the best interest of clients. The term client as used here is broadly applicable to whomever behavior analysts provide services, whether an individual person (service recipient), a parent or guardian of a service recipient, an organizational representative, a public or private organization, a firm, or a corporation.
- 2.09 Treatment/Intervention Efficacy.
  (c) In those instances where more than one scientifically supported treatment has been established, additional factors may be considered in selecting interventions, including, but not limited to, efficiency and cost-effectiveness, risks and side effects of the interventions, client preference, and practitioner experience and training.
- 4.02 Involving Clients in Planning and Consent.
  Behavior analysts involve the client in the planning of and consent for behavior-change programs.

(Q10) In addition to the school personnel, who else might Emily's family ask about the behavioral changes they have seen in Emily? Why is it important to get a well-rounded depiction of Emily's behavior (Reference Ethics Box 2.2, Behavior Analyst Certification Board, 2014)?

Ethics Box 2.2

Professional and Ethical Compliance Code for Behavior Analysts

- 2.09 Treatment/Intervention Efficacy.
  (a) Clients have the right to effective treatment (i.e., based on the research literature and adapted to the individual client). Behavior analysts always have the obligation to advocate for and educate the client about scientifically supported, most-effective treatment procedures. Effective treatment procedures have been validated as having both long-term and short-term benefits to clients and society.
- 3.01 Behavior-Analytic Assessment.
  (a) Behavior analysts conduct current assessments prior to making recommendations or developing behavior-change programs. The type of assessment used is determined by the clients' needs and consent, environmental parameters, and other contextual variables. When behavior analysts are developing a behavior-reduction program, they must first conduct a functional assessment.

Additional Web Links

Kansas Institute for Positive Behavior Support—Data Collection and Measurement Resources:
http://www.kipbs.org/kmhpbs/resources/data-collection-and-measurement.html
The Assessment of Functional Living Skills
https://www.partingtonbehavioranalysts.com/page/afls-74.html
Acceptance and Commitment Therapy
https://contextualscience.org/act

CASE: i-A7

Sam's Struggles with "Real-Life" Friends
Setting: Home/School   Age Group: Adolescence

LEARNING OBJECTIVE:

- Create an event recording data collection process.

TASK LIST LINKS:

- **Measurement**

  - (A-01) Measure frequency (i.e., count).
  - (A-03) Measure duration.
  - (A-05) Measure interresponse time (IRT).
  - (A-12) Design and implement continuous measurement procedures (e.g., event recording).
  - (A-14) Design and implement choice measures.

- **Measurement**

  - (H-01) Select a measurement system to obtain representative data given the dimensions of the behavior and the logistics of observing and recording.
  - (H-02) Select a schedule of observation and recording periods.

- **Intervention**

  - (E-08) Use the matching law and recognize factors influencing choice.
  - (E-09) Arrange high-probability request sequences.
  - (E-11) Use pairing procedures to establish new conditioned reinforcers and punishers.

KEY TERMS

- **Event Recording**

  - Event recording, also referred to as frequency recording, is a direct count of behaviors. This is often used to measure the number of times a specific target behavior occurs during a predetermined observation period (Ault and Bausch 2014, p. 53).

- **Gait**

  - Gait refers to the pattern of limb movement observed in humans and animals. In humans, gait refers to the ways humans move, either naturally (e.g., walking, jogging, running) or specialized through training (e.g., dancing, martial arts, and military marching) (Schwartz et al. 2008).

- **Reliable**

  - In applied behavior analysis, reliability of measurement refers to the consistency of measurement over time, or the extent to which repeated measurement of the same target behavior result in similar values (Horner et al. 2005).

- **Social Skills**

  - Social skills refer to any skills, verbal and nonverbal, that involve interacting or communicating with others. Examples of social skills include interpersonal skills such as sharing and turn-taking, conflict resolution skills such as dealing with winning and losing and apologizing, and problem-solving skills such as asking for help (Reichow and Volkmar 2010).

- **Valid**

  - In applied behavior analysis, validity of measurement refers to the extent to which behavior measurement data are directly relevant and related to the behavior selected for change (Cooper et al. 2007; Horner et al. 2005).

Sam's Struggles with "Real-Life" Friends

Sam, Sam, or "Sam1212" his online persona, thought he had friends. But did he? Thirteen-year-old Sam has always been a huge fan of what his parents call "screen time" but what he calls "life." As soon as he returns home from school—as soon as he leaves the outer door of the school, really—Sam is onto screens. His parents are unaware of some of his screen time, as they simply do not have a chance to see it. As soon as he crashes through the heavy steel doors of the school but before they slam shut heavily behind him, for example, he is onto his first screen. Like all the students in his school, his cell phone is his constant companion, and it is out of his pocket, into his hands, password expertly thumb-keyed in with a one-handed grasp immediately (not only in this situation, but during any potential "down time" at school). Anyone close enough to Sam could have heard him sigh heavily at this moment, annoyed that his battery was almost totally drained. But not wanting to lose a moment of time, he moved ahead, starting his walk home with a steady if awkward **gait,** head down, fingers busy, oblivious to the goings-on of the social world around him.

Though many of his peers were similarly checking their phones, it was without the same purpose and intensity that Sam was utilizing. Most of his peers were gathered in groups, waiting for a bus, a ride, or for extracurricular activities to begin. They would glance down at their cell phone screens, laugh, or share their screen with a friend for a moment, look at one another, and burst into laughter together. Sam was not engaged in this social world—the social world infused with technology—he was engaged only in his screen, scrolling back and forth between programs, texting, commenting, and updating his online life. He had no more of an emotional reaction than the quirk of a raised eyebrow, and no social interaction was possible at the pace of his walking which gave others a strong "Stay away!" message, as clearly obvious as if it were written on a placard being carried through the gathered after-school crowds.

At home, the story was similar. Although Sam's mother—a healthcare professional with varied 12-h shifts on weekdays and often through the weekends—had paid careful attention to screen-time recommendations throughout Sam's childhood she had basically given up at this point, figuring that Sam was doing what the rest of his peers were doing. For a few years throughout grades seven and eight, life at home and school had moved along fairly smoothly while Sam's screen time was not challenged. His teachers, for example, accommodated a variety of needs in his diverse classrooms. For example, they would often display a choice board for major projects, and one of these choices was usually technology-based. Guess what Sam chose? They typically allowed students to work independently, or in pairs or groups. Guess which Sam chose?

But one day when Sam's mother returned home from a long shift at 2 clock in the morning during the school week, weary and ready for bed, she stopped short as soon as she locked the front door of their home behind her. There was Sam, still up, still wide awake, and still buzzing with activity. He had the television going to his favorite 24-h news station, he had his computer on with a video clip playing, he had his cell phone resting against it with some sort of online game on the go, and his earphones trailed to his tablet computer where it was clearly not his homework displayed on the screen. In shock and surprise, she called his name, and tapped his shoulder, and asked Sam "What are you DOING?" To her great dismay, Sam leapt up, screamed at her for interfering, shut and locked his screens, haphazardly stacked them, left the television blaring, and stalked off to his tiny basement bedroom— where Sam was not officially allowed to engage in screen activity. This moment was the moment of change for Sam's mother, where many thoughts and concerns clicked into place, where memories scrolled through her head, and a strong resolve emerged. *This is not good enough to be my son's life,* she thought. *He can't even have a conversation anymore. It's like he has lost every **social skill** I worked so hard to teach him. I know that many children and adults with a slight* *developmental disability like Sam's have a tough time socially, but it has to be better than this. I don't think he even has one real friend anymore.* She quickly scratched down a reminder to call the local treatment center and went to bed, where she spent the remainder of her short night tossing, turning, and worrying.

The next week, Sam's mother arrived at the treatment center, along with the school's vice-principal (also the head of special education) and Sam's geography teacher. The behavior analyst working with Sam's mother greeted them warmly, well-prepared for this conversation, after having spent a lengthy period of time on the phone with Sam's mother following this recent late-night trauma.

It was clear to the behavior analyst that the goal articulated by Sam's mother in a more scattered and emotional manner—not surprising for the situation at hand—was to reduce his use of technology and increase his friendships "in real life." The behavioral analyst, however, was not yet sure how much technology was in use on a day-to-day basis, and how much time Sam spent engaged in real-life friendships. He was also unsure as to where likely gaps in his social skills lay, which could have led to the change from technology as a preference and a reward, to technology as a foundational way of interacting with the world. Perhaps, he thought, technology functioned as a replacement for the complex social situations that emerge in adolescence. Perhaps Sam would benefit from learning some new skills in one of the social skills-focused groups in our center. With these thoughts, notes, and follow-up research in mind, he invited Sam's mother and Sam's teacher to sit down with him.

The behavior analyst addressed Sam's mother first. "You mentioned that you were concerned about Sam's social skills," he reflected. "I agree that social skills are hugely important at any age, but also that they can get really complicated at Sam's age. Before suggesting any next steps to how we can work on some of his areas of need, though, I think it's really important to do an assessment and to collect some data, so his areas of need become very clear to us. We want to be sure that we are accurate about these needs before we move ahead. If we do an assessment and we collect data, we can also see if change is happening quite clearly. It's good that there are three of you here, because this means we have multiple points of view and our conclusions are more likely to be right." Noting that Sam's teacher and mother were both nodding so far, he continued: "While I was preparing for our consultation today, I pulled out an assessment of social skills which I thought would work well for Sam." The behavior analyst displayed "The Social Skills Checklist" (Mackinnon and Krempa 2005), with Sam's name already filled out. "We can use this both before and after any interventions we decide to do, to see whether there is any change in his social skills." The behavior analyst believed that for Sam, they can probably start with Level 3, which looks at more complex skills, like "corrects others nicely or politely overlooks mistakes" (p. 39). The behavior analyst went on to explain "the great thing about this assessment is that not only is it fairly informal —so we can do it together—but also that it looks at social skills in three types of situations: individual situations, in groups, and in the natural setting like the home or classroom. In addition, we need to be sure we really know how often Sam is interacting with friends in real life and how often he is tuning into a screen for interaction. For this data collection, I thought we could use this **event recording** sheet, which will tell us how many times each day that Sam is doing both of those things. Then, we have to make sure we have trained observers to collect this data while making sure it is **valid**—that it measures what it is supposed to measure—and that it is **reliable**—that we all measure the same thing time after time."

"Well, what do you think? Should we give it a go?" Asked the behavior analyst.

Sam's mom was nodding her head rapidly, while Sam was nodding rather sheepishly. The behavior analyst continued, "I want you two to work together to look very closely at screen time at home. For example, I have created some other easy-to-use data sheets for you to observe and record the duration of screen times, and the interresponse times–the amount of time between using one device and another. This will be good for us to set goals from and for you to engage in some self-management as well. Do you think you can do this all day, between the two of you, for the next seven days, until we meet again?" Again, Sam was nodding less than enthusiastically, and he could tell that his mom was very on board with these plans. What could be better?

The Response: Principles, Processes, Practices, and Reflections

Principles

(Q1) Explain the importance of validity, reliability, and accuracy of measurement (Fig. 2.3).
(Q2) Why might indirect and discontinuous measurement pose threats to the validity of the measurement (Fig. 2.4).
(Q3) Why might poor observer training and reactivity pose threats to the reliability of the measurement?

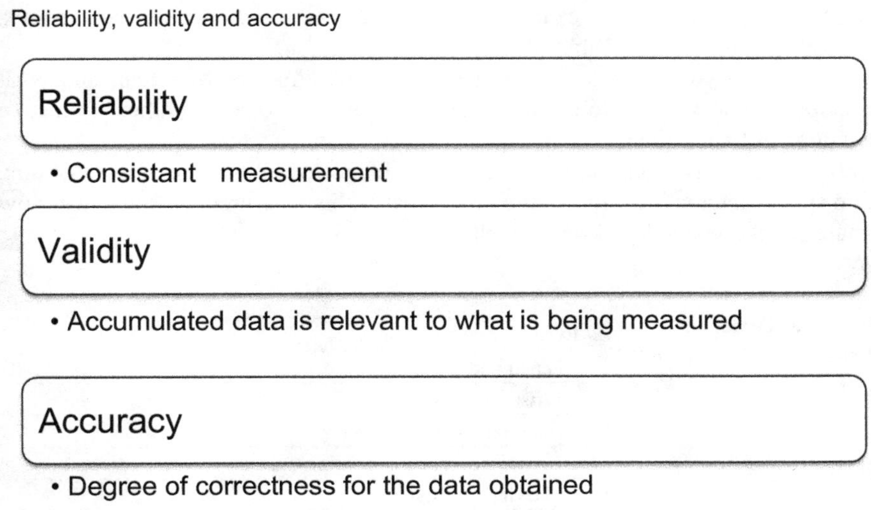

Reliability, validity and accuracy

Reliability

• Consistant   measurement

Validity

• Accumulated data is relevant to what is being measured

Accuracy

• Degree of correctness for the data obtained

Fig. 2.3 Reliability, validity, and accuracy

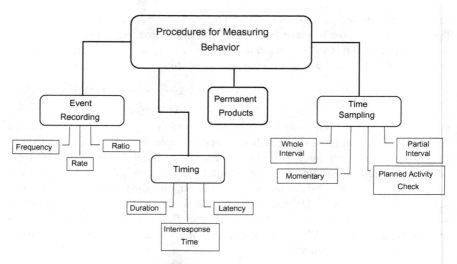

Fig. 2.4 Procedures for measuring behavior

Processes

(Q4) Explain how you would approach observer training with Sam and his parents through the data collection process, ensuring the validity, reliability, and accuracy of the measurement.

(Q5) How could you check for, and maintain, the validity, reliability, and accuracy of the measurement over time?

Practices

(Q6) List at least three types of devices and/or creative strategies you could use for event recording in this case example? For each device listed, identify the strengths and limitations of each (Table 2.3).

(Q7) How do you think a choice board could be effective with Sam and what principles could you use to ensure a balance between choice and other productive activities in Sam's life?

(Q8) As the behavior consultant, you may be interested in the total amount of time Sam spends interacting with technology. What is this measurement called and how would it best be displayed on a graph?

Table 2.3 Devices and strategies for event recording

Event recording devices
• Pencil and paper
• Wrist counters
• Hand-tally digital counters
• Abacus wrist and shoestring counters
• Masking tape
• Pennies, buttons, pebbles, and paperclips
• Pocket calculators

Reflections

(Q9) What are the strengths and limitations of event recording as a method to measure behavior?
(Q10) How might you overcome the limitations you have identified?

Additional Web Links
Social Skills for Adolescents and Adults: http://www.autism.org.uk/socialskills
Building Social Skills: A Resource for Educators:
www.gov.pe.ca/photos/original/BldSocSkills_11.pdf

CASE: i-A8

Olivier's Challenges with Self-Control
Setting: Home/School   Age Group: Adolescence

LEARNING OBJECTIVE:

• Design a mediator-based behavior assessment process.

TASK LIST LINKS

Extinction and plan for extinction

• **Behavior-Change Considerations**

  – (C-02) State and plan for the possible unwanted effects of punishment.
  – (C-03) State and plan for the possible unwanted effects of extinction.

• **Fundamental Elements of Behavior Change**

  – (D-18) Use extinction

• **Assessment**

  – (I-01) Define behavior in observable and measurable terms.
  – (I-03) Design and implement individualized behavioral assessment procedures.
  – (I-05) Organize, analyze, and interpret observed data.

• **Implementation, Management, and Supervision**

  – (K-02) Identify the contingencies governing the behavior of those responsible for carrying out behavior-change procedures and design interventions accordingly.
  – (K-03) Design and use competency-based training for persons who are responsible for carrying out behavioral assessment and behavior-change procedures.
  – (K-05) Design and use systems for monitoring procedural integrity.
  – (K-06) Provide supervision for behavior-change agents.

KEY TERMS

- **Attention Deficit/Hyperactivity Disorder**

  - Attention deficit/hyperactivity disorder (AD/HD) is a brain disorder characterized by difficulty staying focused and paying attention, difficulty controlling behavior, and hyperactivity. The key behaviors associated with AD/HD are inattention, hyperactivity, and impulsivity (National Institute for Mental Health 2012).

- **Extinction**

  - A method whereby a behavior's maintaining reinforcers are withheld. Because of this elimination of reinforcement, behaviors may increase in the form of an extinction burst before the behavior decreases because of no longer having access to reinforcement (Iwata et al. 1994).

- **Mediator Model**

  - A mediator model, or a mediator-based approach to the implementation of behavior interventions, involves a third party or "mediator," such as a parent or a teacher, implementing an intervention program with the individual experiencing the presenting behavior difficulties. In this approach, the behavior consultant or behavior analyst conducts a behavior assessment and develops an intervention program, but does not directly implement the program with their client. Instead, the consultant or analyst focuses on enhancing the knowledge and skills of a "mediator" to implement the program. Behavior change in the individual experiencing the presenting difficulties therefore is mediated by the individual implementing the intervention (Minnesota Northland Association for Behavior Analysis 2012).

- **Procedural Adherence**

  - Procedural adherence, or sometimes referred to as procedural fidelity or treatment integrity, refers to the extent to which an intervention procedure is implemented exactly as planned (Cooper et al. 2007).

Olivier's Challenges with Self-control

"Again? Really?" Olivier's father sighed with frustration, sitting down heavily on the family's living room sofa. "Seriously?" he continued, not noticing that he was shaking his head slowly from side to side, eyes downcast at he looked at what his son had given to him.

He was loosely holding an orange card, a well-used laminated square of construction paper with WARNING written boldly in black marker. "Who exactly gave this to you, and what exactly does it mean, this time?" Olivier's dad asked with sounds of helplessness and hopelessness in his voice.

"It wasn't my fault! You know that!" yelled Olivier, loudly enough to scare the family cat out from under the sofa where the small family was seated. "I was at that basketball game, you know, at the rec center? The ones they have every Friday. We were winning all along, but then we started to lose—of course," he intoned dramatically, rolling his eyes for effect. "It wasn't going well, and we—well I—had to do something, right?"

Olivier's father ignored what seemed to be a rhetorical question, though he had answered many such questions over the last few years of Olivier's adolescence since his diagnosis of **attention deficit/hyperactivity disorder.** Now, with Oliver turning 15, he had hoped things might get better. He tried to bring the conversation along: "And what was that something?" He waited for the answer, cringing inside, already responding emotionally to what he was sure was a repeat of the same issues they had—his son had—been experiencing over and over as of late. While he waited, he thought back to the report they had received about Olivier when he was nine.

"It's AD/HD," the psychologist had said. "I am sure of it. He has all of the symptoms; he is not missing even one. His behaviors that make me think this is the correct diagnosis are happening at home, at school, and sometimes in the community. They have been happening—you said—since he was a toddler. You must be exhausted!"

If I wasn't then, I sure am now! Olivier's dad reflected. *I feel like I have tried to provide punishment with him in every way possible—and consistently—but none of it seems to make even a bit of difference in these types of defiant behaviors.* Frustrated with the lingering few successes and mostly dismal failures, he sorted through the magnets and paper on the fridge and came up with the contact information for a behavior therapist. *Now, this is a call I had hoped to never make*, he thought with disappointment, *but it can't be helped. There is really nothing left to try.* He left a message for the behavior therapist and began the process of waiting, wondering what would come first: a call, a meeting, and a solution, or another warning (or worse) from the basketball coach, the referee, a teammate, or a parent?

"Well, this is quite a disappointment," Olivier's father summed up for the behavior therapist, at the end of their first hour-long consultation, less than two weeks after his initial, inquiring phone call. "I wasn't expecting to have homework. I was expecting a solution to all of this."

"To figure out a solution that is highly likely to be effective," responded the behavior therapist calmly, "we both need to know the whole picture of what is going on. But even before we proceed with collecting data, we have to find out what the most important behavior of interest is: the one that is socially significant for Olivier and needs to decrease the very most of all of the issues you have described for me today. **Extinction** is usually a preferred method, but we need to determine if this is the method we want to take by collecting data to begin. First, talking to everyone involved is a really good idea for us to be able to make sure we are focusing on the right issue. Then, we will work on assessments. After that, we will make a plan and I will work with you in building skills to help change Olivier's challenging behavior. This is called a **mediator model**. It really makes sense, since you are the person who spends the most time with Olivier. One of the first things you said to me when you initially arrived was that you were "done." You said you didn't know what else to try. But you also said you hadn't talked with Olivier's coach, teachers—even his mother—in months. Working through this process, I will give you strategies and skills, but it is a process, and takes time and steps, as well as knowing what is going on with Olivier in all areas of his life right now."

Fast-forwarding yet another few weeks, Olivier's father leafed through the notes scratched into his coil notebook during a variety of hurried conversations about Olivier. He translated his rough comments and read them out loud to the behavior therapist:

- "Olivier's coach said that he has 'frequent outbursts' and argues with pretty much everyone on the team, including him and the assistant coach, but also the parents watching, the other players on either team, and pretty much anyone who interacts with him on or off of the court. He said this happened 'especially when things don't go his way.'"
- "The assistant coach told me that he has actually received quite a few warnings and penalties but this one—the one (the only one) that he brought home that started all this—was the very last one. If he gets one more, the assistant coach assured me that he would be kicked out of the program. He said that he would 'be sure to arrange it.'"
- "His mother said she is seeing the same kind of things when he visits, but she can't really tell what sets him off. She said that his issues come 'out of the blue' these days."
- "Like you suggested, I also talked to Olivier. He told me that he really, really likes playing basketball, and he wants to 'get along with everyone' but he also said that 'people keep doing things to annoy him.'"

Olivier's father closed his notebook, leaned over the behavior therapist's desk, and excitedly said, "That's done. Now what?" The behavior therapist competently and patiently reviewed all the steps in the assessment part of the future intervention plan with Olivier's father. "Now we can carefully define Olivier's behavior that is need of change. That is a huge help! Next, we need to talk about gathering specific information—or data—to help decrease Olivier's challenging behavior. But first, let's go back to what you said when we first met. You told me that you 'provided punishments' for Olivier but that they didn't make any difference. Let's talk about what punishment means, and how we can get some really solid evidence to determine if our interventions are making a difference. The key is to collect some numbers—again, some data—showing when, where, why, and how often, this challenging behavior is happening. Like I said before, extinction, or not providing reinforcement for his behaviors will help to decrease it, but it's a process that takes time, and things may get worse before they get better. We have to plan for what may happen when his behavior no longer gets reinforced. With us all working as a team, we are going to find a way to be successful. With you being really well trained in all of this, we will be able to get really good **procedural integrity**: we are going to be able to do things the right way! I think you are far from 'done' and that there are many reasons to move ahead with this assessment to help Olivier enjoy basketball, his peers, and other social situations with much more success, and many fewer challenging behaviors."

The Response: Principles, Processes, Practices, and Reflections

Principles

(Q1) Explain why the procedure of extinction could be used in this case and comes to the consultant's mind immediately. What are some downfalls of using extinction in this case?

(Q2) Explain why the procedures used by Olivier's father in response to Olivier's behavior may not be resulting in a decrease or increase in the problem behaviors.

Processes

(Q3) In a mediator model, training mediators to correctly implement an intervention program or procedure is critical. Identify how the implementation of extinction needs to be trained to the parents. What warnings do you need to provide them when implementing the procedure (Fig. 2.5)?

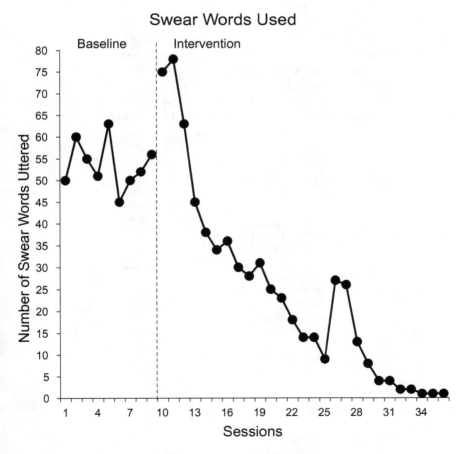

Fig. 2.5 Graph of Oliver's swear word use over time. Graph displays an extinction burst as well as spontaneous recovery

Table 2.4 Sample mastery criteria

Master criteria
• Zero incidences of target behavior over 1 week
• 80 % accuracy over 3 consecutive days
• 90 % accuracy over 2 consecutive days
• 4/5 steps completed accurately
• 5 min over 3 consecutive days

(Q4) Explain how you might know when Oliver's parents have mastered the procedure to be implemented (Table 2.4).

(Q5) What dimension of behavior (frequency, rate, duration, latency, or interresponse time) would you be most interested in Olivier's parents gathering? Why would this data be useful? How could it be used to measure progress in the future?

(Q6) What method of training would you use to train Olivier's parents on data collection? How could you ensure consistency across both parents?

Practices

(Q7) Outline how you would measure procedural adherence over the course of the intervention program? Explain why it is important to measure procedural adherence repeatedly over the course of an intervention program, and not just in the early stages of a program (Table 2.5).

(Q8) What might you do if, based on the data collected, you begin to notice that certain procedures are not being implemented exactly as outlined?

Table 2.5 Sample procedural integrity (treatment fidelity) checklist (Hall et al., 2016)

Stay, play, and talk procedural integrity checklist	Never implemented (0–30 %)	Partially implemented (30–90 %)	Fully implemented (90–100 %)
The program implementer directs the identified child and peers toward one another (physically and in conversation)			
The program implementer prompts peers to use the stay, play, and talk skills and interacts with the identified child in 90 % of situations			
The program implementer prompts the identified child to respond to the peers if necessary or he or she does not respond within 5 s			
The program implementer prompts the peers to reinforce the identified child if the peers do not do it automatically			
The program implementer reinforces the peers for interacting with the identified child in 90 % of situations			
The program implementer provides children with reinforcers for completing the identified skills			

Reflections

(Q9) Forming a cohesive intervention team in which all mediators are implementing the intervention program consistently and correctly is an important part of mediator-based behavior consultation. At times, the way in which a mediator might be interacting with the individual experiencing the behavior difficulties might be contributing to the occurrence of the presenting behavior problems (e.g., unknowingly providing reinforcement in response to a problematic behavior). How might you address this with a mediator without compromising the rapport you have worked to develop?

(Q10) There are different reasons why an individual's motivation might change, for example, establishing operations and abolishing operations. How do these principles differ? Considering Olivier, how might they offer an explanation for his behavior?

Additional Web Links
AD/HD Clinical Practice Guidelines
http://www.cdc.gov/ncbddd/adhd/guidelines.html
Punishment as a component of classroom management: http://www.education.com/reference/article/classroom-management/#C
What Makes Extinction Work?
http://www.ncbi.nlm.nih.gov/pmc/articles/PMC1297782/pdf/jaba00007-0133.pdf

CASE: i-A9

Miguel used to skip to school, but now, he is skipping school
Setting: School   Age Group: Adolescent

LEARNING OBJECTIVE:

- Synthesize behavior and psychoeducation assessment data and formulate a hypothesis about why an identified target behavior is occurring.

TASK LIST LINKS

- **Experimental Design**

  - (B-02) Review and interpret articles from the behavior-analytic literature.
  - (B-10) Conduct a component analysis to determine the effective components of an intervention package.

- **Fundamental Elements of Behavior Change**

  - (D-01) Use positive and negative reinforcement.
  - (D-02) Use appropriate parameters and schedules of reinforcement.

- **Assessment**

  - (I-04) Design and implement the full range of functional assessment procedures.

KEY TERMS

- **Avoidance Contingency**

  - As a form of negative reinforcement, an avoidance contingency occurs when a response prevents or postpones the presentation of a stimulus (Cooper et al. 2007).

- **Escape Contingency**

  - As a form of negative reinforcement, the individual escapes from a stimulus or a response is terminated (Kahng et al. 2003).

- **Establishing Operation**

  - In applied behavior analysis, establishing operations are antecedent variables that alter the effectiveness of behavioral consequences to function as reinforcers or punishers. Establishing operations can increase the probability of a behavior by enhancing the perceived value of a particular outcome and in turn then increase an individual's motivation to display behaviors that will provide access to that outcome (Michael 2000).

- **Intervention Package**

  - Also called a comprehensive treatment model, where a group of practices are strategically designed as part of an approach to specifically highlight and target a specific behavior or disorder (Wong et al. 2014).

- **Learning Disability**

  - Learning disabilities are a group of disorders that are lifelong and are characterized by a gap between a person's expected achievement and their performance. Individuals with learning disabilities may have average or above-average intelligence, but struggle with their performance at school, home, community, or workplace. Learning disabilities can affect areas such as listening, reading, speaking, writing, spelling, and mathematics (National Centre for Learning Disabilities 2014).

- **Negative Reinforcement**

  - In applied behavior analysis, negative reinforcement is said to have occurred when there is an increase in the future frequency of a behavior, following the termination, reduction, or removal of a stimulus (Cooper et al. 2007).

Miguel Used to Skip TO School, But Now He Is SKIPPING School!

Miguel is 17 years old. In the school system, this seems quite mature, but in the context of his entire expected life span, he is still quite young. Miguel, however, is taking decision-making into his own hands much of the time. Just last week, for example, only one short month into the new school year, his parents received a phone call from the principal at Main Street High School, which his father answered with trepidation, in the midst of his busy work day. The principal, Ms. Roberts, jumped right into the conversation, not wasting any time on pleasantries, which immediately raised Miguel's father's level of anxiety. Ms. Roberts expressed concerns about Miguel's recent absences from class. *Absences?* Miguel's father thought, raising one eyebrow while he waited for more.

"Over the last two weeks," Ms. Roberts listed in a dispassionate manner, "Miguel has missed more than seven classes, with most of these absences occurring during Mr. Hill's grade 12 English class." She further noted that on one occasion, she personally witnessed Miguel actually leaving the school at a time when he was expected to be in class. "Even though Miguel is almost 18 and he can soon make his own decisions, we are not there, yet. I would like you, and your wife, to meet me, quite soon, so we can try to figure out how best to support Miguel not only with his impending graduation, but getting the most of this last year that he can. We want him to reach his potential, not just get through the year."

That evening, Miguel's parents did what they used to call "preparing for battle." They sat together at the kitchen table with the last 10 years or so of his assessments, reports, IEPs, and more spread out over their round kitchen table, while Miguel was reportedly "doing homework" in his room. Although their table could hold eight people in a pinch, it was covered from edge-to-edge with paper, often piled up high, as well as spread out wide. Their first area of focus was looking over Miguel's comprehensive psychoeducational assessment that was now a few years old. Its major finding was something they had seen and heard many times before: Miguel had a **learning disability**. While he could express himself well verbally at and often above grade level and was measured as having above-average intelligence, he struggled with written expression: reading, writing, and spelling. In the past, terms such as dyslexia and dysgraphia were used to explain his diagnosis, but his latest report just noted that he has "characteristics that are consistent with a learning disability."

Just last month, his parents moved the family to a new community, after Miguel's mother started a new job. Unfortunately, this coincided with Miguel's final year of high school; however, they made a family decision that the opportunity and the significant pay raise were both too good to give up. Miguel did not know this, but it also allowed his parents to put away even more funds to be available for his future, post-secondary education. But the practical reality was that this meant that Miguel had to leave the school he has become used to (and the school and its faculty that knew him well) and start at a new school for that all-important final year of high school.

Several years ago, at his previous school, Miguel began to display similar behavior difficulties, avoiding work in class and skipping classes altogether. Miguel's parents went over this while leafing through the fairly thick sheaf of disciplinary reports. After many meetings with his teachers, his principal, and the resource staff, including a behavior consultant and the school's guidance counselor, a support plan had been put in place for Miguel and his somewhat challenging behaviors began to improve. This support plan involved a combination of adaptive instruction—through which in-class activities were adapted to draw more on Miguel's areas of strengths and extra supports such as more time to complete assignments were implemented—and changes in the way his teachers interacted with him, such as focusing on increasing positive interactions and offering more praise and encouragement following each of his successes. Combined, this **intervention package** resulted in Miguel enjoying time in class, and his parents had even noticed him becoming more confident in himself, they recalled. However, they never figured out which part of the intervention package was causing the changes or was most effective—they had not completed a component analysis. Miguel was doing so well that when the family moved last month, his parents decided that they would not tell the school about his diagnosis. They felt that Miguel had gained the skills and the confidence he needed to be successful and no longer needed the supports that were in place at his old school. Miguel had agreed, feeling that that he could do it and that he did not want to be singled out in a new school. *Perhaps all of us were wrong.*

Next, they pulled out the notes that had carefully taken at one of his interdisciplinary meetings last year. "Remember," recalled Miguel's mother, "back before we implemented that support plan that worked so well? That behavior consultant had some really good ideas: data-supported ones, of course. She observed so much of Miguel's behavior that we thought she was a going to solve all of our problems at once! She is the one who told us that Miguel's repeated school-skipping could be explained by the principle of **negative reinforcement**." Miguel's mother underlined this phrase with her finger in her notes, tapping it for emphasis. "She told us that there was a very clear pattern, when Miguel was finding certain classes very difficult, not going to class meant the end of that so-called unpleasant experience. She went on to explain that these experiences are acting as an **establishing operation**, increasing the value of escaping, or avoiding the class and the work that went with it and that it is because of this **escape contingency** or **avoidance contingency** that Michael's behaviors are not only continuing, but increasing in frequency. Remember how it was all like a different language then, and we had to practice and learn all of this new vocabulary to understand what was happening?" They stopped reminiscing for a moment, quietly recalling this time of hope and success. Their eyes met as they felt a simultaneous wave of fear and silently wondered: *Is this what is happening all over again? Are we right back to where we started that very long year ago?*

When they arrived at the school meeting together the next day, after both arranging time off work, Miguel and his parents listened carefully and attentively as the principal and his English teacher recited their lists of concerns in a well-practiced way. Mr. Hill noted that each time he assigns a task in class, Miguel is doing other things and not completing assignment. "It's pretty frustrating," Mr. Hill interjected. "Your behaviors are getting in the way and getting my other students off-track, too. I have tried reprimanding you, Miguel, for talking and joking with other students, for playing on your cell phone, for leaving class without permission, and even for tearing up your assignment papers." As he spoke and "ticked off" each of Miguel's offenses on his left hand, his tone rose and became a little aggressive. "Things really escalated last week when you began to tease a peer in class when you were supposed to be writing an essay. When you began hitting and punching each other, which led to wrestling on the floor, I had to call for help from the office to have the two of you physically removed. Never before in my career have I had to do such a thing!" Mr. Hill went on to say that each time these behaviors had been occurring, he had been giving Miguel a verbal reprimand and sending him to the office on his own. He does not understand why these behaviors are not stopping and instead are increasing. "After this particular situation, Miguel, you haven't even come to class anymore. I just do not know why you are choosing to act this way."

Principal Robert smoothly picked up the conversation and said that she would like to call in a behavior analyst to conduct an assessment of Miguel's behavior. Miguel's parents locked eyes and laughed wryly: "That's just what we were *thinking*. But first we do have some information to share with you, that I don't think you have, yet, in your files about Miguel. When we were looking over his documents, we came across this one and thought, *Uh oh!* Because of his problems with reading, he has is used to using assistive technology in class, but is also a little embarrassed about it, and certainly would never ask you for it. Unfortunately, with the move, I think this information didn't get passed on to you. Here, we'll read this bit." Miguel's mother pulled out the much-folded document—a psychoeducational assessment—and read:

It is recommended that Miguel utilize educational software to assist with multiple educational demands that meet his educational and cognitive profile. Text-to-speech software will decrease demands for reading, working memory, comprehension, and processing speed.

With one potential solution on table, the tension in the room dissipated, and, in that moment, those caring for Miguel became a team. Now, willingly—and with new hope—Miguel's parents began to openly share information about Miguel's learning disability, his past assessments, and past behavioral challenges.

The Response: Principles, Processes, Practices, and Reflections

Principles

(Q1) Drawing on a specific example from this case, use the Antecedent-Behavior-Consequence template in Table 2.6 below to illustrate how the principle of negative reinforcement may offer an explanation for the presenting problem behavior (Table 2.6).

(Q2) *Thinking* further about the example that you used in question #1, would you classify this as an escape or attention-seeking contingency? Please explain your selection.

Table 2.6 Antecedent behavior consequence template

Date and Time	Location	Antecedent	Behavior	Consequence

Process

(**Q3**) *Thinking* further about the problem behavior that you outlined in questions #1 and #2, how might the attached psychoeducational assessment in Fig. 2.6 findings inform your hypothesis as to why this behavior may be occurring (Fig. 2.6)?

(**Q4**) Based on the diagram in Fig. 2.7, what pathway do you think the team at the previous middle school had taken when implementing an intervention? Do you think that the intervention they chose was truly based on the function of the behavior? In the current scenario, what could be completed to determine the function of the behavior and ensure the correct intervention is implemented?

Practices

(**Q5**) In this case, what functional assessment procedures would you use to determine what the function of the behavior is and what interventions are effective or ineffective (Fig. 2.8)?

(**Q6**) Once a hypothesis as to why a presenting behavior difficulty may be occurring has been formulated, you must decide whether to proceed with an intervention program, or test the hypothesis through a functional analysis—often by exposing the individual to conditions that might evoke the problematic responses. When a behavior may be occurring due to negative reinforcement, is it ethically justifiable to expose the individual to aversive stimuli in order to test the effects of the removal of the stimulus? Why or why not (Fig. 2.9)?

(**Q7**) In the current case, would you recommend testing of your hypothesis or would you recommend proceeding with an intervention program? Explain your rationale.

A Psychoeducational Assessment - Miguel

Examinee: Miguel Rodriguez

Chronological Age: 12

Referral Question

Miguel was referred by the Office of Student Learning at Eagle Heights Middle School, after the team had suspected educational accommodations were needed for him to achieve in his schoolwork. Miguel's parents reported that he struggled all of his academic life, and took time extra time to complete most things, if they were completed at all--as usually he ran out of time. Miguel's teachers and parents have recently reported falling behind in classes and struggling academically. They reported that he has had difficulty with timed tests and although he can verbally report the information, he often does poorly on assignments. The psychoeducational assessment is requested to determine any learning accommodations that would assist Miguel in his college academics.

Current Assessments Administered

- Wechsler Intelligence Scale for Children – V (WISC-V)
- Wechsler Individual Achievement Test- II (WIAT-II)

Assessment Results

Wechsler Intelligence Scale for Children (WISC-V)

Composite Scores	Percentile	Range
Verbal Comprehension	58th	Average
Visual Spatial	30th	Average
Working Memory Index	30th	Average
Fluid Reasoning	58th	Average
Processing Speed Index	23rd	Low Average
Full Scale IQ	61st	Average

Fig. 2.6 A psychoeducational assessment—Miguel

Wechsler Individual Achievement Test- II (WIAT-II)

Subtest	Percentile	Grade Equivalent
Word Reading	5th	2:6
Mathematics	68th	7:0
Written Language	59th	6:2
Oral Language	68th	7:2

Summary

In combination, the results of this assessment demonstrate that Miguel struggles in reading and writing, and would indicate a Specific Learning Disorder with an impairment in reading (315.00) according to the DSM-5. In combination, it will take Miguel longer to process information. Miguel demonstrates average skills in other areas of written expression, verbal skills, and visual spatial skills.

Based on the results of this assessment, Miguel meets the requirements for educational accommodations. Below are a list of recommended accommodations that would be helpful to assist Miguel in his schoolwork.

Recommendations

1. Double Time with Breaks
   Miguel would benefit from additional time on tests in order to assist him in processing the information according to his cognitive profile. This would ease his anxiety as he watches peers finish before her. Allowing Miguel breaks during testing would also prevent him from becoming taxed in testing situations.

2. Utilizing Educational Computer Software
   It is recommended that Miguel utilize educational software to assist with multiple educational demands that meet his educational and cognitive profile. Text-to-speech software will decrease demands for reading, working memory, comprehension, and processing speed.

Fig. 2.6 (continued)

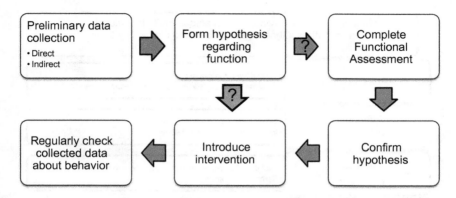

Fig. 2.7 Diagram of the steps towards a behavior intervention plan

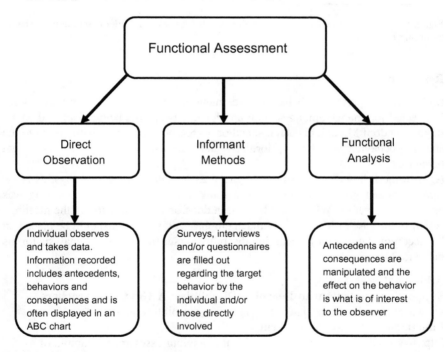

Fig. 2.8 Functional assessment procedures

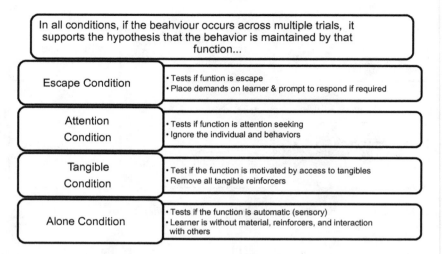

Fig. 2.9 Functional behavior analysis conditions, what it tests and a brief description of what to do during the condition

Reflection

(Q8) Often, as part of the behavior assessment process, a particular target behavior is selected for change among several problematic behaviors being displayed. What might you do if Miguel, his parents, and/or his teachers disagreed with you as to the specific behavior you have prioritized and selected for change as the target behavior?

(Q9) In the following case study, Miguel was included on the meetings, as is his right to attend given his age. Do you think what was said at the meeting was appropriate for him? What could have been done or said differently in the meeting?

(Q10) In the case of Miguel, how much emphasis do you think should be placed on his accommodations for his learning disability versus the functional analysis for his behavior?

Additional Web Links

Supporting Students with Learning Disabilities: A Guide for Teachers
www.bced.gov.bc.ca/specialed/docs/learning_disabilities_guide.pdf

Functional Behavior Assessment
http://www.educateautism.com/functional-behaviour-assessment/example-of-a-functional-analysis.html

Children attending IEP Meetings
https://www.understood.org/en/friends-feelings/empowering-your-child/self-advocacy/should-i-encourage-my-child-to-go-to-iep-meetings

CASE: i-A10

If Jaz can't get here on time, she is fired!
Setting: Work Place   Age Group: Adulthood

LEARNING OBJECTIVE:

- Design a behavior assessment plan.

TASK LIST LINKS

- **Fundamental Elements of Behavior Change**

    - (D-02) Use appropriate parameters and schedules of reinforcement.
    - (D-03) Use prompts and prompt fading.
    - (D-07) Conduct task analyses.

- **Specific Behavior-Change Procedures**

    - (E-03) Use instructions and rules.
    - (E-07) Plan for behavioral contrast effects.
    - (E-08) Use the matching law and recognize factors influencing choice.
    - (E-09) Arrange high-probability request sequences.
    - (E-10) Use the Premack principle.
    - (E-11) Use pairing procedures to establish new conditioned reinforcers and punishers.

- **Behavior-Change Systems**

    - (F-01) Use self-management strategies.

- **Intervention**

    - (J-03) Select intervention strategies based on task analysis.

KEY TERMS

- **Self-Management**

    - Self-management is when an individual themselves applies behavior-change tactics to their own behavior to bring about a desired change in that behavior (Lee et al. 2007).

- **Self-Monitoring**

    - Self-monitoring occurs when an individual observes his or her own behavior and documents the occurrence or absence of an identified target behavior (Ganz and Sigafoos 2005).

- **Visual Schedule**

    - A visual schedule provides a visual sequence of events that tell an individual what will occur, and in what order, using pictures or picture symbols (Dettmer et al. 2000).

If Jaz Can't Get Here on Time, She Is Fired!

Jaz's supervisor glanced quickly at her watch once again, silently noting Jaz's lateness to herself and checking off another issue on her mental list of problems in supervising Jaz's supported work placement. Twenty minutes later or so, she did the same thing, this time unable to suppress her raised eyebrows, pursed mouth, and almost imperceptible shaking of her head from side to side. *She has been late SO much this month. That's just not good enough*, she thought. *I don't think anyone should be working here who can't do the job, no matter how much help that person might have—or not have.* Jaz's supervisor recommenced her current task, moving shampoo bottles from an enormous cardboard box lying on the floor to the shelves of the department store. With a careful eye for detail, she tweaked each one, ensuring that they were lined up with great precision. Moving back with her hands on her hips and her head titled to one side, she examined her work with pleasure. *It looks good*, she judged, *at least until Jaz gets here and takes my work apart. I don't think it's anything to do with any "developmental disability," but more of a way to create chaos wherever she goes, getting the rest of us in trouble. But I guess I need to do my job, too, and my job today is her.* Taking her empty box to the back storage room to break it down with the other recycled products, she continued checking and rechecking her watch. *Jaz is almost an hour late yet again.*

In time—a long time—Jaz appeared, ready for work. Jaz was dressed carefully and neatly in her well-fitting vest with the logo of the department store emblazoned on the back, her name tag clipped securely on the left side of her zipper, and her nonslip black work shoes tightly laced. She stood in front of her supervisor and smiled tentatively, with a soft, "I'm here!"

In turn, her supervisor snorted gently, *thinking, At this point, that's not something to celebrate!* Out loud, she said in return, "Okay, well let's see what's on the list for today." Jaz opened her breast pocket and pulled out her **visual schedule**.

Her schedule of tasks was housed in a mini-binder, with a visual on each page representing one of the tasks that she accomplished at the department store. Every day when she arrives, her first job is to meet with her on-site supervisor of the day and to arrange the visual depictions of her tasks for that shift. Every night when she gets home, she arranges the visuals in order of her personal preference, with her favorites at the front. While riding the bus to the department store, she often takes out the mini-binder and happily gazes at the visual representing her favorite things at work.

When she passed her visual schedule to her supervisor, her supervisor snapped it open and licked her finger in preparation for page-turning. The first visual strategy was a photograph of a small shopping basket with two handles, representing the job of walking through the store in a careful pattern, searching abandoned baskets in the warm, welcoming store, and returning them to the nested stack at the doors to the entrance way. The friendly greeters often gave her a big smile, stopped to say hello, or showed her pictures of their families. The second was a visual of a broom. This task was sweeping the floor of the in-house cafeteria, where Jaz loved to smell the french fries cooking, and was often given a few chicken fingers dipped in honey for her excellent cleaning job. The third visual depicted a spray bottle. This meant that

Jaz was to go to the watch, jewelry, and glasses section to spray and wipe the display cases, where she always enjoying seeing the glass and jewels wink with store lights bouncing off of their surfaces.

But Jaz's supervisor said, "Nope, nope, and nope," as she flicked past those visuals. Then, she snapped open the three tiny metal rings holding them into the binder and put them in the "Done" pocket. "You are late and I already did these jobs," she explained, not unkindly. Rifling through the other choices, she placed these three at front: a photograph of a shopping cart, which meant that Jaz needed to go outside, find stray carts in the parking lot, and push them through the snow, slush, and network of cars to the cart corral; a photograph of the bathroom door, which meant that Jaz must go to the women's washroom and clean up stray bits of paper towel, toilet paper, and garbage and put them away properly; and a visual symbol for "Returns" which means she had to wheel a cart around the store figuring out where returned toys, housewares, and other department store goods belonged.

As soon as she snapped the metal rings shut again and told Jaz, "These are what you need to do today," Jaz snatched the binder, crammed it back in her pocket, and went back to the staff room. She sat down at the staff table nearest to the far, darkened corner of the communal space, and skidded her chair so her knees were touching the wall. "ARGH!" she wailed, rocking rhythmically with her arms clenched around her stomach. This happened to be a day when her support worker was on-site for a visit, which typically happened once every two weeks for Jaz's current needs.

Jaz's support worker was walking from her parked car to the back entrance of the department store, *thinking* about Jaz and Jaz's strengths and needs. *Jaz has done amazingly well*, she thought, *with this work place program. I used to be here every day—really every moment—to help Jaz with the day-to-day tasks of this part-time position. But now, with her **self-management** program and **self-monitoring** process she knows to call me or text me if she has a problem, and when I come in—like today—she is generally pretty happy and engaged in various tasks around the store with which she seems quite comfortable. The visuals have been a huge help to developing independence. Last year, I had to make visual mini-schedules for every "job" she was assigned, but now all she needs are those single visual prompts and she knows the routines of each task. But something has changed*, she pondered. *On my weekly reports sent by store manager, I am seeing that Jaz has been late for all her shifts in the last two weeks. Sometimes, she is almost an hour late! Often, she seems upset, too—out of the blue (they say)—and the staff doesn't know why. But she is at the point where she is disrupting the customers and the other staff, and it is taking some prolonged and intensive help to get her to calm down enough to work. With those two things combined, Jaz is missing a good chunk of her work day.*

How can we solve this problem? Who can help? Do I need to come more often? What is really going on? She knows that at home they have set a no-late rule, where she loses access to reinforcers if she is late. Why was she late here? She knows, however, that at home she access to many choices and reinforcement all the time for the positive things she does. Here, it is not quite as consistent, and she often does not get reinforced for some of the routine things. These were the thoughts going through the support worker's head, when she entered the store and pulled open the heavy steel door to the staff room. She was just in time to see Jaz, once again, pull out her visuals of today's task, stand up with great energy, and throw them angrily into the garbage can. Preparing herself to wail again, she saw the support worker out of the corner of her eye. Although Jaz was not typically physically demonstrative, she raced over to the support worker with her characteristic fast-paced stride and short steps and clasped her in a desperate hug. "What's wrong?" Jaz's support worker asked as she began to wonder how she might assess this situation. She thought about where to begin and remembered reading about the relevance of behavior rule and task analysis. *Those might be the right tools to help Jaz out of this tough spot,* she thought with optimism, as she began to prepare.

The Response: Principles, Processes, Practices, and Reflections

Principles

(Q1) Why might the relevance of behavior rule be an important guide in the assessment of Jaz's behavior?

(Q2) When Jaz' supervisor states that Jaz shows up 30 min late, or 1 h late, what is she measuring (interresponse time, latency, rate)? Would this be an appropriate measure to use to track progress in the case of Jaz and her work? Why or why not?

Processes

(Q3) Behavior analysts utilize a range of assessment methods including interviews, checklists, tests, and direct observation. What method or methods would you recommend be used in the case example of Jaz? Please explain your selection (Fig. 2.10).

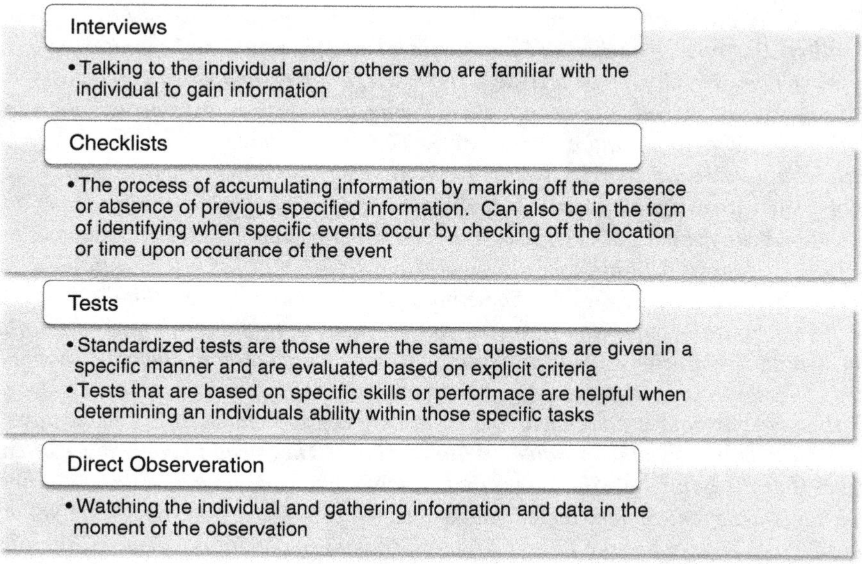

> **Interviews**
> • Talking to the individual and/or others who are familiar with the individual to gain information

> **Checklists**
> • The process of accumulating information by marking off the presence or absence of previous specified information. Can also be in the form of identifying when specific events occur by checking off the location or time upon occurance of the event

> **Tests**
> • Standardized tests are those where the same questions are given in a specific manner and are evaluated based on explicit criteria
> • Tests that are based on specific skills or performace are helpful when determining an individuals ability within those specific tasks

> **Direct Observeration**
> • Watching the individual and gathering information and data in the moment of the observation

Fig. 2.10 Assessment methods

(Q4) Explain how the behavior contrast effect is used in this case study.
(Q5) Explain how the matching law is used in this case study.

Practices

(Q6) Explain how you would carry out the assessment method or methods selected in question #3.
(Q7) Identify and operationally define a target behavior for Jaz and describe the social significance of the selected behavior.
(Q8) Jaz organizes her visual schedule with jobs she seems to enjoy doing. How could these jobs be organized with less preferred jobs such as tidying the women's washroom, or doing returns? What is this behavior principle called?

Reflections

(Q9) Jaz's work supervisor is encouraging you to teach Jaz to mop the store floors as a priority, simply because this is a need that the store requires. You question whether this is in the best interest for Jaz and, wanting to embrace the scientific method, feel as though you should wait for the assessment evidence to guide you in your decision regarding areas of initial concern. Explain how you would respond to the supervisor's request.
(Q10) What would be important to incorporate in Jaz's work day to continue to make it reinforcing for her?

Additional Web Links
Association for Positive Behavior Support–Developmental Disabilities (focus on adults): http://www.apbs.org/new_apbs/adultRef.aspx
Work support:
http://www.worksupport.com/index.cfm
The Matching Law
http://www.ncbi.nlm.nih.gov/pmc/articles/PMC3357095/

References

Ault, M., & Bausch, M. E. (2014). Monitoring assistive technology: Make event-based data recording work for you. *Journal of Special Education Technology, 29*(2), 51–64.
BCOTB. (2012). *Skills assessments for children with autism spectrum disorders.* Retrieved from http://bcotb.com/skills-assessment-for-children-with-autism-spectrum-disorders/
Behavior Analyst Certification Board (2014). *Professional and ethical compliance code for behavior analysts.* Retrieved from http://bacb.com/wp-content/uploads/2016/01/160120-compliance-code-english.pdf
Cooper, J. O., Heron, T. E., & Heward, W. L. (2007). *Applied behavior analysis* (2nd ed.). Upper Saddle River, NJ: Pearson.
Dettmer, S., Simpson, R., Myles, B., & Ganz, J. (2000). The use of visual supports to facilitate transitions of students with autism. *Focus on Autism and Other Developmental Disabilities, 15* (3), 163–169.

Ganz, J., & Sigafoos, J. (2005). Self-monitoring: Are young adults with MR and autism able to utilize cognitive strategies independently? *Education and Training in Developmental Disabilities, 40*(1), 24–33.

Hall, C., Maich, K., Van Rhijn, T., Mallabar, S., Hatt, A., & Ahi, M. (2016). *Stay, play, and talk—Phase IV*. Unpublished manuscript, University of Guelph, Guelph, Ontario.

Hayes, S., & Smith, S. (2005). *Get out of your mind and into your life: The new acceptance and commitment therapy*. Oakland, CA: New Harbinger Publications.

Horner, R., Carr, E., Halle, J., McGee, G., Odom, S., & Wolery, M. (2005). The use of single-subject research to identify evidence-based practice in special education. *Exceptional Children, 71*(2), 165–179.

Iwata, B. A., Pace, G. M., Cowdery, G. E., & Miltenberger, R. G. (1994). What makes extinction work: An analysis of procedural form and function. *Journal of Applied Behavior Analysis, 27* (1), 131–144.

Kahng, S. W., Boscoe, J. H., & Byrne, S. (2003). The use of an escape contingency and a token economy to increase food acceptance. *Journal of Applied Behavior Analysis, 36*(3), 349–353.

Lee, S., Simpson, R., & Shogren, K. (2007). Effects and implications of self-management for students with autism: A meta-analysis. *Focus on Autism and Other Developmental Disabilities, 22*(1), 2–13.

Mackinnon, K., & Krempa, J. (2005). *Social skills solutions: A hands-on manual for teaching social skills to children with autism*. New York, NY: DRL Books.

Mayer, G. R., Sulzer-Azaroff, B., & Wallace, M. (2014). *Behavior analysis for lasting change* (3rd ed.). Cornwall-on-Houston, NY: Sloan Publishing.

Michael, J. (2000). Implications and refinements of the establishing operation concept. *Journal of Applied Behavior Analysis, 33*, 401–410.

Minnesota Northland Association for Behavior Analysis. (2012). *Standards of practice for applied behavior analysis in Minnesota*. Retrieved from http://www.mnaba.org/

National Centre for Learning Disabilities. (2014). *Types of learning disabilities*. Retrieved from http://ncld.org/

National Institute for Mental Health. (2012). *Attention deficit hyperactivity disorder*. United States Department of Health and Human Services. Retrieved from http://www.nimh.nih.gov/health/publications/attention-deficit-hyperactivity-disorder/index.shtml

Pearson Education. (2007). *Chapter 3: Selecting and defining target behaviors*. Retrieved from https://www.google.ca/url?sa=t&rct=j&q=&esrc=s&source=web&cd=1&ved=0ahUKEwjqsKf4gMPJAhXJ6IMKHS35ABsQFgghMAA&url=http%3A%2F%2Fgator.uhd.edu%2F~williams%2Faba%2FCH03.ppt&usg=AFQjCNF_ptvxbbuE-Fo-238B2X3d1Ao1qQ&sig2=53JfJgnl-b1jxjLBI1Ihow

Reichow, B., & Volkmar, F. (2010). Social skills interventions for individuals with Autism: Evaluation for evidence-based practices within a best evidence synthesis framework. *Journal of Autism and Developmental Disorders, 40*(2), 149–166.

Schwartz, M., Rozumalski, A., & Trost, J. (2008). The effect of walking speed on the gait of typically developing children. *Journal of Biomechanics, 41*(8), 1639–1650.

Wong, C., Odom, S. L., Hume, K. Cox, A. W., Fettig, A., Kucharczyk, S., et al. (2014). *Evidence-based practices for children, youth, and young adults with Autism spectrum disorder*. Chapel Hill: The University of North Carolina, Frank Porter Graham Child Development Institute, Autism Evidence-Based Practice Review Group.

Part II
Planning

Chapter 3
Planning-Focused Case Studies for Preschool-Age to School-Age Children

Abstract Section one of this book explores the assessment process throughout childhood, adolescent, and adult years—an imperative first step in beginning any behavior-change program. Section two begins to examine the process of utilizing behavior assessment findings to create intervention programs. The current chapter begins by exploring intervention planning for preschool-age and school-age children. Many of the situations outlined in the case scenarios that are presented involve behavior analysts working as part of multidisciplinary teams, working together with professionals from other disciplines to interpret assessment information, and developing evidence-informed intervention plans. Increasingly, behavior analysts find themselves working alongside and in collaboration with professionals from a range of disciplines (e.g., psychologists, physicians, speech and language pathologists, occupational therapists, and special education teachers). This multidisciplinary team of professionals often strive to adopt a person-centered approach, placing the individual being supported, and their family members, at the center of the decision-making and intervention planning process. At the same time, team members attempt to work together to draw on one another's areas of expertise to develop cohesive and coordinated intervention plans. While a person-centered multidisciplinary approach has tremendous potential to result in comprehensive intervention plans that draw from, and blend, best practices across disciplines, this process is not without its challenges. Professionals attempting to work together may face competing or contradictory views as to the causes and factors contributing to presenting behavior difficulties. This, in-turn, may then translate into conflicting recommendations for behavior-change programming. In this chapter, entitled "Planning-Focused Case Studies for Preschool-Age to School-Age Children," these complex multidisciplinary team dynamics are explored through five case scenarios involving preschool-age and school-age children in home, school, clinical, and community settings.

Keywords Preschool · School-age children · Intervention · Intervention planning · Multidisciplinary teams · Psychologists · Physicians · Speech and language pathologists · Occupational therapists · Special education teachers · Best practices

© Springer International Publishing AG 2016   85
K. Maich et al., *Applied Behavior Analysis*,
DOI 10.1007/978-3-319-44794-0_3

CASE: ii-P1

We all are experts, but none of us alone has all the expertise.
Setting: Home   Age-Group: Preschool
LEARNING OBJECTIVE:

- Determine how to form an interdisciplinary team with a behavior analyst

TASK LIST LINKS:

- **Experimental Design**

    - (B-01) Use the dimensions of applied behavior analysis (Baer et al. 1968) to evaluate whether interventions are behavior analytic in nature.

- **Identification of the Problem**

    - (G-01) Review records and available data at the outset of the case.
    - (G-02) Consider biological/medical variables that may be affecting the client.
    - (G-03) Conduct a preliminary assessment of the client in order to identify the referral problem.
    - (G-04) Explain behavioral concepts using nontechnical language.
    - (G-05) Describe and explain behavior, including private events, in behavior-analytic (nonmentalistic) terms.
    - (G-06) Provide behavior-analytic services in collaboration with others who support and/or provide services to one's clients.
    - (G-07) Practice within one's limits of professional competence in applied behavior analysis, and obtain consultation, supervision, and training, or make referrals as necessary.
    - (G-08) Identify and make environmental changes that reduce the need for behavior analysis services.

- **Intervention**

    - (J-07) Select intervention strategies based on environmental and resource constraints.

KEY TERMS:

- **Developmental Pediatrician**

    - Developmental pediatrics is a specialty field within pediatrics, and these professionals observe, examine, and assess children to find out "'Why is my child developing differently from other children?' and 'What can be done to help my child?'" (McMaster Children's Hospital 2013, p. 5).

- **Interdisciplinary Team**

    - Interdisciplinary (often used synonymously with "multidisciplinary") teams are comprised of multiple team members from varied disciplines (e.g., psychiatry, social work, and behavior analysis) working together for common goals such as effective intervention (Dillenburger et al. 2014).

- **Rapport**
  - Rapport is typically a subjective measure of relationship quality which is essential for many relationships, including therapeutic and/or professional ones, often associated with positive interactions (McLaughlin and Carr 2005).

We All Are Experts, But None of Us Alone Has All the Expertise

Luis, a new behavior consultant with a few years of experience in applying the principles of ABA in school settings, had recently moved to a position that demanded a high level of involvement in varied clinical community settings, including their strength: on-site IBI programs. His responsibilities included visiting home settings, but also demanded attention to these home and community settings across a wide geographical area of mostly rural homes, in areas of low population density. However, he spent most of his time delivering IBI at the clinic. After a few months in this position, he sat down with his supervisor to talk over a few issues. He began, "Remember how you told me that there are 'challenges to rural settings'? I think I finally 'get' what you meant! You know about this three-year-old I have just started to work with this week. Well, I have done my first home visit. He is a very complex child in a complicated home setting. He already has multiple diagnoses and some other queries at such as young age." Gesturing to the thick, heavy file resting on the desk between them. "Look at this—and that's not all. I have a portable drive full of assessment reports and programming recommendations, including IBI. I met with his parents, I mean, his guardians—really his grandparents—who have unexpectedly taken on the responsibility of parenting this little boy. He is not yet walking, he is not yet talking, and he appears to have little means of letting his wants and needs be known to those around him. He is showing some unusual behaviors, such as a grinding his jaw together in a visible manner during most of his waking hours. But his caregivers are already exhausted. They say that they have been to so many appointments that really neither of them can continue to be employed full time; that every appointment leads to a new referral. They are spending hours on the road taking this boy to appointments for what they call 'poking and prodding' but they think all of their time could be used in better ways, such as maybe accessing some type of specialized program. Though they have the assessments in place, they haven't yet started IBI therapy. Yesterday, they received a phone call about an appointment with a pediatric specialist who is a six-hour drive away, or a plane flight that they can't afford. And it's winter!"

"You <u>are</u> getting it for sure," answered Luis's supervisor, who smiled at this learning process happening in front of her eyes. "I think this is a good moment for me to remind you that when you started working here, you mentioned that some of your future goals for your own professional development involved—if I recall correctly—the words leadership, initiative, and creativity."

"Yes, that's right," answered Luis, with trepidation, clearly wondering where this was going.

"It sounds to me like this set of issues you are seeing relates to what a lot of our families complain about, and what we often refer to in the field as 'fragmented services.' I am really glad that you have brought this up. It's very possible that we have sort of become used to this as just the way things are here. But there is one initiative that I think might help this child and family and many more like them: an **interdisciplinary team**. We have quite a few of them in our clinic alone!"

"That's not exactly what came to my mind in this situation," responded Luis. "Tell me a little more."

"In this case, I think that that a focus on early intervention would likely be the right next step for *thinking* about developing a team, since we have so many very young children on our caseloads. It seems that more young families are choosing to move to our rural areas where there is the freedom for movement and certainly a perceived sense of safety that city living might not give them. In any case, such a team would involve many professionals from varied disciplines. For example, we have an occupational therapist on board, who could assess for sensory issues, such as this young boy's jaw grinding. We might have a speech–language pathologist, who would assess his speech, and teach him ways of communicating. We might have a **developmental pediatrician** do a consulting visit, who can diagnose and support any medical issues. Of course, we would have a behavior analyst who, in addition to teaching new skills and planning for behavioral change, might take on the role of team formation and **rapport**-building in the group. But the most important piece of a team is collaborating as equal partners who come to understand and appreciate the perspectives, skills, and strengths that each team member brings to the discussion. So what do you think, Luis? Do you want to be the visionary who pulls all of the pieces of the puzzle together into one picture?"

The Response: Principles, Processes, Practices, and Reflections

Principles

(Q1) In developing a new team, often setting a terms of reference for the team is helpful in learning how to work together. Using the chart below as a guide, determine a terms of reference for the team (Table 3.1).

(Q2) As a behavior analyst on the team, the fourth edition task list item G-06 applies: "Provide behavior-analytic services in collaboration with others who support and/or provide services to one's clients" (BACB, 2012). When planning for the child, potential conflicts between various team members' priorities and the types of intervention methods that are specific to their field may arise. What may some of these be?

Table 3.1 How to develop terms of reference (Divisions of Family Practice, n.d.)

Components of a term of reference	Questions to answer
1. Purpose	• Create the purpose and responsibilities of the committee • Decide the outcomes the committee will accomplish • Determine if the committee is responsible for following up to a need determined by an external group
2. Membership	• Determine membership criteria and committee size • Agree upon committee roles • Determine the term for committee members
3. Meetings	• Agree upon meeting frequency and location • Determine frequency that terms of reference will be reviewed • Determine who will organize meetings and agenda items
4. Minutes	• Determine how and by whom the minutes will be taken and distributed
5. Resources	• List the resources needed to fulfill the purpose of the committee
6. Reporting/relationship	• State who the committee reports to and how the report occurs • Determine the components that need to be reported and the response time required • Determine a conflict resolution strategy

Processes

(Q3) In Luis' case, when working with a speech–language pathologist (SLP), the SLP may approach teaching language differently than a behavior analyst. List 5 ways you could incorporate each profession's methods to teach language in order to work together to develop a language program.

(Q4) In the same situation, when working with an occupational therapist (OT), the OT may suggest working to help Luis develop fine and gross motor skills in a way that is different than you would as a behavior analyst. List 5 ways you could incorporate their teaching methods with those a behavior analyst would use.

Practices

(Q5) A verbal behavior approach is often one way a behavior analyst begins to teach language to a child. However, a popular way that many speech–language pathologists teach language is with core vocabulary. What are the pros and cons to using either approach with a client (Table 3.2)?

(Q6) When planning for someone like the client in the case study who is failing to meet developmental milestones such as walking and talking, behavior analysts usually complete a behavior skills assessment to determine his or her current skill repertoire. What skills assessment could you use that would benefit all members of the team? What assessments would you avoid that may be difficult to share across disciplines?

(Q7) When planning for a young client, as in this case study, it is important to both understand the immediate, short-term goals, including skills that can be obtained, and understand the long-term goals that the family hopes for their child. List short- and long-term goals that you would have that are optimistic and strength-based. (Table 3.3).

Table 3.2 Verbal behavior approach to teaching language compared with the core vocabulary approach to teaching language (Sundberg and Sundberg 1990; Zangari 2013)

Verbal behavior	Core vocabulary
1. Choose method to communicate, including pictures, sign, vocal language, and speech-generating device	1. Learner should have access to core vocabulary. Can be via augmentative and alternate communication (AAC) system that is technology based through a speech-generating device, or low tech through a communication board
2. Based on the foundation that language is learned by altering the environment, cues, and discriminative stimulus (SD), known as the instruction	2. Ensure the AAC system has ample vocabulary, slightly more than what the learner currently knows to ensure they have exposure to future language targets and allows the opportunity to explore these words
3. Based on a function-based view of language (that language is broken into components based on their function)	3. As the learner begins to use the language that are currently being taught, add more vocabulary to the AAC system
4. Often begins by teaching the learner to mand (request) for reinforcers	4. Plenty of opportunities should be contrived to practice the use of core words
5. Learners are also taught to echo and imitate, enabling them to learn new words, signs, etc.	5. Give support, the learner is learning and will need help to use the words
6. Distinctions are made between the speaker and the listener	6. Give access to more words when the learner begins to show signs they are understanding. Mastery is not expected nor is it necessary
7. The learner is also taught to respond to language (listener responding—also known as receptive language)	
8. Tacting is another primary verbal operant where the learner labels items	
9. Learners are taught more difficult functions of language, while programming in generalization and maintenance	

Table 3.3 Short- and long-term goal-setting hierarchy (CornerStone 2008)

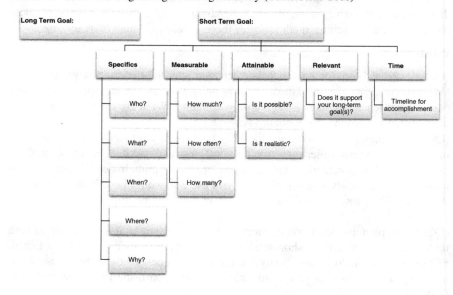

Reflections

(Q8) When planning for a client who is in a rural area, list the factors that you would need to determine with the team before beginning your behavior analyst services. What factors would influence you before you started your assessment? Would you complete your assessment in the same way as you would if there was not an interdisciplinary team?

(Q9) Read the article below. List the benefits of applying ABA services with an interdisciplinary team from the perspective of the therapist. What are the drawbacks? Now list the benefits and drawbacks of the interdisciplinary team from the client's point of view.

http://www.publish.csiro.au/?act=view_file&file_id=AH070330.pdf

(Q10) Some therapists may shy away from an interdisciplinary approach because it makes it more difficult to implement the services that they are familiar with. By adopting this approach or attitude, what may the therapists, other team members, families, and client be prone to?

Additional Web Links

American Speech-Language-Hearing Association:
http://www.asha.org

Canadian Association of Occupational Therapists
https://www.caot.ca

The Role of a Behavior Analyst within an Interdisciplinary Team:
http://www.tbi-sci.org/conference/2012Presentations/Schaub-Peters%20Role%20of %20BA_Feb%2025th%2020%20Min_FINAL_1-13-12.pdf

Collaborative Training in ABA:
http://www.academia.edu/2926867/Collaborative_Training_and_Practice_among_ Applied_Behavior_Analysts_who_Support_Individuals_with_Autism_Spectrum_ Disorder

Verbal Behavior versus Core Vocabulary
http://autism.outreach.psu.edu/sites/omcphplive.outreach.psu.edu.drpms. autismconference/files/32Presentation.pdf

Teaching Language: ABA versus SLP:
http://www.autismtrainingsolutions.com/resources/case-study/aba-training- methods-verbal-behavior-speech-language-pathology

Skills Assessments
http://www.behaviorbabe.com/assessments.htm

CASE: ii-P2 Guest Author: Adam Davies

Guest Author: Adam Davies, Master of Arts Candidate, Ontario Institute for Studies in Education of the University of Toronto

Change is needed, but who is it that has to change?
Setting: Childcare   Age-Group: Preschool
LEARNING OBJECTIVE:

- Implementing the mediator model for change

TASK LIST LINKS:

- **Measurement**

  - (A-12) Design and implement continuous measurement procedures (e.g., event recording).

- **Behavior-Change Considerations**

  - (C-01) State and plan for the possible unwanted effects of reinforcement.
  - (C-02) State and plan for the possible unwanted effects of punishment.
  - (C-03) State and plan for the possible unwanted effects of extinction.

- **Identification of the Problem**

  - (G-01) Review records and available data at the outset of the case.
  - (G-03) Conduct a preliminary assessment of the client in order to identify the referral problem.
  - (G-04) Explain behavioral concepts using nontechnical language.
  - (G-05) Describe and explain behavior, including private events, in behavior-analytic (nonmentalistic) terms.
  - (G-06) Provide behavior-analytic services in collaboration with others who support and/or provide services to one's clients.

- **Measurement**

  - (H-01) Select a measurement system to obtain representative data given the dimensions of the behavior and the logistics of observing and recording.
  - (H-02) Select a schedule of observation and recording periods.

- **Assessment**

  - (I-06) Make recommendations regarding behaviors that must be established, maintained, increased, or decreased.

- **Intervention**

  - (J-06) Select intervention strategies based on supporting environments.
  - (J-07) Select intervention strategies based on environmental and resource constraints.

- **Implementation, Management, and Supervision**

  - (K-02) Identify the contingencies governing the behavior of those responsible for carrying out behavior-change procedures and design interventions accordingly.

- (K-03) Design and use competency-based training for persons who are responsible for carrying out behavioral assessment and behavior-change procedures.
- (K-04) Design and use effective performance monitoring and reinforcement systems.
- (K-05) Design and use systems for monitoring procedural integrity.
- (K-06) Provide supervision for behavior-change agents.
- (K-09) Secure the support of others to maintain the client's behavioral repertoires in their natural environments.

KEY TERMS:

- **Behavior**

  - In applied behavior analysis, this refers to the activity of living beings—the actions of people (the dependent variable) that is observable and measureable (Cooper et al. 2007).

- **Functional Relation**

  - In applied behavior analysis, the relationship between two variables–the dependent (behavior) and independent variables (environment) are related in this regard when the behavior (dependent variable) changes with modifications to the environment (Dixon et al. 2012).

- **Language Delay**

  - A mild-to-severe lag in the development of a child's language capabilities (Bochner et al. 1997).

- **Mediator Model of Behavior Intervention**

  - A model of behavior intervention where individuals in a client's life, such as family members or a professional in their home, school, or work life, are provided with the skills necessary to produce clinically significant behavior change through high-quality treatment plans and behavior analyst's assistance (Minnesota Northland Association for Behavior Intervention 2012).

Change is Needed, But Who Is It That Has to Change?

Ploy, a young three-year-old in a new early learning and childcare center, experiences difficulties while in her childcare environment. Ploy has a **language delay** and is struggling when trying to express her wants and needs to those around her. Ploy tries to communicate with other peers and staff at her center, but is often unable to accurately convey what she means and struggles with peer-to-peer interactions. At one point, last week Ploy grabbed all the crayons off the table and threw them at her peers who were sitting at the table while making sounds that resembled words, but were incomprehensible. Ploy appears to be frequently frustrated; as a result, she bursts out into tantrums that feature frequent crying, verbal aggression, and throwing objects.

Ms. Tracey, Ploy's Early Childhood Educator, has been working in childcare for more than thirty years. Ms. Tracey is very confident in her approach to working with children and feels content with how she interacts with children. She uses a warm, gentle, but firm manner for interacting with children that seems effective. Ms. Tracey is at a state of tribulation with Ploy due to her frustration and anxiety about Ploy's explosions during classroom-wide instructional periods. Ms. Tracey responds to Ploy's verbal and aggressive **behaviors** by verbally reprimanding her, and placing her in a time-out, Ploy is removed from her peers to sit in the corner alone with her back to the other children. Ms. Tracey's reasoning for this form of discipline is that she feels that Ploy will learn that her outbursts are unacceptable and distracting to the other children during her time spent reflecting while isolated from her peers.

Recently, Ms. Tracey has been struggling with Ploy's tantrums in particular within her large class of fifteen other children, with only one assistant and herself as adult figures. With all the diverse needs of all the other children, Ms. Tracey is finding it difficult to attend to Ploy while ensuring that the other children are receiving the appropriate amount of attention. *I don't know what to do with her,* Ms. Tracey thought, *I wish she would listen to me and act just like the other children. I have no idea what she is saying to me most of the time. She needs to smarten up!* After much tension between Ploy and Ms. Tracey, Ms. Tracey places a referral to a local behavioral support agency for assistance with Ploy. Within her referral, Ms. Tracey specifies that she requires behavior consultation in order to ensure that Ploy changes her behavior.

During the initial meeting between Ms. Tracey and the behavior consultant, Ms. Tracey reinforces the idea that Ploy requires alterations in her behaviors. Ms. Tracey conceives that her actions are unrelated to Ploy's outbursts and states that Ploy is almost uncontrollable, as this has worked for many other children she has taught in the past. Ms. Tracey spends the entire meeting discussing Ploy's behaviors and does not provide her own reactions to Ploy's behavior besides stating that she believes that Ploy "needs to stop." Ms. Tracey quickly leaves the meeting soon afterward and does not appear to think that she can do anything else to help Ploy, but instead thinks that Ploy needs an intervention outside of her classroom.

Upon visiting Ms. Tracey's classroom numerous times, it becomes clear that Ms. Tracey may need to try different techniques and that Ploy may be reacting in different ways to the techniques she is currently employing. Ms. Tracey has begun to leave Ploy alone in a corner in the classroom and does not acknowledge Ploy's presence in large group instruction. The behavior consultant attempts to speak to Ms. Tracey several times, and Ms. Tracey either quickly responds, or barely acknowledges the consultant and walks away. During the latest visit, Ms. Tracey responds to the behavior consultant's entrance into the classroom by stating, "I am very busy. Ploy is over there. Please go spend time with her. Let me know what program you have for Ploy and how long it might be until she will begin to change her behavior."

After taking extensive observation data, Ms. Tracey sits down with the behavior consultant to discuss how to assist Ploy. The behavior consultant explains how the environment that surrounds Plot affects her behaviors and reactions; the individuals, objects, and atmosphere around Ploy mould her environment. Thus, Ploy's behavior and her environment have a **functional relationship**, and Ploy's behaviors can change with alterations in her environment. The behavior consultant elucidated how the individuals in Ploy's life impact her behaviors and play a large part in her success at school. The consultant explained, "Ploy requires a **Mediator Model of Behavior Intervention** that provides influential individuals, or mediators in her life, implementing required skills to assist her in managing her behaviors. In other words, she explains that she will not be working individually with Ploy, but would like to take on the role of helping Ms. Tracey implement different strategies with Ploy. "This model involves a high level of interaction between you and I to ensure that Ploy has higher levels of success." The consultant continued to explain how they could work with Ms. Tracey to intervene Ploy's behaviors. This would occur with a formal assessment of Ploy's behaviors, communicating between the consultant and Ms. Tracey to assist in planned interventions, with assessments of progress and regular meetings between Ms. Tracey and the consultant. After explaining this approach to Ms. Tracey, the consultant smiles at her and asks, "How do you feel about this approach? Can we work together to make a successful school environment for Ploy?"

THE RESPONSE: PRINCIPLES, PROCESSES, PRACTICES, AND REFLECTIONS

Principles

(Q1) What factors could be impacting Ploy's behaviors in the classroom?

(Q2) Explain why it is important to directly observe an individual's behaviors in the environment during the assessment and planning process? How is this important to the concept of functional relationships? How could your approach to Ploy's behavior differ if you had just met with Ms. Tracey and completed an indirect assessment of the behavior?

(Q3) Many individuals who are not trained in behavior analysis use punishment to try and change behavior. Indicate any positive and negative punishment Ms. Tracey uses. What is problematic with this? Looking at the Professional and Ethical Compliance Code for Behavior Analysts (2014), what guidelines are relevant to the use of punishment and this case study?

Processes

(Q4) Explain how you would approach Ms. Tracey, and take her through the process of a Mediator Model of Intervention and behavior skills training to ensure the least amount of tension and most successful approach between yourself and the mediator (Fig. 3.1) (Reference Ethics Box 3.1, Behavior Analyst Certification Board, 2014)?

Ethics Box 3.1

Professional and Ethical Compliance Code for Behavior Analysts

- 2.04 Third-Party Involvement in Services.

  (a) When behavior analysts agree to provide services to a person or entity at the request of a third party, behavior analysts clarify, to the extent feasible and at the outset of the service, the nature of the relationship with each party and any potential conflicts. This clarification includes the role of the behavior analyst (such as therapist, organizational consultant, or expert witness), the probable uses of the services provided or the information obtained, and the fact that there may be limits to confidentiality.

  (b) If there is a foreseeable risk of behavior analysts being called upon to perform conflicting roles because of the involvement of a third party, behavior analysts clarify the nature and direction of their responsibilities, keep all parties appropriately informed as matters develop, and resolve the situation in accordance with the code.

  (c) When providing services to a minor or individual who is a member of a protected population at the request of a third party, behavior analysts ensure that the parent or client-surrogate of the ultimate recipient of services is informed of the nature and scope of services to be provided, as well as their right to all service records and data.

  (d) Behavior analysts put the client's care above all others, and should the third party make requirements for services that are contradicted by the behavior analyst's recommendations, behavior analysts are obligated to resolve such conflicts in the best interest of the client. If said conflict cannot be resolved, that behavior analyst's services to the client may be discontinued following appropriate transition.

Fig. 3.1 Model of training a mediator by a behavior analyst

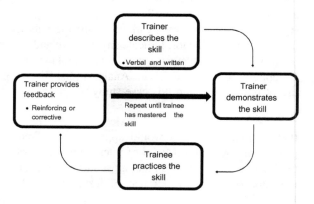

Considerations for Mediator Training

☐ **Motivation:**How motivated is the mediator?

☐ **View of ABA:** Do they think that the Behavior Consultant will fix the individual or are they prepared to take an active role?

☐ **Risk Factors:** Are there risk factors that may indicate the mediator will not follow through?

☐ **Emotional Resources:** Does the mediator have the emotional resources to continue to work with the challenging behaviors?

☐ **Physical Resources:** Is the mediator able to handle the individual physically?

☐ **Secondary Gain:** Is there reasons that the mediator does not wantthe individual to improve?

☐ **Philosophical & Attitudinal Conflict:** Does the mediator believe in the positive approach to behavior or believe that discipline needs to be enforced?

☐ **Personal Emotions:** Does the mediator have biass or dislikes that will influence the approach?

☐ **External Constraints:** Are their constraints such as workload, money, or staffing that can prevent the intervention from continuing?

☐ **Behavioral Characteristics of the Person:** Is therate, duration, and severity of the behaviors too much for the mediator to handle?

☐ **Organizational Structure:** Is structure in place to supervise the intervention and ensure that everyone knows the plan?

☐ **Inter-Personal Issues:** Does the mediator have personal needs and thus the mediator training needs to be adapted?

☐ **Training Issues:** Is there substantial time for adequate training and follow-through?

(Willis & LaVigna, 1998)

Fig. 3.2 Considerations for mediator training

(**Q5**) What may need to be completed before implementing the formal behavior skills training to ensure that this intervention is successful? For example, look at this checklist about considerations for mediator training (Fig. 3.2).

(**Q6**) How would you explain to Ms. Tracey why using punishment could be problematic with Ploy (Table 3.4)?

Practice

(**Q7**) Create a plan that you would formulate with Ms. Tracey to assist Ploy in listening to instructions in the classroom.

(**Q8**) Using the mediator model described above in question 4, describe your plan for teaching Ms. Tracey to implement the above plan.

Reflection

(**Q9**) Identify any strengths and limitations of your above plan and of using the Mediator Model of Intervention for Ploy and Ms. Tracey.

(**Q10**) Do you think the mediator model of implementing a behavior program with Ploy would have the same success as if the behavior consultant implemented the plan? What do you think will be key variables that will influence success for the mediator model implementation of the program?

Table 3.4 Positive and negative punishment and the difficulties with using punishment

Concept	Definition	Example
Positive punishment	The **addition** of a stimulus to an environment after the occurrence of a behavior that reduces the future likelihood of the behavior reoccurring	A child walks from the entrance of the house to the bathroom with muddy shoes. As a result, his mom asked him to wash the floor where he tracked mud • The child's mom is attempting to reduce the child's walking through the house with muddy shoes by **adding** the chore of cleaning up the muddy footprints
Negative punishment	The **removal** of a stimulus to an environment after the occurrence of a behavior that reduces the future likelihood of the behavior reoccurring	A child is playing soccer with her team; after an opponent scores a goal, she removes her shoe and throws it at the opponent. Her coach takes her out of the game • The coach is attempting to alter the players behavior by **removing** her from playing in the game, a preferred activity
Difficulties with punishment	• The individual being punished may respond to the punishment emotionally and/or aggressively • In response to punishment, the individual may attempt to escape the environment or avoid it all together. For example, the soccer player above may stop playing soccer • Environments where the behavior is not punished may experience an increase in the behavior—this is known as behavioral contrast • An individual who receives punishment may imitate this behavior • When an individual provides a reprimand following a behavior, the reprimanded behavior may immediately stop, thereby reinforcing the individuals behavior of providing reprimands, and as a result positive praise and contingent reinforcement for desired behaviors decreases	

Additional Web Links
Mediator Model
http://www.ncbi.nlm.nih.gov/pmc/articles/PMC3592486/
Behavior Skills Training
http://opensiuc.lib.siu.edu/cgi/viewcontent.cgi?article=1728&context=gs_rp
Reinforcement and Punishment
http://bcotb.com/the-difference-between-positivenegative-reinforcement-and-positivenegative-punishment/

CASE: ii-P3

You mean you want to TRAIN my student?
Setting: Home   Age-Group: Preschool
LEARNING OBJECTIVE:

- Understanding the three-term contingency and punishment

TASK LIST LINKS:

- **Fundamental Elements of Behavior Change**

  – (D-16) Use positive and negative punishment.
  – (D-17) Use appropriate parameters and schedules of punishment.

- **Identification of the Problem**

  - (G-03) Conduct a preliminary assessment of the client in order to identify the referral problem.
  - (G-06) Provide behavior-analytic services in collaboration with others who support and/or provide services to one's clients.

- **Assessment**

  – (I-06) Make recommendations regarding behaviors that must be established, maintained, increased, or decreased.

KEY TERMS:

- **Behaviorism**

  – Behaviorism is the philosophy of the science of human behavior (Skinner 1976).

- **Consequence**

  – Anything that occurs after the target behaviors; consequence-based interventions, then, are interventions that occur after the behavior to either increase the target behavior through reinforcement (e.g., token economy) or decrease the target behavior through punishment (e.g., time-out).

- **Experimental Analysis of Behavior**

  – The Experimental Analysis of Behavior (EAB) is a specialization within behaviorism, which focuses on basic research that studies the relationships between behavior and the environment to understand the basic principles of behavior (Skinner 1966, 1976).

- **Punishment**

  - Punishment-based strategies can be controversial and ethically fraught, and are consequence-based interventions utilized to reduce the future occurrence of the target behaviors (DiGennaro Reed and Lovett 2008; Ringdahl and Falcomata 2009).

- **Structure**

  - Providing structure is a pedagogical strategy that provides "clarity, order, and predictability" to an environment such as the classroom. It often includes elements such as careful environmental arrangement (e.g., work stations and dividers), visual cues (e.g., pictures and color-coding), and consistent routines and procedures (e.g., schedules and timers) (Scheuermann and Webber 2002, p. 123).

You Mean You Want to Train My Student?

It was treat day in the staff room. Fridays—staff treat days—were really the only day that everyone tried hard to be in the staff room at the same time. All the teachers, administrators, and other staff members took turns signing up to bring in snacks, beverages, and other essentials to celebrate the end of a busy teaching week and the beginning of the weekend. This particular day was a school-wide professional development day, and nobody had yard duty or lunch duty. Therefore, the staff room was busy and loud, and everyone delighted in the whole hour available for lunch, treats, and most important—conversation.

The grade one teacher, Mr. Sato laughingly commented to one of her colleagues who teaches the Kindergarten program as she chose from the assortment of baked goods, "This is just like some of us do with our students: giving a treat for good behavior! I wish it were that easy. Remember Sandy from last year? He sure is a handful, now. What was he like last year?"

The Kindergarten teacher licked her finger and pursed her lips while she thoughtfully considered her response. "Well, he was up and down, really. I specifically remember that he had a really tough time on Mondays and Fridays—just like we do sometimes." She laughed and continued, "I also remember that we had to provide him with a lot of **structure** or he struggled with his behavior. You never know at that age, though. Sometimes it just takes a while to get adjusted to the school system. I don't think he spent much time out of the home before coming here."

Mr. Sato considered this new information. "Well, I am really looking forward to this afternoon's workshop on applied behavior analysis. I need some new tricks for Sandy. I seem to be doing okay with the rest of the class, but I just don't get him at all. And once he starts acting up, he gets a lot of the other boys riled up too. If I can't break this pattern, I am going to have a really big problem getting through

June." He glanced at the wall. "It looks like our time is almost up. Do you want to head down together?"

The Kindergarten teacher and Mr. Sato joined what looked like about fifty other staff members, happily taking some social time together. The room was quite full. *This must be a really popular topic*, Mr. Sato thought. *I just hope it is something that works.*

The workshop began with Mr. Sato carefully listening to the presentation and taking notes on his laptop, which was balanced on his knees. After about an hour, Mr. Sato sighed quietly and shut its lid. Unable to stay engaged and listen any longer, he took the opportunity to fill out a sticky note that audience members were encouraged to use for questions and/or comments to be addressed following afternoon break. On it, he wrote, *I don't get it. Giving treats for good behavior? I don't want to train my student like I trained my puppy, and the students should do it as good citizens because they want to, not because they will get something for it.* He signed his name. His comment was not read aloud in the problem-solving session, but the speaker—a private behavior consultant—came up to him after the break and offered to come in and meet with him after school on Monday to further discuss strategies.

On Monday, Mr. Sato tried to explain what he didn't like about the behavior consultant's presentation. "I just don't believe in training children this way. If a student has a bad behavior, I provide a **consequence** to that student. Right now, I have a student called 'S.' S has a current trick that he does which is tossing things out of his desk, and I don't mean in a gentle way. One by one, he takes things like erasers, pencils, balled-up pieces of paper, and he tosses them towards the front of the classroom. I can usually ignore him for a while, and so can the other students in the class. But after a while, he takes out bigger, heavier, and louder things—like this giant book on dog breeds he likes to keep around—and proceeds into tossing those. It seems like he is trying to hit the ledge where I keep our whiteboard markers. And when this starts happening, other students get involved, and giggle, and imitate him. Then I have to give a consequence to him, so at this point, either I call the office or I send him to the office. Then I send home a note in his agenda. Luckily, the office is right across the hall from my classroom. So I guess that's his punishment. I keep telling him 'Be good, and good things happen,' and 'Be bad, and bad things happen.' I have noticed this tends to be during French class, but I don't know what that has to do with anything. I also can't see how giving him a treat will help!"

"That's quite a bit of information, so thank you for that. An important part of the field of applied behavior analysis, or ABA is that each child—each case—is unique. But it also means that we follow scientifically based patterns of behavior. So we are all alike—but we are also different. This means that, in this field, we carefully assess each student and then apply the principles of **behaviorism**. In my case, all my practice in the field—it is an applied science—is guided by behavior analysis. Way back, it started with a wider field called the **Experimental Analysis of Behavior**. But I apologize. You probably don't want to know all of that! We are not completing ABA for scientific reasons, such as the original animal studies were, ABA is applied in practical settings like yours. My point is that it is a very well-established field that really works and we have decades of careful research that shows that this. Sometimes, though, we have to back up a little bit and look at how we understand different terms that sometimes have different meanings in the clinics where I work with children and the schools where I work with students. For example, in schools, I hear the terms reward, consequence, but the word 'punishment' is really not used and is thought of as a hurtful practice. But in ABA, we use the terms reinforcement, consequence, and punishment, but they have quite different meanings, which makes things difficult and we often have to spend some time separating fact from fiction."

"What do you mean? Can you give an example? And you are quite right. If the school district heard me mentioning punishing a student, they would be all over me!" Mr. Sato widened his eyes with the thought of it.

"Let's talk about that, then. In ABA, punishment is what we do that decreases a behavior. So, if a student is talking way too loudly in class during group work, you go over and quietly put your finger to your lips in a 'Shh!' motion, and that student stops yelling, that's actually working as a punishment for that student. But you are not being angry or mean or inappropriate in any way to that student, which are some of the meanings we sometimes attach to the word '**punishment**.'

"Hmm," responded Mr. Sato. "That kind of explains a lot. So, what do you think we can do with my student 'S'?"

The Response: Principles, Processes, Practices, and Reflections

Principles

(Q1) Define, in appropriate professional manner, how you would explain the three-term contingency (ABC sequence) to Mr. Sato (Fig. 3.3).

(Q2) List the times that Mr. Sato used the term "consequence" correctly and incorrectly. What was he really describing?

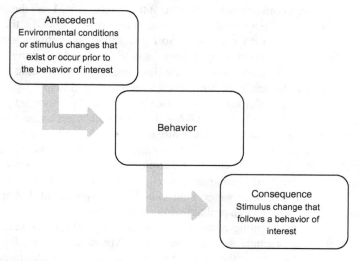

Fig. 3.3 The three-term contingency (Doher, n.d.)

Processes

(Q3) Examine how the Experimental Analysis of Behavior is different than applied behavior analysis utilizing Baer et al. (1968).

(Q4) List the reasons that punishment can be ineffective or lead to other ethical concerns. Read the article: http://help4teachers.com/punishment.htm

Practice

(Q5) What would you suggest as a behavior plan for student "S" that could replace Mr. Sato's current behavior strategies?

(Q6) Develop a script of how you could convince Mr. Sato that you are not "training" his student but rather providing him with structure and other alternative behaviors. What differential reinforcement strategies from the chart below would you use (Fig. 3.4)?

Differential Reinforcement of Incompatible Behavior

- Reinforcement is provided after the occurance of a behavior which is impossible to occur at the same time as the behavior targeted to replace
- e.g. The behavior to replace is spitting, the individual will recieve reinforcement for engaging in drinking, talking, and having their lips closed because all these behaviors are incompatible with spitting.

Differential Reinforcement of Alternate Behavior

- Reinforcement is provided after the occurace of a behavior that is an acceptable replacement for the behavior targeted to reduce or replace. This behaviour is not necessarily incompatible with the targeted behavior
- e.g. The function of the behavior to eliminate is escape, the individual will be provided with reinforcement anytime he requestes a break.

Differential Reinforcement of Other Behavior

- Reinforcement is provided for any behavior that is not the target behavior. Reinforcement could also be provided if the behavior does not occur within a specified interval.
- Sometimes called, 'reinforcement of zero rates of responding' because it is reinforcement for the absense of the behavior
- e.g. Each recess that the child does not engage in kicking her peers, she will recieve reinforcement.

Differential Reinforcement of Low Rates of Responding

- Reinforcement is provided when the learner engages in a behavior less frequently than they have in the past. The goal is to reduce the number of times a behavior occurs, not to eliminate the behavior
- e.g. A student who frequently requests the teacher check his work while he is working on it. The teacher will provide reinforcement if he only asks work to be checked over twice before submitting it.

Fig. 3.4 The types of differential reinforcement procedures

(Q7) A goal of many behavior plans is to reduce extrinsic reinforcers such as edibles and tangible items. Create a plan to completely eliminate the use of extrinsic reinforcers, while ensuring that intrinsic motivation and social reinforcement would be effective as reinforcement.

Reflection

(Q8) What ethical safeguards do you also need to implement when using punishment strategies (Reference Ethics Box 3.2, Behavior Analyst Certification Board, 2014)?

Ethics Box 3.2

Professional and Ethical Compliance Code for Behavior Analysts

- 4.08 Considerations Regarding Punishment Procedures.
  (a) Behavior analysts recommend reinforcement rather than punishment whenever possible.
  (b) If punishment procedures are necessary, behavior analysts always include reinforcement procedures for alternative behavior in the behavior-change program.
  (c) Before implementing punishment-based procedures, behavior analysts ensure that appropriate steps have been taken to implement reinforcement-based procedures unless the severity or dangerousness of the behavior necessitates immediate use of aversive procedures.
  (d) Behavior analysts ensure that aversive procedures are accompanied by an increased level of training, supervision, and oversight. Behavior analysts must evaluate the effectiveness of aversive procedures in a timely manner and modify the behavior-change program if it is ineffective. Behavior analysts always include a plan to discontinue the use of aversive procedures when no longer needed.

(Q9) People often misuse the word consequence for the word punishment. Do you think that people would use punishment strategies as frequently if they used the correct wording? Why do you think that people may rely on punishment strategies versus reinforcement strategies when they are not informed of ABA strategies? See Fig. 3.1 for a reference.

(Q10) Can you think of an instance where punishment strategies could be used incorrectly and lead to the unfortunate harm of a client?

Additional Web Links

Experimental Analysis of Behavior

http://www.ncbi.nlm.nih.gov/pmc/articles/PMC1338181/pdf/jeabehav00169-0039.pdf

Some current dimensions of applied behavior analysis (Baer et al. 1968)

http://www.ncbi.nlm.nih.gov/pmc/articles/PMC1310980/

The Good, The Bad, The Ugly: Punishment
http://www.iloveaba.com/2011/12/good-bad-ugly-punishment.html
Thinning Reinforcement
http://www.ncbi.nlm.nih.gov/pmc/articles/PMC3196205/
The Association for Behavior Analysis International Position Statement on Restraint and Seclusion
http://www.ncbi.nlm.nih.gov/pmc/articles/PMC3089400/

CASE: ii-P4

Zara's Ounce of Prevention
Setting: Community   Age-Group: School Age
LEARNING OBJECTIVE:

- Describing functional communication, choice, and visual strategies

TASK LIST LINKS:

- **Measurement**

  – (A-14) Design and implement choice measures.

- **Fundamental Elements of Behavior Change**

  – (D-01) Use positive and negative reinforcement.

- **Specific Behavior-Change Procedures**

  – (E-09) Arrange high-probability request sequences.
  – (E-10) Use the Premack principle.

- **Behavior-Change Systems**

  – (F-01) Use self-management strategies.
  – (F-07) Use functional communication training.
  – (F-08) Use augmentative communication systems.

KEY TERMS:

- **Choice Board**

  – A choice board structures choices available for a period of time (e.g., before bedtime) or activity (e.g., recess) by providing a visual organizer of preferred and possible options for children or adults who have difficulty with open-ended choice (Rao and Gagie 2006).

- **First/Then Board**

  – A first/then board is a visual depiction of a less preferred activity (first) followed by more preferred activity (then) (ErinoakKids Centre for Treatment and Development 2012). It is built on the Premack principle, which stipulates that a more preferred activity will be a reinforcer for a less preferred activity (Geiger 1996).

- **"I want …" Board**
  - "I want …" boards are types of communication boards to encourage requesting (also called manding), with a communication partner using nonverbal language in an organized and efficient way (Special Education Technology British Columbia 2015).

Zara's Ounce of Prevention

Zara, an eight-year-old girl with a developmental delay, sat down to breakfast at one of the long, busy tables provided by the city's summer day camp that she was attending. In the middle of the table rested a syrup bottle, salt-and-pepper shakers, paper napkins, jugs of water and juice, and bins of cutlery. Every morning for the past four mornings camp had started out exactly in the same manner. Day camp staff—mostly young students in the first summer after their first year of post-secondary studies in various community services programs—placed large platters of breakfast on each table. Each morning, breakfast consisted of whole wheat buttered toast, scrambled eggs, bacon, and a selection of fruit. After breakfast was placed on the table, Zara immediately stood up, howled in anger, and ran out of the room. One of the staff members of the camp would find her in the cloakroom, sitting on the bench in the corner of the room, yelling and crying, using vocalizations they could not quite understand. The camp's inclusion counselor would come into the cloakroom and spend most of the morning trying to help Zara to calm down, coaxing her into joining the rest of the group for the morning's planned activities. The inclusion counselor would talk using a soft and calm voice, pointing out the benefits of swimming, crafts, and even snack time. The inclusion counselor never felt like her interventions did much good, but eventually Zara would respond, and follow the inclusion counselor to the day camp's planned activities and Zara would join in with campers. Today had been no exception to any of these events, breakfast was as usual, Zara responded in her typical manner, she hid where she had the previous four mornings, the inclusion counselor responded in her characteristic fashion, and eventually Zara got up and followed her to the activity the rest of the campers were engaged in.

During the regularly scheduled get-together of staff members after the campers left on the refurbished school bus for homes near and far throughout the city, the director expressed this about Zara, their biggest camp problem: "Every day we go through the same routine. Every time, she comes here and reacts exactly like this. When is she going to stop already?" He was obviously frustrated. As a young staff with few similar experiences to draw on for support, the director and the inclusion counselor decided to call head office of summer camps, hoping that they would have ideas. And they did have some luck with this strategy.

"Check with her parents," suggested one staff member at head office. "Always check with parents—they are the experts. Look at her intake form and see what it says. Many children with communication challenges use some sort of alternate communication methods to get what they want and need: maybe visuals, sign, or some sort of technology. If those strategies don't work, get back to me and I will drive out to your site and help you plan some next steps."

Right away, the camp staff headed to the small, rarely used office beside the first aid building, and pulled out Zara's forms from this week's enrollment. *Zara has a developmental disability*, they read, and nodded. They already knew this. *Please use the visuals in her knapsack for communication. These are the only way she has of expressing her wants and needs to you.* Following an arrow to the back of the form, they continued to read, *I will send them in her backpack each morning. I have added many camp-related graphics. If you need anything else, just send me a note.*

The next morning, the inclusion counselor met Zara as she stepped off the bus and before she entered the dining hall for breakfast. She followed Zara to the dining hall, sure (from her observations) that Zara would like to stay with her routines and stay with the other students at camp. Once Zara was seated, she asked Zara if she could check her knapsack. Zara shrugged her shoulders and shrugged off her knapsack—which she generally kept with her the whole day. *Now maybe we know why*, the inclusion counselor pondered. Reaching in, her fingers touched what felt like small plastic bags and also what felt like a binder. The inclusion counselor pulled out these items and set them on the bench beside Zara. She noticed a **choice board**, and **first/then board**, and what looked like a board for a **visual schedule**. Leafing further through the binder into which all of these visual strategies were organized, she came across an **"I want ..." board** that had a few stripes of what looked like part of the hook-and-loop tape. Unsure what to do, she turned it over and found that Zara's mother had written helpful directions on the back:

- Hook no more than three choices to the board. Be sure to use choices that Zara can have at the time. REAL choices.
- Ask Zara, "What do you want?"
- Zara will choose what she wants and hook it beside "I want ..."
- Praise Zara and give her the item.

This is fantastic, she thought. *I am going to try it for breakfast if I can get it ready before they serve the food.* The inclusion counselor told Zara that she would be right back, went to the kitchen to consult about the breakfast menu, and added visuals for cereal, eggs, and pancakes to the menu. She took it back to Zara and carefully followed the prompts indicated: "Zara, what do you want for breakfast?"

Zara threw up her hands and then cocked her head to one side with her finger on her lips, appearing like she was carefully considering her options. But it was not more than a brief moment until she tore off the "pancakes" picture, and stuck it onto the correct place on the board. The inclusion counselor was excited and praised Zara with, "Good choosing!" As the inclusion counselor was providing praise, the breakfast platters were being placed down, she quickly passed her the pancakes and exclaimed, "Pancakes are yummy!"

Breakfast went smoothly and Zara was happy for the first morning ever at day camp. *Clearly,* thought the inclusion counselor, *an ounce of **prevention** is better than a pound of cure! My grandmother was right!*

The Response: Principles, Processes, Practices, and Reflections

Principles

(Q1) Describe how the first/then board uses the principles of a high-probability request sequence and the Premack principle.

(Q2) Describe how choice boards can change behavior for clients such as Zara?

Processes

(Q3) How was functional communication and augmentative communication used for Zara in the above case? What behavior did it replace (Fig. 3.5)?

(Q4) Using the instructions for the choice board that Zara's mother created, describe why the instructions and number of choices were laid out in this manner. Describe how you, the behavior analyst teaching Zara to use a choice board, would have initially introduced the system. How many choices would you have provided?

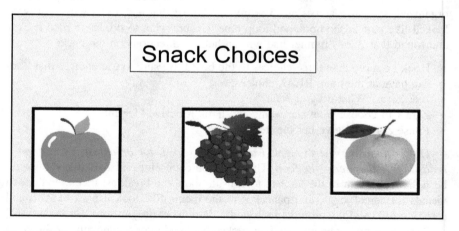

Fig. 3.5 Sample choice board. Pictures would be affixed to the page with hook-and-loop tape, this way the learner can remove the picture indicating their choice

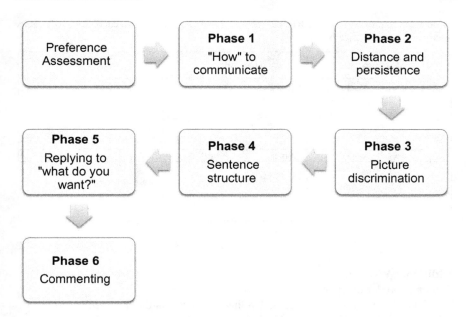

Fig. 3.6 Phases of the Picture Exchange Communication System (Boster and Haghighi, n.d.)

Practice

(Q5) The "I want…" board is a functional communication method, whereby Zara can demand or request what she wants. Describe the steps to implementing a more complex augmentative communication system with Zara. An example of a systematic approach to this is the Picture Exchange Communication System (PECS), as displayed in Fig. 3.6.

(Q6) Based on the information about Zara, what type of visual schedule would you design for Zara? How would you implement it?

Use the following Web site as a resource: http://www.iidc.indiana.edu/pages/Using-Visual-Schedules-A-Guide-for-Parents

(Q7) Using the following worksheet, indicate the way that Zara was communicating without her "I want" board and with it (Table 3.5).

Reflection

(Q8) In what way can functional communication training enhance the quality of life for individuals without speech?

(Q9) In the above case study, Zara's counselors were not using her augmentative communication system or other visual strategies when they began interacting with her. What difficulties do you think individuals might face when using augmentative communication?

(Q10) How do visual strategies act as self-management strategies?

Table 3.5 Chart to document ABC data from the above case study in two conditions, with choice board and without choice board

Antecedent	Behavior		Consequence
With	Choice	Board	Unavailable
With	Choice	Board	Available

Additional Web Links
Choice Board Tip Sheet
http://visuals.autism.net/tipsheet/en/TipSheet-ChoiceBoardandChoiceBoard%
28Iwant%29-final.pdf
First/Then Board
http://connectability.ca/visuals-engine/firstthen-board-popup/
PictureSET (Special Education Technology British Columbia)
https://www.setbc.org/pictureset/
Functional Communication Training Tip Sheet
http://autismpdc.fpg.unc.edu/sites/autismpdc.fpg.unc.edu/files/FCT_Steps_0.pdf
Picture Exchange Communication System
http://www.pecs.com

CASE: ii-P5

Let's just make Zara stop.
Setting: Home   Age-Group: Preschool

LEARNING OBJECTIVE:

- Forming an interdisciplinary team to decrease behaviors

TASK LIST LINKS:

- **Assessment**

  - (I-03) Design and implement individualized behavior assessment procedures.

- (I-04) Design and implement the full range of functional assessment procedures.
- (I-06) Make recommendations regarding behaviors that must be established, maintained, increased, or decreased.

- **Behavior-Change Considerations**

  - (C-03) State and plan for the possible unwanted effects of extinction.

- **Intervention**

  - (J-02) Identify potential interventions based on assessment results and the best available scientific evidence.
  - (J-04) Select intervention strategies based on client preferences.
  - (J-05) Select intervention strategies based on client's current repertoires.
  - (J-06) Select intervention strategies based on supporting environments.
  - (J-07) Select intervention strategies based on environmental and resource constraints.
  - (J-08) Select intervention strategies based on the social validity of the intervention.
  - (J-12) Program for maintenance.

KEY TERMS:

- **Functionally Equivalent**

  - Behaviors that are functionally equivalent are "alternative, desired behaviors that the person should perform instead of the problem behaviors," in essence, making the problem behaviors less desirable, ineffective, inefficient, and irrelevant (O'Neill et al. 1997, p. 71). These are also termed *replacement behaviors* as they have the same function and result in the same reinforcer being delivered (Cipani and Schock 2011).

- **Interviews**

  - Interviews—part of the assessment process—are structured meetings with those exhibiting problem behaviors and/or those supporting them (e.g., parents and therapists), in order to "collect information about events that influence problem behaviors" to identify relevant variables that may lead to effective intervention strategies (O'Neill et al. 1997, p. 9).

- **Maintenance**

  - Maintenance is continuing to independently perform a behavior over time beyond its initial skill training (Miller et al. 2014).

- **Natural Environment Teaching**

  - Natural environment teaching, commonly recognized by its 'NET' acronym, simply references "instruction that can occur throughout the day at opportune moments in naturally occurring contexts" (LeBlanc et al. 2006, p. 50).

- **Observations**

  - Observations are direct, structured, data-based viewings in order to "validate and clarify summary statements about what predicts and maintains problem behavior" (O'Neill et al. 1997, p. 35), an essential step in behavioral assessment.

- **Questionnaires**

  - Questionnaires are one potential part of the assessment processes using structured, written tools. They typically follow interviews and extend and refine information gathered through interviewing (Cooper et al. 2007).

- **Resistance**

  - Resistance refers to opposing, rejecting, or sabotaging future directions, such as recommendations for treatment (Bailey and Burch 2010; Block 2011).

Let's Just Make Zara Stop

It was Zara's second summer at day camp. Zara, the camp counselors, and the inclusion counselor consistently used Zara's visuals to help her communicate her wants, needs, and preferences. For example, after lunch at craft time, Zara used her choice board to choose among that day's offering of crafts, like making a bracelet, tie dying a shirt, or sewing a leather wallet. Things were going fairly smoothly with Zara, compared to the first week of camp last year!

One problem behavior does seem to be rearing its head, though, thought the inclusion counselor. She thought back to Zara's relationships with her peers. *Last year, you wouldn't even have really known that Zara had peers—much less friends. She didn't protest at sitting with her peers, even in noisy settings. For example, she sat at the long benches at the dining hall where the campers were singing loud songs and playing those repetitive cup games. She seemed to enjoy the camp-wide games on the acre of lawn and dirt outside. She didn't mind the laughing, yelling, and splashing that happened at the pool. But now she seems to be aware of her peers, and is starting to get into trouble with them …*

"So, what's really going on?" said the staff member from head office, conveniently, also expected to perform consultation duties at the local camps due to her Board Certified Behavior Analyst (BCBA) designation.

"Zara is doing really well with almost everything, now that she is able to express her wants and needs. We are continuing to use her visual strategies, and we have trained all of our new staff to use them, too. So that's not a problem. In fact, we are all really pleased at our smooth start this year after such a troublesome beginning next summer. But I wanted to chat with you about a problem that seems to be growing right before our eyes. Zara has taken to creating some troublesome interactions with her peers. She is doing things like poking other campers with her fingers, pulling on their shirts, and walking up and putting her face in their face. And it's really annoying the others. They have taken to either ignoring her or telling her to go away, depending on the day. Of course, like you told me last year, I checked her intake sheets and I spoke with her mother, but I couldn't find any information related to these particular behaviors. Zara's mom says that Zara has never had many peer interactions because she spends so much time with adults."

The BCBA responded with a two-part plan for moving forward: "It sounds like what we want to do is teach some new skills. That would be part of a plan. She might not have the social skills she needs to interact effectively with her peers."

"Seriously?" interrupted the inclusion counselor, speaking without quite *thinking* it through, "Teach a new behavior? I called out you here to help me get rid of this problem."

"I get it," responded the BCBA, used to various forms of **resistance**. "But that would only be one part of a plan. And it might not be you teaching these new social skills. But don't forget that summer camp is an inherently social context and is obviously great for **natural environment teaching**. But let me tell you another important piece, before we get into details of teaching new skills. We also need to figure out the function of Zara's behavior. Every behavior has a function—including problem behavior like Zara's. We need to find out that function. To do this, we will need to complete what is called a functional behavior assessment. I am sure you have heard of this."

"Heard of it, yes." The inclusion counselor said, intrigued. "But that is about the extent of my experience."

"You are going to know a lot more pretty soon! For example, it's important to know that is commonly understood that there are four functions, and Zara's is likely one of these, or some kind of combination of a need for attention, tangibles, sensory, or escape/avoidance."

"Oh, it's definitely escape. I am pretty sure that Zara is just trying to get away from the other campers," enthused the inclusion counselor.

"That may be true, but behavior analysis is based in science," answered the BCBA. "So we need to do an assessment for sure, with **observations**, **interviews**, and **questionnaires**. You can definitely help with this, as you know Zara well and see her here at camp every day. But we will ask others at camp to help, too, like her group counselor and the craft counselor who has also supported her regularly. Once we know the function, then we can teach her specific skills: ones that are **functionally equivalent**. In other words, it will provide her with the same thing, but in a socially acceptable manner. These more socially appropriate behaviors will replace her problem behavior, so Zara won't have to do it anymore. The new behavior will get her what she needs more easily and effectively."

"I can't possibly argue with that, I guess," said the inclusion counselor, in return, "but I'm still telling you that I really think it would be best if the poking and other problem behaviors would just stop."

"Agreed! But behavior change is a process, and we want to make changes that are appropriate, and ones that will stick long-term, in the world of behavior analysis, after a new skill is taught, we would have a **maintenance** program to ensure that skill continues to be displayed. So if Zara is doing this poking, pulling, and, well, 'getting in the faces' of her peers, we might teach her how to get attention using one of her visuals, for example. We would also have to teach the other campers about how the visuals work and how to respond to Zara when she uses them. Then, Zara would get attention from her peers and she will have no need to engage in those problem behaviors. But that is just an example how it might play out. What do you think? Just say the word and—quite importantly parent willing—we can get it started in the next few days. But let's put the question of the function aside, now, and talk about the skills-building piece. You mentioned poking other campers with her fingers, pulling on their shirts, putting her face in their faces. These are indeed problem behaviors, but they are giving us an important message that Zara is not getting this quite right. If she is seeking a connection with her peers, she is indeed getting one. But I wonder what would happen if we taught her a more effective way to get their attention: better than pulling on shirts and those other disruptive behaviors you mentioned." The BCBA paused, looking up pointedly.

"I guess I can see your point. If she could get their attention by, like, waving hello, then she wouldn't NEED to poke them. So how on earth do we teach that when everyone is running all over the camp all the time?" The inclusion counselor managed to look both pensive and skeptical.

"I though you might ask me that," responded the inclusion counselor. "How about we use what is in your back pocket?"

Puzzled now, the inclusion counselor patted her own pocket and pulled out her phone. "You mean we should call her mother if this stuff happens?"

"Not quite! I mean that we should record the other campers getting attention the socially appropriate way! They tend to love being in the spotlight, and since they aren't allowed to use technology in the camp experience, they will be even more interested. Of course, you will have to get permission from their parents, but I think we can start teaching this to Zara using video modeling from her peers. What could be better?"

The Response: Principles, Processes, Practices, and Reflections

Principles

(Q1) List the reinforcers that are currently maintaining the behavior and given the definition of extinction, list the feasibility of them being withheld in the current setting.

(Q2) In the following case study, what are two or more reasons that video modeling might be effective to teach new skills?

Processes

(Q3) Describe what the BCBA means by resistance in this case. Then, research one or more strategies that would be effective to overcome resistance when working with staff who are implementing behavioral strategies.

(Q4) Observations, interviews, and questionnaires were used in the following case to get initial data on the behavior and begin to understand patterns. In the figure below, indicate benefits and downfalls to using these different strategies (Table. 3.6).

Table 3.6 Functional Assessment Strategies (O'Neill et al. 1997)

Functional Assessment Strategy	Benefits	Barriers
1. Functional Assessment Interview: A conversation with persons who witness the challenging behavior to determine variables that influence problem behaviors that cannot always be directly observed or manipulated		
2. Direct Observation: Through observing and collecting data, using such forms as the Functional Assessment Observation (FAO) form or ABC data collection, predictors, consequences, and perceived functions can be determined as they occur in the environment.		
3. Functional Assessment Questionnaires: Pre-made questionnaires such as the Functional Analysis Screening Tool (FAST) or Motivation Assessment Tool (MAS) help to determine the function based on how persons in the environment respond to function-based questions about the behavior.		

Practice

(Q5) Based on the following functional assessment interview excerpt, what do you think the function of the behavior is? Why? What further information do you need to collect? (Fig. 3.7).

(Q6) Based on the following information from the direct observation, do you still believe the behavior is the result of the same function as in question 5? (Table 3.7) .

(Q7) List five generalization and five maintenance strategies that would be effective in helping Zara continue to use the socially appropriate behaviors with peers in the future.

Reflection

(Q8) Below are four sample functionally equivalent social behaviors that could be used for Zara. List both possible benefits and any potential downfalls of teaching each behavior. Why do you need to be conscious of the alternative behaviors when teaching social skills?

- Saying "Hi,"
- Shaking peers' hand,

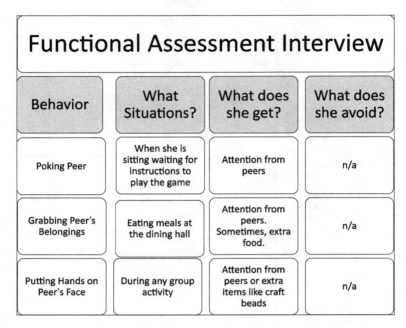

Fig. 3.7 Functional Assessment Interview Excerpt for Zara

Table 3.7 Direct Observation of Zara's behavior data (O'Neill et al. 1997)

Time	Antecedents						Consequence	Perceived Function					
	Transition	Interruption	Demand/Request	Being Alone	Hard Task	Other		Get Attention	Escape/Avoid	Get Tangible	Sensory	Other	Don't Know
9:03 AM			X				- Peer attention - Extra bacon	X		X			
10:15 AM			X		X		- Peer attention	X	X				
10:36 AM					X		- Peer attention	X					
11:17 AM	X		X				- Peer attention						
11:56 AM	X		X				- Peer attention - Extra bun	X		X			

- Bringing a toy up to peers to play, and
- Tapping a peer on the shoulder

(Q9) These alternative behaviors can be taught to Zara by an adult. Why is it appropriate or inappropriate to have an adult teach these skills? What skills could a peer teach and what benefits would this approach have?

(**Q10**) In this situation, what other considerations need to be made for Zara when teaching her social skills? What ways could you determine if her skills are age appropriate? How could you determine what age appropriate skills to teach her?

Additional Web Links
Contingency Pathways Charting
http://www.pent.ca.gov/beh/path/path.html
Functional Behavior Assessment
http://cecp.air.org/fba/
Teaching Functionally Equivalent Behaviors
http://nyspbis.org/RF1415/Research%20Articles/Teaching%20Functionally%20Equivalent%20Replacement%20Behaviors%20to%20Students.pdf
Functional Behavior Assessment Questionnaires, Checklists, Observations, and Interviews
http://www.specialconnections.ku.edu/ ~ kucrl/cgi-bin/drupal/?q=behavior_plans/functional_behavior_assessment/teacher_tools

References

Baer, D. M., Wolf, M. M., & Risley, T. R. (1968). Some current dimensions of applied behavior analysis. *Journal of Applied Behavior Analysis, 1*(1), 91–97. http://doi.org/10.1901/jaba.1968. 1-91

Bailey, J. S., & Burch, M. R. (2010). *25 essential skills & strategies for the professional behavior analyst: expert tips for maximizing consulting effectiveness.* London: Taylor & Francis.

Behavior Analyst Certification Board (2014). *Professional and ethical compliance code for behavior analysts.* Retrieved from http://bacb.com/wp-content/uploads/2016/01/160120-compliance-code-english.pdf

Block, P. (2011). *Flawless consulting* (3rd ed.). New York, NY: Pfeiffer.

Bochner, S., Price, P., & Jones, J. (1997). *Child language development: Learning to talk.* London: Whurr.

Boster, J., & Haghighi, M. (n.d.). *PECS assignment.* Retrieved from: http://pecsassignment. weebly.com/uploads/3/1/8/0/31808553/2792793. png?663

Cipani, E., & Schock, K. M. (2011). *Functional behavioral assessment, diagnosis, and treatment: A complete system for education and mental health settings.* New York, NY: Springer.

Cooper, J. O., Heron, T. E., & Heward, W. L. (2007). *Applied behavior analysis* (2nd ed.). Upper Saddle River, NJ: Pearson.

CornerStone. (2008). *Smart goal setting worksheet: With guidance notes.* Retrieved from: https:// www.ndi.org/files/Handout%203%20-%20SMART%20Goal%20Setting%20Worksheet.pdf

DiGennaro Reed, F. D., & Lovett, B. J. (2008). Views on the efficacy and ethics of punishment: Results from a national survey. *International Journal of Behavioral Consultation and Therapy, 4*(1), 61–67.

Dillenburger, K., Röttgers, H., Dounavi, K., Sparkman, C., Keenan, M., Thyer, B., et al. (2014). Multidisciplinary teamwork in autism: Can one size fit all? *Australian Educational and Developmental Psychologist, 31*(2), 97–112. doi:10.1017/edp.2014.13.

Divisions of Family Practice. (n.d.). *How to develop terms of reference.* Retrieved from: https:// www.divisionsbc.ca/CMSMedia/Divisions/DivisionCatalog-provincial/R%20and%20R% 20Toolkit/recruit-how-to-develop-terms-of-reference.pdf

Dixon, D., Vogel, T., & Tarbox, J. (2012). A brief history of functional analysis and applied behavior analysis. In *Functional assessment for challenging behaviors*. New York: Springer Publishing.

Doher, P. (n.d.). *Three term contingency*. Retrieved from: http://abaappliedbehavioranalysis. weebly.com/three-term-contingency.html

ErinoakKids Centre for Treatment and Development. (2012). *'First-then' board*. Retrieved from https://www.erinoakkids.ca/getattachment/Resources/Growing-Up/Autism/Visual-Supports/ First-Then-Board.pdf.aspx

Geiger, B. (1996). A time to learn, a time to play: Premack's principle applied in the classroom. *American Secondary Education, 25*(2), 2–6.

LeBlanc, L. A., Esch, J., Sidener, T. M., & Firth, A. M. (2006). Behavioral language interventions for children with autism: Comparing applied verbal behavior and naturalistic teaching approaches. *The Analysis of Verbal Behavior, 22*, 49–60.

McLaughlin, D. P., & Carr, E. G. (2005). Quality of rapport as a setting event for problem behavior: Assessment and intervention. *Journal of Positive Behavior Interventions, 7*(2), 68–91.

McMaster Children's Hospital. (2013). *Welcome to DPR: Developmental pediatrics and rehabilitation services*. Retrieved from http://www.hamiltonhealthsciences.ca/documents/ Patient%20Education/DPR-lw.pdf

Miller, I., Crosland, K. K., & Clark, H. (2014). Behavioral skills training with teachers: Booster training for improved maintenance. *Child and Family Behavior Therapy, 36*(1), 19–32. doi:10. 1080/07317107.2014.878176.

Minnesota Northland Association for Behavioral Analysis. (2012). *Standards of practice for applied behavioral analysis in Minnesota*. Retrieved from: http://behavioraldimensions.com/ wpcontent/uploads/2012/11/MNABA-Standards-9-12.pdf

O'Neill, R. E., Horner, R. H., Albin, R. W., Sprague, J. R., Storey, K., & Newton, J. S. (1997). *Functional assessment and program development for problem behavior: A practical handbook*. Belmont, CA: Wadsworth Cengage Learning.

Rao, S. M., & Gagie, B. (2006). Learning through seeing and doing: Visual supports for children with autism. *Teaching Exceptional Children, 38*(6), 26–33.

Ringdahl, J. E., & Falcomata, T. S. (2009). Applied behavior analysis and the treatment of childhood psychopathology and developmental disabilities. In J. L. Matson et al. (Eds.), *Treating childhood psychopathology and developmental disabilities* (pp. 29–54). doi: 10.1007/ 978-0-387-09530-1

Scheuer, B., & Webber, J. (2002). *Autism: Teaching does make a difference*. Boston: Wadsworth.

Special Education Technology British Columbia. (2015). *I have something to say sample*. Retrieved from https://www.setbc.org/pictureSET/Resource.aspx?id=455

Skinner, B. F. (1966). What is the experimental analysis of behavior? *Journal of the Experimental Analysis of Behavior, 9*(3), 213–218.

Skinner, B. F. (1976). *About behaviourism*. New York, NY: Vintage Books.

Sundberg, C. T., & Sundberg, M. L. (1990). Comparing topography-based verbal behavior with stimulus selection-based verbal behavior. *The Analysis of Verbal Behavior, 8*, 31–41.

Zangari, C. (2013). *Teaching core vocabulary*. Retrieved from: http://praacticalaac.org/strategy/ teaching-core-vocabulary/

Chapter 4
Planning-Focused Case Studies from Adolescence to Adulthood

Abstract Building on chapters one through three, the current chapter (chapter four) focuses on utilizing behavior assessment findings to create intervention programs to support adolescents and adults. Emphasis continues to be placed on working within multidisciplinary teams; however, in these stages of the life span, transition planning—from school to employment to independent living—becomes an increasingly critical area of focus. These transitions can be particularly complex for individuals with ASD and other developmental disabilities. The case scenarios presented in this chapter explore complex and sensitive dynamics often experienced during the adolescent, adult, and senior years. Considerations such as independent work and living, social skills, relationships with colleagues at work, with friends and neighbors, and with intimate partners are explored. The cases presented in this chapter challenge learners to consider the interplay of biological, psychological, and social factors that contribute to the onset and maintenance of behavior difficulties. These cases will further highlight the importance of positive and strength-based interventions along with the complex ethical considerations associated with developing the least intrusive, yet evidence-based, behavior support programs. In Chapter 4, entitled "Planning-Focused Case Studies for Adolescents and Adulthood," these complex considerations are explored through five case scenarios involving adolescents, adults, and seniors in home, school, work, and community settings.

Keywords Planning · Intervention programs · Adults · Adolescents · Life span · Transition planning · School · Employment · Independent living · Autism · Biological factors · Psychological factors · Social factors

CASE: ii-P6

Why Does Jana Struggle in Some Places, and Not Others?
Setting: Home   Age Group: Preschool

LEARNING OBJECTIVE:

- Determine the behaviors for change by operationalizing them and collecting data

© Springer International Publishing AG 2016   119
K. Maich et al., *Applied Behavior Analysis*,
DOI 10.1007/978-3-319-44794-0_4

TASK LIST LINKS:

- **Measurement**

  - (A-13) Design and implement discontinuous measurement procedures (e.g., partial and whole interval, momentary time sampling).

- **Behavior-Change Considerations**

  - (C-02) State and plan for the possible unwanted effects of punishment.

- **Identification of the Problem**

  - (G-04) Explain behavioral concepts using nontechnical language.
  - (G-05) Describe and explain behavior, including private events, in behavior-analytic (nonmentalistic) terms.
  - (G-06) Provide behavior-analytic services in collaboration with others who support and/or provide services to one's clients.
  - (G-07) Practice within one's limits of professional competence in applied behavior analysis, obtain consultation, supervision, and training, or make referrals as necessary.

- **Measurement**

  - (H-01) Select a measurement system to obtain representative data given the dimensions of the behavior and the logistics of observing and recording.
  - (H-02) Select a schedule of observation and recording periods.
  - (H-03) Select a data display that effectively communicates relevant quantitative relations.
  - (H-05) Evaluate temporal relations between observed variables (within and between sessions, time series).

- **Assessment**

  - (I-01) Define behavior in observable and measurable terms.
  - (I-02) Define environmental variables in observable and measurable terms.
  - (I-03) Design and implement individualized behavioral assessment procedures.

KEY TERMS:

- **Environment**

  - The construct of environment is essential to ABA, where "emphasis is placed on the functional relationship between human behavior and the environment" (Hernadez and Ikkanda 2011, p. 283). The environment is a setting or place that "lie[s] beyond the individual" (Neal and Neal 2013), each with distinct features (e.g., school, home, and community), often where social interactions happen.

- **Gender Identity**

  - Gender identity can be defined as "one's innermost concept of self as male, female, a blend of both or neither—how individuals perceive themselves and what they call themselves. One's gender identity can be the same or different from their sex assigned at birth" (Human Rights Campaign 2016)

- **Operationalize**

  - To operationalize a behavior is to provide a carefully developed definition that is not only observable, but also measurable: "a clear, precise description of the events or items being measured" (Mayer et al. 2014, p. 134).

- **Paraprofessional**

  - In the ABA field, a paraprofessional can be described as a trained employee of a school or agency typically responsible for the provision of direct service, such as "the day-to-day implementation of one-on-one treatment" (Serna et al. 2015, p. 2) and who "carries out intervention methods under the direct supervision of a BCBA" (p. 3).

- **Unstructured Time**

  - Unstructured times in the school environment are typically thought of as periods of time in the school day where minimal or no external structure is provided (e.g., lunch period) by school personnel (e.g., teachers); instead, students focus on socialization (Koegel et al. 2014).

Why Does Jana Struggle in Some Places, And Not Others?

Fifteen-year-old Jana is a complex high school student attending a large, urban high school, spread over three floors containing hundreds of classrooms. She is an adolescent girl—complicated all on its own—in an academic program for high-achieving students, with a diagnosis of Autism Spectrum Disorder. During the second term of class this year, her average hovers around 93 %, which is typical for her. Jana excels in Math- and Science-based courses (of which she takes plenty) but struggles in courses that are heavily based on language and literature—and social understanding. Without these latter courses, her average would be closer to 97 %. She is already planning to apply for post-secondary programs that will fit with her areas of strength. But in the high school setting, she still sometimes struggles when high school life moves beyond the academics and into its social components.

Over a brief moment of break time in the high school's large staff room, the guidance counselor, various subject teachers, and/or some of the school's **paraprofessionals** (both on Jana's IEP team) often chat. Today, their conversation was about next steps for Jana. "I just do not quite get what is going on with Jana these days," said one of the paraprofessional. "Although I am only 'officially' with her to check in a few times a day to see if she has any outstanding needs, I often bump into her when I am called to deal with issues concerning other students. I am focusing on the issue I have been called in to deal with but there are times when I hear quite a bit of yelling and even growling—and see some shoving—coming from Jana but I can't hear enough of the conversations, nor pay enough attention to figure out exactly what is going on between her and the other students."

"And I just never see this, ever," replied her Calculus teacher. "She is fine in class. She works hard, she gets everything done (usually early). She listens to lectures. She will even show her calculations up front to share with the class. Granted, she is fairly quiet and doesn't interact much with others. But I would be completely shocked if I heard her ever *growl* in my class. This doesn't make sense to me. I just don't see it. Is this kind of behavior happening in her other classes?"

The paraprofessional consulted her notes: "Not that I can see, no. It is like there is a different world going on behind the scenes in the washrooms, in the hallways, by the lockers, and probably in the cafeteria, too. Maybe even outdoors. I think we'd have quite the story about what really happens in high school if we paid more attention to these **environments**. It is kind of scary how different it is. And I don't mean just for Jana. I think it's time for a meeting so we can stop this in its tracks. Let me chat with the guidance counselor and see what she can pull together. Okay?"

Luckily, Jana's father—her primary, custodial caregiver—was available quite quickly, and the IEP team came together. For the first time, the school's behavior counselor also attended the meeting regarding Jana. They began by addressing Jana's father. First, the guidance counselor spoke, "As we have talked about on the phone, Jana has run into some difficulties this year. It seems like these problems are not related to her academics or anything that happens inside the classroom, in that sense. From our informal notes that we have gathered so far, and in consultation with one another, it seems that she is struggling in what we would call "**unstructured**" time. So, socially-based times like hanging out by the lockers, chatting in the hallways and washrooms, and eating lunch together in the cafeteria. She is often seen slamming lockers, punching her fist into the wall, and yelling. Her subject teachers express great surprise that she is having difficulty anywhere (like what happened earlier today, where she threw a peer's gym shoes out the window), because they see none of it in class time, even in her less-preferred classes like Advanced Placement English."

Jana's father, looking comfortable, but concerned, answered, "Yes, I am not surprised. Keep going: tell me more."

The behavior counselor took a turn, "While I have just joined Jana's team—it's nice to meet you and I have some paperwork for you to complete—it sounds like we should do a few things next. One, we should **operationalize** Jana's challenging behavior so we all know exactly what the behavior is that is causing difficulties and so we would all describe it in the same manner. Then we need to gather some formal data. I suggest a scatterplot that will show us exactly when these incidents are occurring. I also suggest that we talk to Jana about all of this, including the data collection. She might have some insight into what is going on behind the scenes where we cannot see what is happening ourselves. I was hoping that she would attend today, actually, but I hear she is not feeling well. Before I let the next person speak, I want to emphasize that every person is complex, and depending on diagnoses, skills, strengths, and needs—as well as the environment—behaviors can be quite different. And environment doesn't need to mean home versus school versus community settings; it can also mean the classroom versus the hallway versus the cafeteria. There might be variables happening in those latter places that we may not know, see, or understand—yet."

Jana's father nodded throughout, "And you are right on that last one for sure. I can actually provide some insight into that. Jana wasn't willing to share this information before, but since the "cat is out of the bag" so to speak with her peers, she asked me to tell you too. That is actually the reason she didn't come to the meeting. She has been struggling with her gender identity lately, and some of the boys in her grade have "caught her"—this is what Jana says—in the boys' washrooms where she says she is more comfortable. So you can imagine the gossip that is happening. I am afraid she is taking a lot of teasing and mocking from pretty much everyone. It would be my prediction that this isn't happening when teachers are around. So, how are we going to find out what's happening when teachers aren't there, and how are we going to stop it, before it stops her from being such a successful student?"

The Response: Principles, Processes, Practices, and Reflections

Principles

(Q1) List three advantages and three disadvantages to using a scatterplot in this situation with Jana to determine when the behaviors are occurring.

(Q2) Referencing the Web site below, indicate the types of measurement systems that could be used with Jana with the scatterplot (i.e., frequency and duration). What measurement system would be most advantageous in this situation to give the team the information that they need.
http://www.specialconnections.ku.edu/?q=behavior_plans/functional_behavior_assessment/teacher_tools/scatter_plot

Processes

(Q3) Social interactions and unstructured time is difficult for many individuals with ASD. Indicate if there is a different data collection method that you could utilize with Jana other than the scatterplot that would provide you with additional or different information, especially given the information Jana's father shared regarding her gender identity.

(Q4) In this situation you are trying to measure unstructured periods of time, would you use an observational method of data collection having someone else collect data, or would you use a self-management strategy? Why or why not?

Practice

(Q5) Create an operational definition of Jana's behavior that you will measure. You may need to create more than one.

(Q6) Looking at the scatterplot below, what does the data indicate is occurring? What other information would have been helpful if a different data collection method was used (Table 4.1)?

Table 4.1 Example scatterplot of Jana's challenging behavior at school

Time Interval	Class/Activity	Date: Oct 1	Oct 2	Oct 3	Oct 4
8:15–8:29 AM	Arrival	▓	▓	▓	
8:30–8:44 AM	Chemistry				
8:45–8:59 AM	Chemistry				
9:00–9:14 AM	Chemistry				
9:15–9:29 AM	Chemistry				
9:30–9:44 AM	Chemistry				
9:45–9:59 AM	1st Break	▓	▓	▓	▓
10:00–10:14 AM	Calculus				
10:15–10:29 AM	Calculus				
10:30–10:44 AM	Calculus				
10:45–10:59 AM	Calculus				
11:00–11:14 AM	Calculus				
11:15–11:29 AM	2nd Break	▓		▓	▓
11:30–11:44 AM	Lunch	▓	▓	▓	
11:45–11:59 AM	Lunch	▓	▓	▓	
12:00–12:14 PM	Lunch	▓	▓	▓	
12:15–12:29 PM	Lunch		▓	▓	▓
12:30–12:44 PM	Lunch				▓
12:45–12:59 PM	3rd Break	▓	▓	▓	▓
1:00–1:14 PM	Biology				
1:15–1:29 PM	Biology				
1:30–1:44 PM	Biology				
1:45–1:59 PM	Biology				
2:00–2:14 PM	Biology				
2:15–2:29 PM	4th Break	▓	▓	▓	▓
2:30–2:44 PM	Literature				
2:45–2:59 PM	Literature				
3:00–3:14 PM	Literature		▓		
3:15–3:29 PM	Literature				
3:30–3:44 PM	Literature				
3:45–3:59 PM	Wait for bus	▓	▓	▓	▓

Legend:

▓ Occurrence of Behavior

(Q7) Develop a data collection method using a self-management strategy that you could create with Jana to help understand what is occurring in her environments to help plan for the intervention. Use the steps in the Web site below to help guide your practice.
http://www.iidc.indiana.edu/pages/Dont-Forget-About-Self-Management

Reflection

(Q8) Why is it important to design a program for unstructured periods for individuals with ASD? How does this help with quality of life or social validity?
(Q9) How does Jana's current struggle with gender identity influence the intervention planning process? What other supports or strategies may be warranted?
(Q10) Guideline G-07 on the *Tasklist* (BCBA, 2012) indicates that behavior analysts are to practice within their own limits of professional competence. In this situation, do you think that a behavior analyst in a school setting has the necessary professional development to deal with someone who is facing gender identity issues? Do other fields besides behavior analysis need to be involved, if so which ones and how (Reference Ethics Box 4.1, Behavior Analyst Certification Board, 2014)?

Ethics Box 4.1

Professional and Ethical Compliance Code for Behavior Analysts

- 1.02 Boundaries of Competence.
  (a) All behavior analysts provide services, teach, and conduct research only within the boundaries of their competence, defined as being commensurate with their education, training, and supervised experience.
  (b) Behavior analysts provide services, teach, or conduct research in new areas (e.g., populations, techniques, behaviors) only after first undertaking appropriate study, training, supervision, and/or consultation from persons who are competent in those areas.
- 1.05 Professional and Scientific Relationships
  (c) Where differences of age, gender, race, culture, ethnicity, national origin, religion, sexual orientation, disability, language, or socioeconomic status significantly affect behavior analysts' work concerning particular individuals or groups, behavior analysts obtain the training, experience, consultation, and/or supervision necessary to ensure the competence of their services or they make appropriate referrals.

Additional Web Links
Self-Management
http://www.asatonline.org/for-parents/learn-more-about-specific-treatments/
applied-behavior-analysis-aba/aba-techniques/self-management/

Defining Behavior
http://iris.peabody.vanderbilt.edu/wp-content/uploads/2013/05/ICS-015.pdf
Scatterplot Data Collection
http://www.autismoutreach.ca/elearning/applied-behaviour-analysis-aba/
scatterplot-data-collection
Data Sheets
http://www.behaviorbabe.com/datasheets.htm
Interventions for Unstructured time for Individuals with ASD
http://www.hdc.lsuhsc.edu/lasard/presentations/workgroups/2012%201213%
20Success%20at.%20Recess%20and%20Other%20Unstructured%20Times.pdf

CASE: ii-P7

Changing Ilyas's Outcomes by Changing his Environment
Setting: Home   Age Group: Adulthood

LEARNING OBJECTIVE:

- Determining strengths and skill building necessary for an adult transitioning into a supported living environment

TASK LIST LINKS:

- **Behavior-Change Considerations**

  - (C-01) State and plan for the possible unwanted effects of reinforcement.

- **Behavior-Change Systems**

  - (F-06) Use incidental teaching.

- **Identification of the Problem**

  - (G-01) Review records and available data at the outset of the case.
  - (G-03) Conduct a preliminary assessment of the client in order to identify the referral problem.
  - (G-06) Provide behavior-analytic services in collaboration with others who support and/or provide services to one's clients.
  - (G-08) Identify and make environmental changes that reduce the need for behavior analysis services.

- **Measurement**

  - (H-01) Select a measurement system to obtain representative data given the dimensions of the behavior and the logistics of observing and recording.
  - (H-02) Select a schedule of observation and recording periods.
  - (H-03) Select a data display that effectively communicates relevant quantitative relations.

- **Intervention**

  - (J-14) Arrange instructional procedures to promote generative learning (i.e., derived relations).

KEY TERMS:

- **Deficits**

  - In the field of developmental disabilities and education, a person's deficits in skills are often the focus of assessment and intervention, focusing on their weaknesses in order to qualify them for additional supports or special education services in the school system (Cosden et al. 2006).

- **Group Homes**

  - Residences for groups of individuals with similar difficulties that arose after the deinstitutionalization movement, whereby individuals had homes in the community with a group of other individuals which are staffed to provide the support and care that is individualized to each individual (Felce et al. 2008).

- **Independent Living**

  - Independent living focuses on the self-determination of individuals with disabilities and the belief that they have the right to live as independently as possible. Independent living skills are the skills that individuals need to live a more independent life, including anything from meal preparation, to making choices, to living in a supportive living arrangement (Ritchie and Blanck 2003).

Changing Ilyas's Outcomes by Changing His Environment

The parents of 30-year-old Ilyas were feeling tired. Having waited until later in life to have a family in the first place, and then after three lusty boys making their way into the world barely two years apart each, Ilyas was born on his mom's 42nd birthday. Of course he was a welcome delight, but now things are complicated as they continue to care day-to-day for him, a now full-grown son with a developmental disability, while they themselves started to feel the effects of aging as they entered their seventh decade of life. "There is also that little part of me," intoned Ilyas's mother, quietly, "that says that it should be my time at some point. All of our friends are long retired, taking cruises, vacations, and doing house exchanges all over the world. I feel like we have earned that turn, too." As grandparents to six grandchildren of various ages who were growing up very quickly and still-involved parents to their three other, older children, they longed to visit more regularly, without upsetting Ilyas's schedule.

"Perhaps," mused Ilyas's father, "it is really time to explore ours—and Ilyas's—options for more **independent living**. At least, more independent from us. And we need to update our wills, too. We must make sure that Ilyas's future is always protected, even if we are not here or he is not with us, just as we have always done. Maybe it's time to involve 'the professionals' once again."

Frustrated by what always seemed to be a focus on diagnoses and **deficits** from the time that Ilyas was young and involved clinicians confirming his developmental disability, his parents had gradually moved away from what they called "the professionals," and typically taught and supported Ilyas on their own. After he left school at the age of 20, this became even more true. His parents developed a small business from the basement of their home, delivering healthy food from the local farmers' markets to senior citizens with low mobility. After 10 straight years in this routine, Ilyas did almost everything except the complex accounting and taxes, and drive the van. "We need to ensure that wherever Ilyas is in the future, he is able to maintain his working life, and the self-esteem we know he derives from contributing to our community," added his mother. Ilyas parents were quite ready for a second retirement from this second career which was developed around Ilyas's skills and needs.

In the following weeks, they visited at least a dozen **group homes** in their sprawling city, from smaller, downtown locales near all sorts of services and entertainment venues, to larger homes with more live-in clients in serene, suburban settings. In addition to viewing each venue, they kept detailed notes on each one, much like they did when their purchased their own home, decades ago. They also met with the staff and talked about the unique context of each group home. Some were run with state-funded money, and many others were run with private funds, supplemented by rental and care fees paid by the clients, the parents of clients, or trust funds carefully set up by parents or guardians *thinking* about—and planning for—future needs.

Narrowing down their choices after lengthy and difficult family conversations during this major time of transition for Ilyas and his family, they set appointments with the directors of three of the potential group homes that they had earmarked as best possibilities for his present and future needs. Following these meetings, they gathered their notes again and considered their choices with a friend who had known the family for nearly all of Ilyas's life and always showed a special interest in Ilyas. Ilyas parents discussed the group homes a little less optimistically than before. "It seems," started Ilyas's father, "that everyone we have spoken to focuses on his developmental disability. Not only that, they seemed to speak barely of anything else but the potential difficulties he might have in their homes: in the environments. It really wasn't all that positive. I don't understand why they don't want to first get to know Ilyas before they make judgments and recommendations. It's not like every person with a developmental disability is alike. And it's not like every person with a developmental disability has only needs and no strengths and no possibilities and no potential for learning."

Ilyas's mother responded, "True, both you and I realize that Ilyas does need a number of independent living skills which are hard for us to teach and encourage when he is living at home and dependent on us. But he does have many skills that are very positive, including excellent **social skills**. They don't seem to be taking this into account—they don't ask. They haven't met him. They haven't observed him going about his day. So how do they really know?"

The family friend had been following the conversation, but hadn't really contributed anything more than some nods and brief interjections. "I wonder," she suggested, "if the problem is not that you have turned to some professionals to help you through this transition. But perhaps you have turned to the wrong set of professionals. Have you thought about seeking out a professional in applied behavior analysis? Those with ABA expertise will focus on arranging the environment for success and teaching new skills for success in that environment." Ilyas's parents, cautiously optimistic, prepared to reach out to a behavior analyst.

The Response: Principles, Processes, Practices, and Reflections

Principles

(Q1) One definition of social validity includes: "A feature of measured results that includes (1) the social significance or importance of the goals, (2) the social appropriateness of the procedures, and (3) the social importance of the effects" (scienceofbehavior.com, n.d.). Keeping this in mind, how does social validity play a role or how is it defined in Ilyas's case?

(Q2) What is the difference between looking at a strength-based approach versus a skill-deficit approach? How does this work with the principles of applied behavior analysis? Use the chart below to help guide your answer (Table 4.2).

Table 4.2 Strength-based approach versus skill-deficit approach (Luong 2013)

Strength-based concepts	Deficit-based concepts
At-potential	At-risk
Gifts	Weaknesses
Participate	Exclude
Determined	Stubborn
Understand	Diagnose
Opportunity	Ineligible
Applaud (i.e., successes)	Punish (i.e., noncompliance)
Time-in	Time-out
Empower	Control
Process-focused	Behavior-focused
Flexible	Rigid
Unique	Abnormal
Person first	Professional first
Finds, builds, and utilizes strengths	Ignores or minimizes strengths
Client-centered	Mandate-focused

Processes

(Q3) What would be one of the first things that you would do when meeting Ilyas and his family to understand his current skills and goals for future skill building?
(Q4) How would the below checklist assist in determining a plan for Ilyas in his choosing a supported living environment for him? Determine how you would use the checklist with Ilyas (Council Bluffs, n.d.)?
https://docs.google.com/file/d/0BxGP4iWt8SZ_SlFtcENZS3VuVUk/edit

Practice

(Q5) Based on the skills checklist on page 15 of the *Transition Health Care Checklist* at the link below, what would be some preliminary, achievable goals that you could present to the team?
http://www.waisman.wisc.edu/wrc/pdf/pubs/THCL.pdf
(Q6) What observation schedule and type of data collection would you use in Ilyas's case when planning for his goals?
(Q7) Create a data collection sheet to measure Ilyas's current level of independence in the home and in his business. Create a sheet that would assist you in explaining Ilyas's current skills and skills that would lead to future success.

Reflection

(Q8) What could group home personnel change in order to indicate to the family that they were interested in Ilyas as an individual person and understood his strengths? How did language play a role?
(Q9) What are some benefits of a strength-based approach and what are some difficulties with it?
(Q10) Create 10 questions that you would ask Ilyas to determine skills that he would like to develop based on a strength-based approach (Table 4.3).

Table 4.3 Case examples using strength-based approach (ResearchGate, 2006)

Potential areas of strength	Example of strength	How to use the strength in an intervention
Interests—Does the learner have any special interests or favorite characters?	Gloria knows a lot about cellphones. She can talk about many the different makes and models, the differences between the various operating systems, and will spend hours looking at pictures of cellphones	Gloria is struggling to learn to identify numbers when they are presented in an array on the table. Her clinical supervisor suggests the team try presenting numbers on cellphones and having her identify which cellphone is displaying the target number
Routine and Rules—Consider how the learner acts when it comes to rules or routines	Arden learns routines quite quickly, once he is walked through something once or twice he gets the routine down and is able to complete it independently	Arden's teachers were struggling to get Arden to independently pack his backpack and the end of the day. When they asked his mom how she is able to get him doing so many tasks independently she explained that it helps to do it the same way a few times with Arden, then he will know what the routine is

Additional Web Links
Strength-Based Perspective with Families and People with Disabilities
http://familiesinsocietyjournal.org/doi/abs/10.1606/1044-3894.636
Effective Communication with Adults with Developmental Disabilities
http://vkc.mc.vanderbilt.edu/etoolkit/general-issues/communicating-effectively/
Independent Living
http://www.cilt.ca/documents%20of%20the%20cilt%20website/ind_living_
medical_model.pdf

CASE: ii-P8

Shape up, Cris, or ship out!
Setting: School   Age Group: Adulthood

LEARNING OBJECTIVE:

- Determine a team-based approach to creating an intervention plan

TASK LIST LINKS:

- **Fundamental Elements of Behavior Change**

  - (D-15) Identify punishers.
  - (D-19) Use combinations of reinforcement with punishment and extinction.

- **Behavior-Change Systems**

  - (F-01) Use self-management strategies.

- **Identification of the Problem**

  - (G-01) Review records and available data at the outset of the case.
  - (G-03) Conduct a preliminary assessment of the client in order to identify the referral problem.
  - (G-06) Provide behavior-analytic services in collaboration with others who support and/or provide services to one's clients.
  - (G-08) Identify and make environmental changes that reduce the need for behavior analysis services.

- **Measurement**

  - (H-01) Select a measurement system to obtain representative data given the dimensions of the behavior and the logistics of observing and recording.

KEY TERMS:

- **Bio-psycho-social Model**

    – A bio-psycho-social model is an integrated, interdisciplinary approach to support, intervention, and treatment utilized for complex conditions with influences in multiple domains (e.g., medical, psychological, and social) (Griffiths and Gardner 2002).

- **Dual Diagnosis**

    – A dual diagnosis refers to a combination of a substance use disorder and a psychiatric disorder (World Health Organization 2015). Dual diagnosis can also be used to refer to an individual having both a psychiatric disorder and a development disability (Centre for Addiction and Mental Health 2016).

- **Text-to-Speech**

    – Text-to-speech is an example of an assistive technology software that uses "computer-generated speech as a tool for individuals who learn more effectively and efficiently through a multimodal experience and is becoming more commonly available (e.g., in cell phones, tablet computers, and websites).

- **Word Prediction**

    – Word prediction software programs are assistive technology tools that typically work in conjunction with word processors, providing lists of contextual, semantically correct word possibilities predicted from only one or a few typed letters. This allows its users to recognize potential choices read aloud through text-to-speech technology and make word choices, rather than writing and spelling individual words. Users often struggle with print-based reading and writing.

Shape Up, Cris, Or Ship Out!

Crisanto, known to his friends as Cris, was working toward his education degree at a small college focused only on teacher education programs. Most of his classes were capped at 35 students, and often only 18 or 20 were enrolled in each one. At 20 years of age and into the second term of his third year of courses, he thought he had it all figured out. He met with the department of student services and his disability consultant at the college regularly to ensure he was coping well, and using

—or learning—strategies to cope with his **dual diagnosis** of AD/HD and a Specific Learning Disorder which has a noted impact on his ability to process and create print-based information. One of the strategies he figured out how to use early on (with a significant number of individualized supports) in his first year was technology. He started using the electronic planner on his phone with great discipline and care as soon as it became clear (to him and his professors) that he needed it, and took a number of recommended evening classes to learn visual organizational tools, **word prediction** programs, and **text-to-speech** technology. His essays became well formulated, once he could focus on his ideas and not worry about his struggles with transferring his ideas from his brain to a pen, pencil, or the looming blank screen of his laptop. By his second year of classes, most of his grades were in the A and B ranges, with a few of what he called "hiccups" in his language-based classes, like the mandatory French he was taking for his second language requirement. After years of struggle both before high school and in high school, he was pretty impressed with himself.

In this third year, Cris was confident enough to transfer to a larger college, and also registered for some practicum courses in addition to his first term course load. He silently cheered himself with *"I got this!"* as he waded his way through the online registration system. He made sure he had an academic advisor, which was mandatory for all students in the education program, but he didn't bother to find the student services office to register as an exceptional student. Confidently again, he strode into his first class of the fall after a few test runs with a campus map, but stopped short when he realized he was in a large, multilevel lecture hall rather than the small seminar rooms to which he had become accustomed. He settled himself at the far back of the room, laptop open, textbook ready, but found it quite difficult to attend in this very busy, quite noisy—and crowded—learning environment.

Five weeks into his term, with assignments mounting up and due dates fast approaching, other projects overdue, and midterm exams looming, Crisanto flicked through his electronic scheduler, growing more despondent with each look at busy days with multiple expectations. He logged onto his college email, almost too afraid to open it, but more afraid not to after a registered letter showed up at his apartment with a return address from the "Office of Academic Advisement" emblazoned in its top left corner. Scanning his email list for problems, he could see a number of emails from the same source. It had been quite some time since he had checked his email, for important messages, notifications of his grades, or for complaints from his practicum supervisor noting his many unexplained absences at the school. Sighing, he thought, *"I might as well just read the one that came by mail ... it is likely the worst ..."*

He quickly scanned to the main body of the letter, which read:

We are concerned about your grades and your absences this term so far. In a professional program, we are all held to a particularly high standard. Our concerns are listed as followed:

- Poor attendance in a professional program, both in classes and at practicum site.

- Many failing and/or borderline grades in a professional program (minimum acceptable grade is 75 %).
- Poor assignment quality, not reflecting new learning in a professional program (e.g., pedagogical strategies).
- Lack of engagement in the school life of practicum placement (e.g., extracurricular activities).

Please call our office and arrange for a meeting in the next two days. If you do not comply with this emergency meeting, you are at least temporarily un-enrolled from your education degree program. Please note: you are still responsible for this term's fees.

"*Well, at least that's not so bad,*" he considered, quickly picking up his phone to make that so-called very urgent call from his favorite seat at the college's busiest bar, where everyone knew him by name.

Two days later, he sat at the Office of Academic Advisement, awaiting his appointment, rising regularly from his seat to check out the view, the pamphlets, the magazines, and to chat with the administrative personnel. While he was engaged in these activities, his academic advisor was reviewing his file. Shaking his head, he muttered to himself on the way to greet Cris, "I kind of agree with his practicum supervisor. We need to give this guy a few tough consequences, and either he is going to shape up—or ship out. We can't have slackers like him in the education field." However, after his initial consultation with Cris—who provided documentation of his exceptionality to the college for the first time—the advisor could see that the situation was a little more complex than simply a student who was spending too much time at the bars and not enough time at the books. With Cris's consent, he arranged a meeting with a disability consultant, Cris, his practicum supervisor, and of course, a representative from the Office of Academic Advisement. The disability consultant took on the case, responding that, "Clearly, we need to look at this young man from a **bio-psycho-social** perspective. For him, it can't be just about the marks. I think we need to dig a little more deeply into what's going on with Cris."

The Response: Principles, Processes, Practices, and Reflections

Principles

(Q1) Explain what the bio-psycho-social perspective of assessing individuals with disabilities entails.

(Q2) In cases such as Cris, he is entitled to certain accommodations as a result of having an identified disability at college. Looking at the following testing accommodations checklist at the web link below, what are accommodations and how would they have assisted Cris in his term at the college? (INS@NPC, 2015) https://ilsnpc.wordpress.com/category/iep504-plan/

Processes

(Q3) In ABA, the term consequence is used to describe anything that occurred after the behavior happened and is contingent on a behavior (Alberto and Troutman

Table 4.4 Definitions for the four consequences to behavior and corresponding examples

Consequences to behavior	
Positive reinforcement	Positive punishment
Definition: After a behavior stimuli is *added* which causes an *increase* in the future likelihood of that same behavior occurring again **Example**: If Joey hands in his homework on time, his teacher gives him 3 extra marks **Behavior**: handing in homework on time **Consequence:** bonus marks added **Impact**: more likely to hand homework in on time	**Definition**: After a behavior stimuli is *added* which causes a *decrease* in the future likelihood of that same behavior occurring again **Example**: Monique is talking while the teacher is explaining the assigned questions; the teacher assigns extra questions to Monique **Behavior**: talking while teacher is talking **Consequence**: teacher adds more questions on for Monique **Impact**: less likely to talk while teacher is talking
Negative Reinforcement	Negative Punishment
Definition: After a behavior stimuli is *removed* which causes an *increase* in the future likelihood of that same behavior occurring again **Example**: Mr. Mensen's Science class has been quietly working hard at their assigned questions for the entire science period. At the end of class, Mr. Mensen announces to the class that whatever they completed during class time was to be handed in now; the remaining questions would not be homework **Behavior**: Quiet on-task work completing questions **Consequence**: Removal of homework **Impact**: Students will be more likely to work quietly in the future	**Definition**: After a behavior stimuli is *removed* which causes an *decrease* in the future likelihood of that same behavior occurring again **Example**: During lunch break Max shakes his bottle of soda and sprays it toward the cheerleading squad. A teacher walks in as this is occurring, Max has to eat lunch in the guidance counselors office for the remainder of the month **Behavior**: Spraying cheerleaders with soda **Consequence**: Removed from reinforcing environment (cafeteria and peers) **Impact**: Max will be less likely to spray soda in the cafeteria

2009). How was the word consequence used in this case study? What principle was the teacher referring to (Table 4.4)?

(Q4) Look up sample text-to-speech and word prediction software programs that Cris could use at college. What type of prompts are these to help him in school? Label each prompt that would be used in both of these software programs (Table 4.5).

Table 4.5 Types of stimulus and response prompts (Gulick and Kitchen, 2007)

Stimulus Prompts

Prompt	Topography/Method	Common Application	Prerequisites	Limitations
Positional prompt	Placing target object closer to the student	Receptive selection (point/touch/give) tasks	Basic attending skills	Not applicable when drill involves verbal responses
Proximity prompt	Positioning the instructor's body closer to or farther from the student	Receptive pronoun drills ("touch my nose")	Student must be able to verbally imitate	Limited to pronoun or possession drills
Voice inflection prompt	Magnifying or reducing the volume of the instructor's voice for a specific word	Magnification—Receptive selection (point/touch/give) tasks; Reduction—Preventing echolalia	Basic attending skills	None encountered
Gestural (tap/point)	Tapping or pointing to target object	Discrimination tasks; Visual performance tasks	Basic attending skills	Highly imitative students may mimic the tap/point
Gestural (hand placement)	Placing the instructor's outstretched hand nearer to the target object	Receptive selection (giving) tasks	Basic attending skills	None encountered
Gestural (blocking)	Shielding the nontarget object or otherwise blocking access to it	Receptive selection (point/touch/give) tasks	Basic attending skills	None encountered
Gestural (eye gaze or head nod)	Directing instructor's eye gaze or nodding head toward the target object	Receptive selection (point/touch/give) tasks	Well-developed attending skills	Requires student to be aware of subtle body cues
Highlighting	Placing brightly colored paper or other marking on or in close proximity to the target object or location	Receptive selection (point/touch/give) tasks; Receptive placement tasks (prepositions)	Basic attending skills	None encountered

(continued)

Table 4.5 (continued)

Stimulus Prompts

Prompt	Topography/Method	Common Application	Prerequisites	Limitations
Size	Increasing the size of the target object relative to the nontarget object	Receptive selection (point/touch/give) tasks	Basic attending skills	None encountered
Templates	Placing paper templates on the table to indicate specific locations for placement of objects	Sequencing and seriation tasks	Basic attending skills	None encountered
Dotted line prompt	Providing dotted line or lightly drawn figures as guides for the student to complete a written or drawn response	Graphic imitation (drawing/copying/writing) skills	Basic attending skills; Correct grasp of writing implement	None encountered

Response prompts

Prompt	Topography/Method	Common application	Prerequisites	Limitations
Verbal prompt (procedural)	Providing verbal directions to inform the student what they must do to complete the task. Provided either partially (in steps) or whole task	Tasks that have a physical/nonverbal response	Student must have sufficient receptive understanding of the words and concepts used	Can be confusing to prompt verbal responses—especially with echolalic students
Verbal prompt (questioning)	Asking the student specific questions to prompt the completion of a (typically) complex task e.g., "what's missing?" "What did you forget to add?"	Complex verbal and nonverbal tasks	Student must have sufficient receptive understanding of the words and concepts used and in most cases, should have question-answering skills	May evoke distracting verbal responses to the questions that could compete with completion of the physical task
Echoic prompt (whole word/phrase/sentence)	Instructor models the entire verbal response—typically using the sentence form "say (target verbal response)"	Verbal response tasks—tact or intraverbal	Student must be able to imitate the target verbal responses	Student may echo the prompt "say"

(continued)

Table 4.5 (continued)

Echoic prompt (partial word or phoneme)	Instructor models a portion of the target word or the beginning sound (phoneme) of the target word	Single word echoic, tacting or simple intraverbal (fill-in) tasks	Student must be able to imitate the target phoneme or word	None encountered
Physical modeling (whole task)	Instructor models the entire physical response—can be paired with the phrase "do this"	Receptive commands (simple to complex)	Students must be able to imitate motor movements of similar complexity	None encountered
Physical modeling (partial)	Instructor models a portion of the physical response—typically the beginning of the movement cycle	Receptive selection (point/touch/give) tasks	Students must be able to imitate simple motor movements	None encountered
Physical prompt (whole task)	Instructor uses hands-on guidance to walk the student through the entire physical response	Receptive commands (simple to complex) Imitation tasks	None	Generally limited to physical actions Can be used for some rudimentary oral motor actions and phonemic production
Partial prompt (partial)	Instructor provides varying degrees of touch to facilitate the completion of a physical response	Receptive commands (simple to complex) Imitation tasks	None	Same as whole task physical prompt limitation
Peer modeling	Instructor has a peer or sibling physically or verbally model the target response in the presence of the student	Wide variety of verbal and nonverbal tasks	Students must be able to imitate similar verbal or nonverbal movements May be helpful to have the peer model be of similar age and gender as the student	Must establish compliance and interest of the peer Might require separate reinforcement contingency to motivate the peer
Time delay prompt	Instructor provides a short period of time (often paired with reinforcement) between steps of a multistep task	Multistep receptive commands Multistep imitation tasks	Student must be skilled in the completion of component steps of multistep task	None encountered

Practice

(Q5) What type of initial assessment would you complete with Cris to determine his current skills and areas where he could use a skill building program in order to learn additional skills to attend college?

(Q6) Identify a data observation and measurement system that could be used to identify Cris' current skills and areas for growth. What schedule of observation would you use? What dimension of behavior would you measure (Fig. 4.1)?

(Q7) What type of self-management strategies could be implemented with Cris? List three and describe how you would implement them.

Reflection

(Q8) In Cris' situation, what would be some environmental variables that you could change to assist Cris with his success at college (Reference Ethics Box 4.2, Behavior Analyst Certification Board, 2014)?

Ethics Box 4.2

Professional and Ethical Compliance Code for Behavior Analysts

- 4.06 Describing Conditions for Behavior-Change Program Success. Behavior analysts describe to the client the environmental conditions that are necessary for the behavior-change program to be effective

(Q9) In seeing the reaction of the team members in response to Cris' performance in college, what do you think could have been done differently? Do you think this would have been avoided if he was registered as a person with a disability?

(Q10) Knowing Cris was transferring to another college, what types of supports would you have put in place to ensure a seamless transition for Cris?

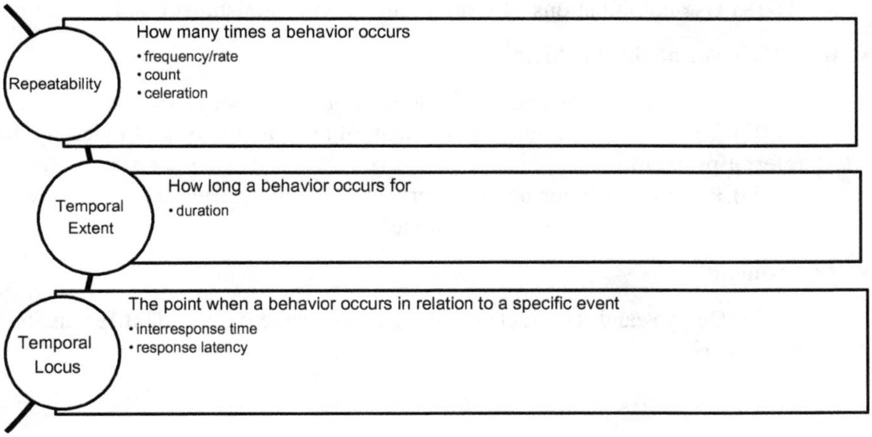

Repeatability
How many times a behavior occurs
- frequency/rate
- count
- celeration

Temporal Extent
How long a behavior occurs for
- duration

Temporal Locus
The point when a behavior occurs in relation to a specific event
- interresponse time
- response latency

Fig. 4.1 Dimensions of behavior and corresponding recording systems

Additional Web Links
Common Misuses of ABA Terms
http://www.wisaba.org/about-behavior-analysis/common-misrepresentations-of-behavior-analysis/misrepresentation-10-terminological-notes-this-area-covers-common-misuses-of-behavior-analytic-vocabulary/
Prompting Learning Module
http://afirm.fpg.unc.edu/prompting
Speech-to-Text Software
http://www.brainline.org/content/2010/12/speech-recognition-for-learning_pageall.html
Word Recognition Software
http://mason.gmu.edu/~aevmenov/Portfolio/Growth/Word_prediction.pdf
Assistive Technology
http://ldatschool.ca/technology/assistive-technology/

CASE: ii-P9 Guest Author: Christina Belcher

Is Garth's Experience Enough?
Guest Author: Dr. Christina Belcher, PhD, OCT
Professor, Redeemer University College
Setting: Community   Age Group: Adult

LEARNING OBJECTIVE:

- Determining behavior principles to apply to a workplace setting utilizing the mediator model

TASK LIST LINKS:

- **Fundamental Elements of Behavior Change**

  - (D-19) Use combinations of reinforcement with punishment and extinction.

- **Identification of the Problem**

  - (G-01) Review records and available data at the outset of the case.
  - (G-03) Conduct a preliminary assessment of the client in order to identify the referral problem.
  - (G-06) Provide behavior-analytic services in collaboration with others who support and/or provide services to one's clients.

- **Assessment**

  - (I-07) Design and conduct preference assessments to identify putative reinforcers.

KEY TERMS:

- **Culture**

  - Culture is a complex, context-bound construct with variable definitions related to both beliefs and its related actions. In the context of behavior, it can be defined as "the extent to which a group of individuals engage in overt and verbal behavior reflecting shared behavioral learning histories, serving to differentiate the group from other groups, and predicting how individuals within the group act in specific setting conditions" (Sugai et al. 2012, p. 200).

- **Progressive Discipline**

  - Progressive discipline is terminology typically found in places of employment and the field of human resources. Progressive discipline "increases the severity of a penalty each time an employee breaks a rule. Typically, a policy progresses from oral warnings to written warnings, suspensions and then termination. That way, employees are not surprised when they reach the end and are fired" (Business Management Daily 2013, p. 6).

- **Rewards**

  - The term reward is often used synonymously with reinforcer (ErinoakKids Autism Services 2012). It is more common outside clinical environments, such as home, school, and work.

Is Garth's Experience Enough?

At 50 years of age, Garth's 30 years of experience at his place of employment had taught him ways to positively enhance–or positively avoid–any workplace conflicts. Garth was an experienced worker and currently held the position supervisor. Garth was well appreciated by his peers for his knowledge and experience in his field, but was also known both in his profession and in his office to be resistant to change. He arrived at his desk with his morning coffee and donut; he had his day neatly ordered into four parts. In the morning, he almost always reviewed his agenda for the day, reviewed his tasks in order of priority, answered his email, and then had a break at 10:30. On Monday, he had weekly meetings beginning with the staff promptly at 11:00 a.m. to address any concerns in the workplace, to commend staff on accomplishments, and to outline new business arising, ending precisely at noon. Lunch consisted of his usual sandwich, fruit, and a paper copy of the local newspaper. In the afternoon, he continued with his files and personal service to customers. In the last half hour of the day, Garth ordered his files for the following day, reviewed any new email, made any required phone calls, slotted in any conference calls, and prepared his task list for the next morning's arrival. Garth functioned like a man on a mission. He took care of business. He was content and satisfied with his performance.

In Garth's supervisory capacity, the ideal employee was one who maintained the agenda and rules of the company. Successful practice leads to success in the future. And that required experience.

Recently, an issue of a member of the staff brought to the table on Monday morning had failed to be resolved during the hour meeting time slot. Garth had implemented company policy by contacting the organization's human resources department to begin the process of addressing the concerns through their **progressive discipline** process regarding an employee who was not meeting the company's expectations in areas of punctuality, which fell into the category of general performance. The human resources professional contacted an internal colleague specializing in workplace behavior: a Board Certified Behavior Analyst (BCBA).

In an initial meeting with the Garth, the BCBA noted that she would like to take some time to consult the literature about what the available evidence suggests might be effective in addressing the difficulties with punctuality. From there, a behavior-change program would be developed. She would monitor progress by collecting data to ensure that behavior-change goals and objectives would be met. She explained that these are all parts of adopting an evidence-informed approach.

Garth immediately had an issue with this idea, and responded by stating: "I have more than 30 years of experience. I do not need to look to some research done elsewhere, or even collect data. I know what to do when things are or are not working. Doesn't my experience count?" This response displayed insight into understanding Garth's behavior across his career span. Although Garth did well maintaining the company processes, he was not innovative in learning new approaches to understanding or mediating the personal habit reformation of those in his care. The BCBA consultant could see that both Garth and the employee in question posed problems for planning this intervention. It appeared obvious to her that both had different views toward business and what was valued in their positions.

The BCBA consultant was concerned with Garth's resistance to change, reliance on experience and habits, and his dismissal of the need for exploring current research on institutional matters. For example, at a recent staff meeting, when staff first raised discomfort with the unreliability of "a staff member" coming to work on time, and suggested some possible interventions, Garth responded by naming such innovation and intervention a waste of time. He believed experience already had shown what worked through what had been maintained and left unchanged. He proceeded to expand his statement by saying that in his experience, it had been suggested that "in the past" those who did not work "did not eat," and that the answer to this young person's noticed behavior of being late for work at the beginning of the day should be, without question, termination. The majority of the staff, however, felt this young man had the potential to be a valued employee, despite his frequent tardiness in arrival to the office or job sites. They liked him. They recognized a sharp mind, personable wit, and a helpful and innovative interpersonal work posture. He often worked later—right into the evening—and that too, was a point of concern for Garth.

Garth liked his timetable to be one that reflected a traditional nine A.M. to five P.M. timeline. He was accustomed to working independently and often could justify his decision making. He was a faithful company employee and was of good value to company history and frequent customers. And his employees liked him as a person. He was just and fair in his dealings: a straight shooter. As a result, the employees—as a group—found themselves in a lock-down as to what to do about Garth's views and their hopes for the employee in question. This issue of resolution was divided. To this end, Garth did not feel that exploring research to change the less-than-desirable habits of employees or to understand the root of this so-called bad habit was necessary.

The BCBA consultant suggested to Garth that in the area of work-related complaints, research showed that different concerns required different views on what made a company successful, and that interpersonal considerations, lifelong learning, and company policy need also be considered. In the current cultural workplace, she explained, a focus on mentoring and guidance for grooming potential success in employees was valued. For growth of the company, it would be helpful to create the conditions in which a younger person could be successful in the workplace in order to continue having the company flourish. Yes, most employees had some flaws in certain areas, but what else could they offer? Positive focus and **rewards** in the workplace were also required. For example, in cases of late arrival to work, there may be other extenuating circumstances in the larger picture of an employee's life that may mitigate that outcome–beyond the first instinct that the employee was lazy, negligent or just indifferent to opportunities. Had the reason for this employee's late arrival ever been addressed? Had his tardiness been addressed individually?

The BCBA consultant suggested that in this case, failure for being to work on time may have been reinforced in other working environments, or individual employment tasks. Like Garth, *experience* in other work situations may have served to reinforce this habit of nonpunctuality as being acceptable, just as punctuality had served to reinforce Garth's own behavior in the workplace. For example, in some venues, punctuality was essential to the job. For example when he was a student, and classes started at 9:00 A.M., a teacher needed to be present by 8:30 at the latest to prepare for the arrival of her charges. Students could not arrive to an absent teacher. However, if someone had a meeting at ten and was already prepared, arriving at 9:45 rather than 9:30 A.M. may not be problematic, depending on the role the individual played.

The BCBA consultant brought to Garth's attention that in a digital age, time and location did not have the cultural implications as they did 30 years ago (nor are parts of the same **culture**). If employees could have the ability to work at home as well as to work face-to-face on tasks, this would raise new ways of "minding the clock" depending on the innovative possibilities of the workplace. If that proved to be the case, some short-term outcomes to address the behavior that has been found wanting by this employee in Garth's current work environment may be helpful to the company as well as illuminating to the employee. It would be helpful to all concerned to consider a "big picture" regarding the employee's late arrival across the broader scope of his life, behavior, and performance as a complex set of events, and not just as an isolated incident unrelated to anything else. His desire to work later may prove to be admirable, and not realistically represent a way "to get out of being on time" or to "make up hours on the clock." Although, if the company had specific reasons for punctuality in this particular employee's work task to be mandatory, (like having a machine ready and safety checked for use in a factory or having shelves stocked with produce before business opened), short-term goals and interventions could be helpful to decrease the problem of tardiness.

In hopes of changing Garth's mindset, the BCBA consultant suggested the process of addressing the concerns through their progressive discipline process (i.e., beginning with letters documenting concerns, frequent meetings, progressing to verbal and written warnings, suspensions, and even dismissal). This initial meeting also shed light on the reality that both Garth and his young employee may see what is valued at work from a different experiential lens, and that lifelong learning for Garth in understanding current research may also be valuable to the future of the company.

The Response: Principles, Processes, Practices, and Reflections

Principles

(Q1) Identify which behavioral principles are involved in progressive discipline. Which principles align with reinforcement and which align with punishment?
(Q2) In this situation, what effects would reinforcement have on behavior as compared to punishment? What would be some of the downfalls of implementing a pure punishment-based procedure as Garth is suggesting (Reference Ethics Box 4.3, Behavior Analyst Certification Board, 2014)?

Ethics Box 4.3

Professional and Ethical Compliance Code for Behavior Analysts

- 4.08 Considerations Regarding Punishment Procedures.
  (a) Behavior analysts recommend reinforcement rather than punishment whenever possible.
  (b) If punishment procedures are necessary, behavior analysts always include reinforcement procedures for alternative behavior in the behavior-change program.
  (c) Before implementing punishment-based procedures, behavior analysts ensure that appropriate steps have been taken to implement reinforcement-based procedures unless the severity of dangerousness of the behavior necessitates immediate use of aversive procedures.
  (d) Behavior analysts ensure that aversive procedures are accompanied by an increased level of training, supervision, and oversight. Behavior analysts must evaluate the effectiveness of aversive procedures in a timely manner and modify the behavior-change program if it is ineffective. Behavior analysts always include a plan to discontinue the use of aversive procedures when no longer needed.

Processes

(Q3) Although the behavior analyst in the case would prefer to use reinforcement-based procedures, she decides to go with the progressive discipline system at the workplace that is already in place. What effect do you think this approach will have in changing Garth's behavior and implementing a different approach to dealing with difficult staff behavior? Use the behavior skills training model as a guide. http://www.bsci21.org/behavior-skills-training-in-4-steps/

(Q4) What changes could you make to each component the progressive discipline approaches to make them more highly based on the principles of reinforcement instead of punishment?

Practice

(Q5) Based on the behavioral skills training approach, list your strategy to teach Garth how to implement the progressive discipline approach with the employee. See Fig. 4.2 (Parsons et al., 2012)

(Q6) What data would you collect before you started the procedure about the current discipline techniques and reinforcement occurring at the workplace? Who would you collect it from?

(Q7) What type of data collection system would you use to track the adherence with the progressive discipline system across the management team?

Reflection

(Q8) Looking at the way that the behavior analyst approached the situation above with Garth, what would you have done differently? Why?

(Q9) When planning with the team on implementing the progressive discipline intervention, what must you consider? What duties and information are you providing to the person who hired you or Garth's boss? What information are you required to keep confidential?

(Q10) In this situation, who is your client? Looking at the Professional and Ethical Compliance Code for Behavior Analysts (2014), are there any potential conflicts of interest (also consider third parties)?

Additional Web Links
Organizational Behavior Management Network
http://www.obmnetwork.com
Discipline without Punishment
http://www.watson-training.com/blog2/46-discipline-with-punishment-a-best-practices-approach-to-disciplining-employees.html
Behavior Skills Training
http://www.bsci21.org/behavior-skills-training-in-4-steps/

CASE: ii-P10

Is Daisy's Behavior a Message in Disguise?
Setting: Home   Age Group: Adulthood

LEARNING OBJECTIVE:

- Determine a team-based approach for understanding the biological causes and communication of behavior.

TASK LIST LINKS:

- **Identification of the Problem**

  - (G-01) Review records and available data at the outset of the case.
  - (G-02) Consider biological/medical variables that may be affecting the client.
  - (G-03) Conduct a preliminary assessment of the client in order to identify the referral problem.
  - (G-06) Provide behavior-analytic services in collaboration with others who support and/or provide services to one's clients.
  - (G-07) Practice within one's limits of professional competence in applied behavior analysis, obtain consultation, supervision, and training, or make referrals as necessary.
  - (G-08) Identify and make environmental changes that reduce the need for behavior analysis services.

- **Measurement**

  - (H-01) Select a measurement system to obtain representative data given the dimensions of the behavior and the logistics of observing and recording.
  - (H-02) Select a schedule of observation and recording periods.
  - (H-03) Select a data display that effectively communicates relevant quantitative relations.
  - (H-04) Evaluate changes in level, trend, and variability (Fig. 4.2).

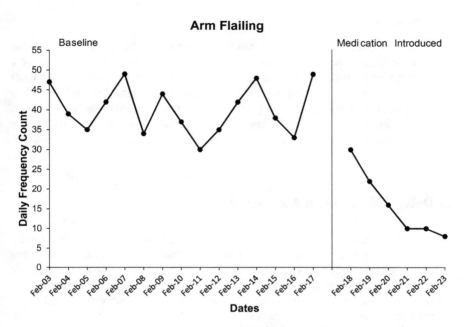

Fig. 4.2 Figure displaying frequency data on Daisy's arm flailing behavior collected by Daisy's nurse before starting medication and after the medication was introduced on the evening of February 17

KEY TERMS:

- **Family Conference**

  - Family conferences typically focus on partnering with the wider family and empowering that family unit in decision making for positive change, rather than supporting an individual in isolation (Hayden, 2009).

- **Functional Perspective**

  - Analyzing behavior from a **functional perspective** means examining behaviors and their environmental consequences to explain why behaviors begin, are maintained, and increase (or decrease over time): "research in laboratory and real-life settings has demonstrated that problem behaviors produce environmental functions that maintain such behavior" (Cipani 2014, p. 78).

- **Medical Causes**

  - Some problem behavior may be related to complex underlying medical causes or conditions (e.g., pain) (Guinchat et al. 2015).

- **Safe Space**

  - A safe space is an antecedent-based environmental adaptation, established as a designated area to go during times of stress or emotional distress, for a break and relaxation. Safe spaces can include elements such as sensory tools (e.g., stress balls), preferred items (e.g., family photographs), and reminders of strategies for self-calming (e.g., visual task analysis), as well as soft, comfortable, and comforting furnishings (Geiger et al. 2010; The Psychology Foundation of Canada, n.d.)

Is Daisy's Behavior a Message in Disguise?

Daisy had reached the magnificent age of 72 while happily living in her family home where she and her late husband had raised their five children. Luckily, this home was a bungalow, allowing her to access every area of functional living space even with some mobility issues. Her children—all adults scattered across the country and around the globe—had moved her fairly ancient washer and dryer upstairs so that she could continue doing her laundry independently, and they took on the job of cleaning the finished basement when they came for their rare visits, since the guest rooms were on this floor. Their visits, however, were becoming quite sparse as they were feeling collectively unwelcome.

The last time that her son visited with his children, Daisy's two oldest grand-children aged 14 and 16 visited; Daisy's behavior was quite unusual—for Daisy. She yelled at them every time they entered the kitchen. When they went out the mall together, she was rude to anyone who asked her a question or held out the door for her. She said things like, "I don't need your help!" in a loud and querulous voice. Her son called his big sister—Daisy's oldest child—and described her as "cantankerous," telling her she better "watch out" next time she visited. When Daisy's daughter did visit the next month, along with Daisy's youngest grandchild, an infant, Daisy's behavior seemed to have escalated. During this visit, whenever Daisy found items of baby care around the house, like her granddaughter's toys, board books, or stuffed animals, she threw them out the back door into the back-yard. Daisy's daughter wanted to retrieve them, but was feeling a little frightened to leave her baby in the house with Daisy. *Would Daisy throw the baby outdoors, as well?* Daisy's daughter was not quite sure what to do, so she gathered her baby's belonging from the yard after her mother went to bed for the evening.

Disturbed by the latest chain of events on each of their visits, Daisy's son and eldest daughter held a **family conference**, with the three other siblings joining in remotely via the computer. After a long and emotional discussion, Daisy's children decided to pay for a day companion for Daisy: a practical nurse with (obviously) experience in working with elderly clients. Daisy's son was given the tough job of convincing Daisy that this would be a good idea, and he managed to pull it off, including obtaining her written permission. However, this did not stop Daisy's new nurse from being the target of her now-sharp tongue and other unusual behaviors, growing in frequency. Daisy's nurse/companion, happily, had taken more than a few professional development events about challenging behavior in aged clientele, and took careful descriptive logs and frequency counts about each day's events. In the following weeks, the nurse used a variety of strategies: She carefully moved herself and any visitors away from Daisy, and if Daisy engaged in any aggression, such as flailing her arms, and snapping her fingers in the faces of her friends, she verbally calmed Daisy with a soft voice and provided helpful suggestions. If necessary, she guided Daisy to a **safe space**, such as her soft, comfortable couch or her rocking chair that faced the window.

"According to my logs," the nurse concluded at the most recent family conference, "these troubling incidents are not decreasing—they are increasing. I think we are going to have to look beyond my services, and plan to engage support from a behavior consultant, as well as a visit back to Daisy's physician. All the data I have collected in these past weeks with Daisy should really help with our planning." Daisy's children agreed, the geographically closest sibling set up the relevant appointments and brought the recommendations back to the next family conference.

"Here are my notes," he began, and read the relevant points to the group, including Daisy's daily nurse:

- Her physician wants to trial her on some different medication to see if they have any effect on her. She says problems like this are common in older people, and that medications tend to keep the worst symptoms under control.
- The physician wants her to have a full physical checkup from head-to-toe. She says it has been close to five years since Mom has done this.
- She also wants us to think about referring Mom to a psychiatrist for an evaluation.
- The behavior consultant agreed that it is very important to examine any **medical causes** for behavior change before looking at them from a behavioral perspective.
- He also said that when the time is right, that we should think about focusing on understanding mom's behavior from a **"functional perspective."** In other words, we should figure out if there her behavior is a message in disguise. He says that all behavior is communication and we need to figure out what mom is trying to tell us. He said that he can help with all of this, and that this is a first step to planning a successful program of behavior change.

He continued, "That's all of it! What do we want to do?"

The Response: Principles, Processes, Practices, and Reflections

Principles

(Q1) What does the team mean when they indicate that they want to look at Daisy's behaviors from a functional perspective? Based on some of the behaviors described in the case, what is the functional perspective for those behaviors?

(Q2) When the nurse guided Daisy to her "safe space," what was the resulting consequence in each of those instances? What behavior principle was at work here?

Processes

(Q3) Daisy's nurse took frequency counts of her behavior. This let the family know the behavior was increasing. What other types of data could she have taken that would have provided the family with more information at this meeting?

(Q4) The next steps, after ruling out any underlying medical factors, that the team is planning is to conduct a functional behavior assessment for Daisy. What could be done before conducting a full observation of Daisy's behavior to start the functional behavior assessment process? Explain the tools that you would use and an explanation of why you would use them (Reference Ethics Box 4.4, Behavior Analyst Certification Board, 2014). Use the following tools as a guide:
https://sites.google.com/a/ghaea.org/challenging-behavior-team/data-collection-resources-1

Ethics Box 4.4

Professional and Ethical Compliance Code for Behavior Analysts

- 3.02 Medical Consultation
  Behavior analysts recommend seeking a medical consultation if there is any reasonable possibility that a referred behavior is influenced by medical or biological variables.

Practice

(Q5) Look at the graph below of the frequency data that the nurse collected and the changes that were tracked once Daisy started the prescribed medication. Explain the level, trend, and variability.

(Q6) Based on the graph above, do you think there is a clear functional relationship between the medication and the behavior change? Why or why not? What data would you take to determine if there was a clear functional relationship?

(Q7) What design could you use to now implement a behavior technique into the intervention with Daisy with the medication alone? What is this type of single-subject design called? How could you design it so you could determine if there was a functional relationship?

Reflection

(Q8) The Professional and Ethical Compliance Code for Behavior Analysts (2014) state that biological and medical factors for behavior change should be considered. At this point, do you think they have been considered to the point that a behavior intervention can begin? What are the risks of waiting for the medical screening? What are the downfalls of not starting the behavior techniques immediately?

(Q9) In the current situation with Daisy, you are hearing information second hand from the doctor through the nurse. Are there any ethical dilemmas by completing your intervention with this communication method? What could you do differently (Reference Ethics Box 4.5, Behavior Analyst Certification Board, 2014)?

Ethics Box 4.5

Professional and Ethical Compliance Code for Behavior Analysts

- 2.04 Third-Party Involvement in Services.

  (a) When behavior analysts agree to provide services to a person or entity at the request of a third party, behavior analysts clarify, to the extent feasible and at the outset of the service, the nature of the relationship with each party and any potential conflicts. This clarification includes the role of the behavior analyst (such as therapist, organizational consultant, or expert witness), the probable uses of the services provided or the information obtained, and the fact that there may be limits to confidentiality.

  (b) If there is a foreseeable risk of behavior analysts being called upon to perform conflicting roles because of the involvement of a third party, behavior analysts clarify the nature and direction of their responsibilities, keep all parties appropriately informed as matters develop and resolve the situation in accordance with the code.

  (c) When providing services to a minor or individual who is a member of a protected population at the request of a third party, behavior analysts ensure that the parent or client-surrogate of the ultimate recipient of services is informed of the nature and scope of services to be provided, as well as their right to all service records and data.

  (d) Behavior analysts put the client's care above all others and, should the third party make requirements for services that are contradicted by the behavior analyst's recommendations, behavior analysts are obligated to resolve such conflicts in the best interest of the client. If said conflict cannot be resolved, that behavior analyst's services to the client may be discontinued following appropriate transition.

(Q10) What other factors must be considered for Daisy? Consider environmental variables as well.

Additional Web Links
ABA in the Elderly
http://www.ncbi.nlm.nih.gov/pmc/articles/PMC2078575/
ABA and Behavioral Medicine
http://www.academia.edu/13279646/Applied_Behavior_Analysis_and_
Behavioral_Medicine_History_of_the_Relationship_and_Opportunities_for_
Renewed_Collaboration
Level, Trend, and Variability
http://www.educateautism.com/applied-behaviour-analysis/visual-analysis-of-aba-
data.html

References

Alberto, P. A., & Troutman, A. C. (2009). *Applied behavior analysis for teachers.* Upper Saddle River: Merrill/Pearson.

Behavior Analyst Certification Board (2014). *Professional and ethical compliance code for behavior analysts.* Retrieved from http://bacb.com/wp-content/uploads/2016/01/160120-compliance-code-english.pdf

Business Management Daily. (2013). 5 steps toward a fair–and firm–progressive discipline policy. *HR Specialist: North Carolina Employment Law, 7*(10), 6.

Centre for Addiction and Mental Health (2016). *Dual Diagnosis.* Retrieved from: http://ontario.cmha.ca/mental-health/mental-health-conditions/dual-diagnosis/

Cipani, E. (2014). Comorbidity in "DSM" childhood mental disorders: A functional perspective. *Research on Social Work Practice, 24*(1), 78–85.

Cosden, M., Koegel, L. K., Koegel, R. L., Greenwell, A., & Klein, E. (2006). Strength-based assessment for children with autism spectrum disorders. *Research and Practice for Persons with Severe Disabilities, 31*(2), 134–143.

Council Bluffs (n.d.). *CBCSD social/emotional skills checklist.* Retrieved from: https://docs.google.com/file/d/0BxGP4iWt8SZ_SlFtcENZS3VuVUk/edit

ErinoakKids Autism Services. (2012). *ABA for families: Reinforcement.* Retrieved from http://www.erinoakkids.ca/Resources/Autism/Applied-Behaviour-Analysis.aspx

Felce, D., Perry, J., Romeo, R., Robertson, J., Meek, A., Emerson, E., et al. (2008). Outcomes and costs of community living: Semi-independent living and fully staffed group homes. *Journal Information, 113*(2).

Geiger, K. B., Carr, J. E., & Leblanc, L. A. (2010). Function-based treatments for escape-maintained problem behavior: A treatment-selection model for practicing behavior analysts. *Behavior Analysis in Practice, 3*(1), 22–32.

Griffiths, D. M., & Gardner, W. I. (2002). The integrated biopsychosocial approach to challenging behaviours. In D. M. Griffiths, C. Stavrakaki, & J. Summers (Eds.), *Dual diagnosis: An introduction to the mental health needs of persons with developmental disabilities* (pp. 81–114). Sudbury, ON: Habilitative Mental Health Resource Network.

Guinchat, V., Cravero, C., Diaz, L., Périsse, D., Xavier, J., Amiet, C., et al. (2015). Acute behavioral crises in psychiatric inpatients with autism spectrum disorder (ASD): Recognition of concomitant medical or non-ASD psychiatric conditions predicts enhanced improvement. *Research in Developmental Disabilities, 38,* 242–255. doi:10.1016/j.ridd.2012.020

Gulick, R. F., & Kitchen, T. P. (2007). *Effective instruction for children with autism: An applied behavior analytic approach.* Erie, PA: The Dr. Gertrude A. Barber National Institute.

Hayden, C. (2009). Family group conferences–are they an effective and viable way of working with attendance and behaviour problems in schools? *British Educational Research Journal, 35*(2), 205–220.

Hernandez, P., & Ikkanda, Z. (2011). Applied behavior analysis. Behavior management of children with autism spectrum disorders in dental environments. *The Journal of The American Dental Association, 142*(3), 281–287. doi:10.14219/jada.archive.2011.0167.

Human Rights Campaign. (2016). *Sexual orientation and gender identity definitions.* Retrieved from http://www.hrc.org/resources/sexual-orientation-and-gender-identity-terminology-and-definitions

ILS@NLC. (2015). *Testing accommodations checklist.* Retrieved from https://ilsnpc.wordpress.com/category/iep504-plan/

Koegel, R. K., Kim, S., & Koegel, L. (2014). Training paraprofessionals to improve socialization in students with ASD. *Journal of Autism and Developmental Disorders, 44*(9), 2197–2208. doi:10.1007/s10803-014-2094-x.

Luong, E. (2013). *Empowering our students: Strength based approaches and self direction.* Retrieved from: https://erinluong.wordpress.com/2013/04/11/empowering-our-students-strengths-based-approaches-and-self-direction/

Mayer, G. R., Sulzer-Azaroff, B., & Wallace, M. (2014). *Behavior analysis for lasting change* (3rd ed.). Conwall-on-Hudson, NY: Sloan Publishing.

Neal, J. W., & Neal, Z. P. (2013). Nested or networked? Future directions for ecological systems theory. *Social Development, 22*(4), 722–737. doi:10.1111/sode.12018.

Parsons, M., Rollyson, J., & Reid, D. (2012). Evidence-based staff training: A guide for practitioners. *Behavior Analysis in Practice, 5*(2), 2–11.

S Ritchie, H., & Blanck, P. (2003). The promise of the internet for disability: A study of on-line services and web site accessibility at centers for independent living. *Behavioral Sciences and the Law, 21*(1), 5–26.

Science of Behavior. (n.d.). *ABA glossary*. Retrieved from http://www.scienceofbehavior.com/lms/mod/glossary/view.php?id=408&mode=letter&hook=S&sortkey=&sortorder=&fullsearch=0&page=13

Serna, R. R., Lobo, H. E., Fleming, C. K., Fleming, R. K., Curtin, C., Foran, M. M., et al. (2015). Innovations in behavioral intervention preparation for paraprofessionals working with children with autism spectrum disorder. *Journal of Special Education Technology, 30*(1), 1–12.

Sugai, G., O'Keeffe, B. V., & Fallon, L. M. (2012). A contextual consideration of culture and school-wide positive behavior support. *Journal of Positive Behavior Interventions, 14*(4), 197–208. doi:10.1177/1098300711426334.

The Psychology Foundation of Canada. (n.d.). Toolbox activities: Quick ways to relax. *Kids Have Stress Too*. Retrieved from http://www.psychologyfoundation.org/files/5714/2288/9989/KHST_Toolbox_Activity_3_Quick_Ways_to_Relax.pdf

World Health Organization. (2015). *Lexicon of alcohol and drug terms published by the World Health Organization*. Retrieved from http://www.who.int/substance_abuse/terminology/who_lexicon/en/#

Part III
Implementation

Chapter 5
Implementation-Based Case Studies for Preschool-Age to School-Age Children

Abstract Applied Behavior Analysis (ABA) focuses on implementing procedures derived from the principles of behavior (e.g., reinforcement and punishment) to improve the quality of people's lives (Baer et al. in J Appl Behav Anal 1:91–97, 1968; Cooper et al. in applied behavior analysis. Pearson, Upper Saddle River, 2007). This "application" of behavioral principles is one of the seminal indicators of the field of ABA, as first described and still referenced by Baer et al. (J Appl Behav Anal 1:91–97, 1968) in their article, *Some Current Dimensions of applied behavior analysis*. The current chapter (Chap. 5) explores the guiding dimensions of ABA (applied, behavioral, analytic, technological, conceptual systems, effective, and generality) as the foundation for the implementation of behavior-change programs. Building on Section 1 (assessment) and Section 2 (planning), Section 3 begins to examine considerations surrounding the implementation of ABA programs to support preschool-age and school-age children. Often, behavior analysts are not directly implementing a behavior-change program and, instead, must teach, support, and guide other mediators (e.g., parents, teachers, and caregivers) to effectively utilize behavior-change strategies. This "mediator model" is a key area of focus when implementing ABA programs. Additional areas of consideration include behavior measurement, visual analysis and interpretation of graphed data, data-based decision-making, and maintaining a dual focus on reducing the frequency of problematic behaviors while introducing functionally equivalent, yet socially appropriate, replacement behaviors. In this chapter, entitled "Implementation—Based Case Studies for Preschool-Age and School-Age Children," these complex considerations are explored through five-case scenarios involving children in home, school, and community settings.

Keywords Implementation · Preschool · School-age children · Reinforcement · Punishment · Technology · ABA · Behavior-change programs · Parents · Teachers · Caregivers · Mediator model · Data-based decision-making · Problematic behaviors · Replacement behaviors

© Springer International Publishing AG 2016   157
K. Maich et al., *Applied Behavior Analysis*,
DOI 10.1007/978-3-319-44794-0_5

CASE: iii-I1

Important for ME, or important for YOU?
Setting: Community   Age-Group: Preschool

LEARNING OBJECTIVE:

- Analyze data to determine the function of a behavior.

TASK LIST LINKS:

- **Measurement**

  - (A-01) Measure frequency (i.e., count).
  - (A-03) Measure duration.
  - (A-12) Design and implement continuous measurement procedures (e.g., event recording).

- **Assessment**

  - (I-04) Design and implement the full range of functional assessment procedures.
  - (I-05) Organize, analyze, and interpret observed data.
  - (I-06) Make recommendations regarding behaviors that must be established, maintained, increased, or decreased.

- **Intervention**

  - (J-01) State intervention goals in observable and measurable terms.
  - (J-02) Identify potential interventions based on assessment results and the best available scientific evidence.
  - (J-14) Arrange instructional procedures to promote generative learning.

- **Fundamental Elements of Behavior Change**

  - (D-03) Use prompts and prompt fading.
  - (D-08) Use discrete-trial and free-operant arrangements.
  - (D-09) Use the verbal operants as a basis for language assessment.
  - (D-14) Use listener training.

KEY TERMS:

- **ABC Chart**

  - A chart that tracks a direct observation technique whereby the antecedent (A), the behavior (B), and the consequence (C) are recorded as they occur in the context which are later analyzed for trends and patterns which can help to determine the function of the behavior and is often part of a functional behavior assessment (Alberto and Troutman 2013).

- **Duration**

  – A dimension of behavior that examines how long a behavior persists (Mayer et al. 2014).

- **Frequency**

  – A dimension of behavior that examines how often a behavior occurs (Mayer et al. 2014).

- **Function-Based Definition of Behavior**

  – Involves defining the behavior based on the function of the behavior (consequences or outcomes) or why the behavior is occurring. Traditionally, the method to discern this information is through a functional behavior assessment or functional analysis (Filter and Nolan 2012).

- **Intensity**

  – A dimension of behavior that examines the forcefulness of the behavior (Mayer et al. 2014).

- **Time-Out**

  – Contingent on the display of a challenging behavior, time-out is a punishment technique that involves the withdrawal of an opportunity to gain access to positive reinforcement or access to positive reinforcers themselves (Cooper et al. 2007).

- **Topography-Based Definition of Behavior**

  – A description of the behavior that involves describing what is occurring rather than why it is occurring, including the movements that comprise the behavior (Alberto and Troutman 2013).

- **Verbal Operants**

  – The principles of applied behavior analysis apply to all human behavior, including verbal behavior. In his book, Verbal Behavior, B.F. Skinner outlined a group of verbal operants, or units of language that each serves a different function. They are mand (i.e., asking for reinforcers that you want), tact (i.e., naming or identifying objects, actions, or events), echoic (i.e., repeating what is heard), intraverbal (i.e., when words are controlled by other words such as when answering questions or having conversations), textual (i.e., reading written words), and transcription (i.e., writing and spelling words spoken to you) (Kelly et al. 2007).

Important for ME, Or Important for YOU?

Tracey has been an Early Childhood Educator for more than 30 years and is well known and well respected as an educator in her community. Year after year she leads teams of educators at the local early learning and childcare center "Great Beginnings," rotating between the preschool-age and school-age classrooms.

In her preschool class this year is Sarah, an energetic three-year-old. Sarah joined the class only a few weeks ago after her family moved into the community. During an initial interview with Sarah's parents, Tracey learned that Sarah has a language delay which causes her to have difficulty expressing herself. Her parents explained to Tracey that because of this, Sarah is often frustrated, and this frustration often escalates into crying, temper tantrums, throwing objects, and, at times, even hitting others.

Tracey has a warm, gentle, but firm approach to managing the behavior of the children in her class. It did not take long before she began to see Sarah's frustration. Last week, Sarah wanted to join two other children, Aiden and Noah, who were busy playing pretend dress up. Tracey watched as Sarah approached the two children and appeared to try to join their play. Having difficulty expressing herself, she had trouble keeping up with their fast-paced dialogue and conversation. After a few minutes, Aiden and Noah began to ignore Sarah, causing Sarah to become very upset. It did not take long before this escalated to Sarah crying and ripping a piece of the dress-up clothing Aiden and Noah were playing with.

Tracey has been responding to Sarah's behavioral outbursts as she always has for all of the children in her classes each year—with a stern verbal reprimand followed by a brief **time-out**, often in the corner of the room, facing the wall. Tracey believes that Sarah has to learn that her outbursts are not acceptable in the classroom.

After about a week of this recurring pattern of Sarah's frustration and behavioral outbursts, Tracey reprimanded and gave Sarah a time-out. Tracey also decided that a referral to a local early intervention program is needed. With only herself and one assistant, and a class of 15 preschoolers, Tracey was struggling to both respond to Sarah and support the other children in the class.

During her initial phone conversation with Rachel, a Board Certified Behavior Analyst, Tracey noted that she would like behavioral consultation because Sarah's behavior has to change, and further thought that Sarah would benefit from one-to-one intensive behavioral intervention (IBI) to teach her social skills. "I can't have these types of outburst in my classroom" Tracey told Rachel. Rachel listened carefully and supportively to Tracey and, after more than 20 min, asked whether she could come in to classroom to see what was happening.

Rachel was looking forward to meeting Tracey and supporting her to develop a supportive intervention for the difficulties that Sarah has been experiencing. She was particularly interested in guiding Tracey to think about both the **topography** and **function** of Sarah's problematic behaviors and to develop habilitation-based goals and objectives. When she arrived at the center, Rachel was greeted by Tracey.

After a warm welcome, Tracey said, "I am very busy, Sarah is over there, please go spend your time with her. Let me know what program you have for Sarah and how long it might be until she will begin to change her behavior. I can't have those outbursts in my classroom."

Rachel was stunned. As she sat in the corner and began to observe Sarah in the classroom, she had a recurring thought: *Who was it that really had to change here, Sarah or Tracey?* In the meantime, Rachel began to collect data on the **frequency** of the behavior, including when it happened, the **duration**, and the **intensity**. She collected **ABC data** for that first morning and asked Tracey whether she could come back each morning during the week. During her observations, Rachel also noted Sarah's use of **verbal operants** such as mands, tacts, echoics, and intraverbals, along with textual and transcription operants. Later the next week, in her office, Rachel analyzed her data and started to complete a **functional assessment**. After looking at the data, a pattern appeared. In the antecedent column, Tracey had placed a demand on Sarah, such as asking her to put away a toy. Afterward, Sarah engaged in the behaviors that Tracey described as an "outburst." Following this, Tracey usually ignored her and moved onto what she had to do with the rest of the children, and usually did the task herself, as she was busy and needed to move on. Rachel looked and thought, *I think I know what is happening here!*

The Response: Principles, Processes, Practices, and Reflections

Principles

(Q1) Describe how Rachel would have collected frequency, duration, and intensity data in the classroom. Which information did each dimension give her for her analysis?

(Q2) Describe Sarah's "outbursts" in terms of function-based and topography-based descriptions.

Processes

(Q3) What other components or information would Rachel need to complete to ensure that her functional assessment is accurate?

(Q4) Score the FAST to see the results from the Web site below. Is this consistent with the information that Rachel found in the ABC data?
https://depts.washington.edu/dbpeds/Screening%20Tools/FAST.pdf

Practice

(Q5) Based on the information in the case study, what is the function of Sarah's behavior (Fig. 5.1)?

(Q6) Determine two intervention goals based on the information received from Sarah's ABC data and the FAST (in question 4).

(Q7) What intervention strategy would you implement with Sarah based on the function of her behavior? What does Tracey need to change as well? Ensure that it is a functionally equivalent behavior in that the replacement behavior meets the same function and consider teaching her alternative behaviors as well (Reference

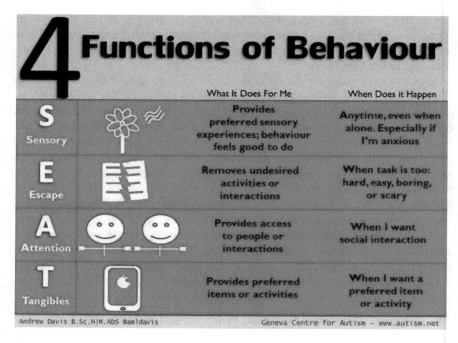

Fig. 5.1 The four functions of behavior (Davis, n.d.)

Ethics Box 5.1, Behavior Analyst Certification Board, 2014). Use this Web site for assistance: http://www.apbs.org/files/competingbehav_prac.pdf

Ethics Box 5.1

Professional and Ethical Compliance Code for Behavior Analysts

- 4.07 Environmental Conditions that Interfere with Implementation.
  (a) If environmental conditions prevent the implementation of a behavior-change program, behavior analysts recommend that other professional assistance (e.g., assessment, consultation, or therapeutic intervention by other professionals) be sought.
  (b) If environmental conditions hinder implementation of the behavior-change program, behavior analysts seek to eliminate the environmental constraints or identify in writing the obstacles to doing so.

Reflection

(Q8) Looking at the assessments that Rachel implemented, is there any other assessments that you would include?

(Q9) Now that the results of the assessment are present, indicate how you will work with Tracey to develop the intervention goals and implement the program.

(Q10) As a Board Certified Behavior Analyst, how might you respond to Tracey's request for an IBI program for Sarah? Could the behavioral supports offered by Rachel include both a one-to-one IBI program and broader behavior consultation? If so, how? If not, why not?

Additional Web Links
Functional Behavior Assessment
http://www.ped.state.nm.us/RtI/behavior/4.fba.11.28.pdf
Positive Behavior Support
https://www.pbis.org
Dimensions of Behavior
http://www.aisd.net/aisd/Portals/14/Definitions%20and%20Examples%20of%20Dimensions%20of%20Behavior.pdf
Target Intervention Goals
http://bringingaba.com/2012/08/27/first-things-first-initial-goals-to-target-when-beginning-an-aba-intervention-program-for-young-children-with-asd/
Data Collection Forms
https://sites.google.com/a/ghaea.org/challenging-behavior-team/data-collection-resources-1

CASE: iii-I2

Robina's Data are WRONG; My EXPERIENCES are right
Setting: Community   Age-Group: Preschool

LEARNING OBJECTIVE:

- Recognize the important role of data collection in the behavior consultation process, and critically evaluate the trustworthiness of measures of behavior.

TASK LIST LINKS:

- **Measurement**

    – (A-01) Measure frequency (i.e., count).

- **Identification of the Problem**

    – (G-04) Explain behavioral concepts using nontechnical language.
    – (G-06) Provide behavior-analytic services in collaboration with others who support and/or provide services to one's clients.

- **Measurement**

    – (H-01) Select a measurement system to obtain representative data given the dimensions of the behavior and the logistics of observing and recording.
    – (H-02) Select a schedule of observation and recording periods.

- (H-03) Select a data display that effectively communicates relevant quantitative relations.
- (H-04) Evaluate changes in level, trend, and variability.
- (H-05) Evaluate temporal relations between observed variables (within and between sessions and time series).

- **Fundamental Elements of Behavior Change**

  - (D-04) Use modeling and imitation training.

- **Specific Behavior-Change Procedures**

  - (E-12) Use errorless learning procedures.

KEY TERMS:

- **Empiricism**

  - In the field of ABA, empiricism refers to objectively gathering and examining evidence about the behavior under study, free of any influence from one's own beliefs or opinions. For example, when selecting an intervention to support a behavior-change program, empirically supported interventions —treatments that have been demonstrated to be effective in rigorous peer-reviewed research—should be selected. Similarly, when implementing a behavior-change intervention, the effects of that intervention should be determined based on rigorous, reliable, and valid data collection and analysis methods. Any conclusions drawn about the effects of the intervention should be based on the data collected and not on the subjective opinions of those involved (Mesibov and Shea 2011).

- **Repeatability**

  - Also referred to as "countability," repeatability refers to measuring how many times a behavior is repeated within a period of time, for example, counting the number of time a behavior is displayed (Bicard et al. 2012; Johnston and Pennypacker 1993).

- **Science**

  - Attempts to empirically gather and organize knowledge about a specific phenomenon under study. As a science, subjective hypothetical constructs from the explanations are removed (e.g., personal experience, the mind, and cognitive explanations) and instead use scientific processes of inquiry such as objective data collection and experimentation to empirically demonstrate relationships between variables (Fryling 2011).

- **Temporal Extent**

  - When measuring behavior, temporal extent refers to recording the elapsed time of a response or the duration of the behavior (Springer et al. 1981; Johnston and Pennypacker 1993).

- **Temporal Locus**

  - When measuring behavior, temporal locus refers to when, during a period of time, and in relation to other events, a behavior occurs, for example, recording response latency—how long after exposure to a certain event a behavior begins to occur; or measuring inter-response time—the elapsed time between instances of behavior (Springer et al. 1981; Johnston and Pennypacker 1993).

Robina's Data Are WRONG; My EXPERIENCES Are Right

"Not again ..." sighed Robina's mother. "I don't know what is wrong with these people," she said sharply to Robina's dad, waiting by the phone to hear the news of the day from their recorded messages. "Seriously, I really question their judgment. We haven't even been back to the after-school program to pick her up today, and they have left ... not one ..." she continued to listen to the recorded messages, "but THREE messages in the meantime. The program's only TWO HOURS long! We haven't seen ANY messages from the school in her knapsack, we haven't had ANY problems with her at home. Her dance instructor never says a word about any so-called 'behavior' problems. Her respite program only has good things to say. I just don't get it! Do you?" Robina's father shrugged, *thinking* back to how difficult the preschool years had been for 6-year-old Robina, wondering if her mother had really forgotten what it was like. *When Robina was first diagnosed,* he recalled, *with not only a likely cognitive delay, but also an Autism Spectrum Disorder, it was one thing after another at her day care. I never want to go back to those days. But it seems like once everyone got used to her—and she got used to them—everything really settled down. Where we used to see screaming and lying on the floor and refused to do anything she was asked, we now get laughing and nods and that wonderful word, "Okay." Even the transition to our school was fine. Given that it's just down the street, Robina can get back and forth with just a little bit of help, and she loves the walk, her teachers, and the other students in her class ... the same kids she has grown up with around here. I kind of thought that this easy pathway for all of us would just keep on from here, but it seems like there is more than one bump in the road.*

"Well," he responded aloud, "let's see what they have to say face-to-face. You can tell me all the details of the phone messages as we walk."

And when they entered the child-sized gates of the after-school program's dedicated entrance area, one of the supervisors was waiting for them, with a very unhappy-looking Robina collapsed on the asphalt, legs in a vee, folded over face to the ground, hands over the back of her head. Robina's parents locked eyes, knowing that the long day was not yet over.

Robina's mother walked Robina home to get supper started—one of Robina's favorite activities at home—and Robina's dad stayed on site to meet with the after-school supervisors for a meeting that was clearly going to happen right then. Seated together on the child-sized chairs around a small, round table, the childcare supervisor began: "Well, as you know from our messages, the main issue we are having with Robina's behavior here in after-school care is her pushing. I am sure you see this at home, as well. She has pushed at least half of our group of 12, and not just pushed the others, but literally pushed them over. She used to just put her hands on their chests and shove a little, but now she is pushing harder and more often. We are getting crying children, plus the other parents are calling with complaints. One of the things that happened after school today was that Robina pushed one of the other so hard that he fell backwards and landed right in our large bucket of building blocks. He is definitely going to be bruised, and we had to fill out an incident report, and of course call the other parents, too. I know we don't have much time, but we are really hoping that you will sign this referral today to get someone in from our head office to start helping Robina out with this very challenging behavior of hers."

Trying repeatedly to break into the ongoing diatribe and having no success, Robina's father took advantage of the pause, here, and attempted to respond in a way that would work for everyone, without showing his likely obvious and growing annoyance. "I agree with you that Robina should not be pushing, but we have actually not witnessed her pushing anyone at home or at respite care or even in her dance classes. So you are telling me this, and I believe you that there are probably problems, but I haven't yet seen any evidence of this. I don't think that you should be telling me about what other parents are saying, either. What I would like to see is something you can show me that proves this is happening. How about some **science**? I was taught in our parenting classes that the best way to tell future behavior is from past behavior. And we aren't having any problems with Robina. I think signing your paperwork today is probably a little premature, but I will take it home and talk it over with my family."

Feeling like they were left with little choice, the after-school care workers nodded their assent, smiled, and shook hands. The next day, though, they started to collect the evidence that they thought Robina's dad was seeking, hoping to show the frequency of Robina's problem behavior. Without a behavioral consultant to help them and to educate on important information and terms such as **temporal locus** and **temporal extent** and **repeatability,** they simply searched online and printed off some ready-made data collection charts. All staff members were shown this chart and were told all that they had to do was put a checkmark on the time and day that Robina pushed one of the other children—or an adult, and it was placed on the supervisor's desk so anyone could access it at any time. After a week, they had collected five sheets of paper, and each day had between three and nine checkmarks. They added up each day's number of pushes, wrote it at the top of each page, and circled it. This is what they presented to Robina's parents at their next meeting together.

Both of Robina's parents took these sheets of data, looked through them one by one, and then carefully laid them down back in order. "This is all very nice," responded Robena's mother, with some not so carefully disguised frustration evidence on her face and in her voice tone, "but it really doesn't tell me very much. Isn't pushing rather a normal thing for energetic young children? How much did the others push? I know you are trying hard, but this really doesn't convince me that there is a problem, or that I should sign your papers. I think that, just maybe, just maybe, we know our child better than you know how to collect data."

The Response: Principles, Processes, Practices, and Reflections

Principles

(Q1) Outline one measure based on repeatability, one based on temporal extent, and one based on temporal locus for the behavior difficulty displayed by Robina. Please explain what type of information each measure would provide and the strengths and limitations of each.

(Q2) If you were consulting to Robina's after-school care workers and her parents, which measure from those that you listed in question #1, would you recommend be implemented? Explain why.

Processes

(Q3) Outline at least two strengths and two limitations of the data collection process implemented by the after-school staff.

(Q4) Describe how you would address the limitations you identified in question#3?

Practice

(Q5) How would you respond to the question posed by Robina's parents: *"Isn't pushing rather a normal thing for energetic young children?"* Using the data sheet below, how might a data collection process with peers help you respond? Complete the form and present a response to the parents (Table 5.1).

(Q6) Attached is a graph of the data collected by Robina's after-school care workers. How might you interpret these data? What conclusions might you draw from the data? What questions does the data raise (Fig. 5.2)?

(Q7) How would you respond to the differences in perceptions of Robina's behavior held by her parents and her after-school program workers? How might a data collection process help you respond?

Table 5.1 Example peer comparison chart for interval recording

Peer Comparison Data Collection Sheet

Date:							
Observer:							
Observe both student and peer, if either of the target behaviors occurs in, check off the corresponding behavior under the specific individual 's column. Check off "none" if neither behavior is observed during that interval							
Interval:		Student:				Peer:		
From:	To:	Behavior 1:	Behavior 2:	None	Behavior 1:	Behavior 2:	None

Summary

Count the number of intervals where the behavior was observed and divide by the total number of intervals. Multiply that number by 100 to get the percent of intervals where the behavior occurred

Student:
Behavior 1: _____/_____ = _____x100=_____%

Behavior 2: _____/_____ = _____x100=_____%

Peer:
Behavior 1: _____/_____ = _____x100=_____%

Behavior 2: _____/_____ = _____x100=_____%

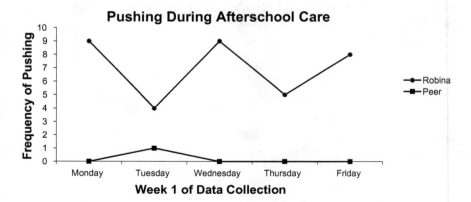

Fig. 5.2 Line graph comparing Robina's same-aged peer's pushing behavior over one week

Reflection

(Q8) Addressing a behavior difficulty without first collecting data on the behavior in question poses a number of risks. Please identify at least two.

(Q9) The after-school workers were collecting data to prove that Robina's behavior is a problem. Does this raise any ethical concerns? Please explain? What type of data collection process would you recommend so that the data are trustworthy and free from any biases (Reference Ethics Box 5.2, Behavior Analyst Certification Board, 2014)?

Ethics Box 5.2

Professional and Ethical Compliance Code for Behavior Analysts

- 2.11 Records and Data.

  (a) Behavior analysts create, maintain, disseminate, store, retain, and dispose of records and data relating to their research, practice, and other work in accordance with applicable laws, regulations, and policies; in a manner that permits compliance with the requirements of this code; and in a manner that allows for appropriate transition of service oversight at any moment in time.

  (b) Behavior analysts must retain records and data for at least seven (7) years and as otherwise required by law.

Look at the IOA calculator as a tool: https://www.abainternational.org/journals/behavior-analysis-in-practice/supplemental-materials.aspx

(Q10) How might a data collection process be a helpful tool in forming a cohesive team between Robina's parents and her after-school workers?

Additional Web Links
Measuring Behavior
https://iris.peabody.vanderbilt.edu/wp-content/uploads/pdf_case_studies/ics_measbeh.pdf
Calculating IOA
https://www.abainternational.org/media/31416/examplespreadsheet.pdf
Data Collection Sheets
http://www.behaviorbabe.com/datasheets.htm

CASE: iii-I3

Let's just get moving along!
Setting: Home   Age-Group: School Age
LEARNING OBJECTIVE:

- Recognize the importance of both short-term behavior tactics to efficiently reduce problem behavior and longer-term programs focused on developing new skills.

TASK LIST LINKS:

- **Measurement**

  - (A-01) Measure frequency (i.e., count).
  - (A-03) Measure duration.

- **Experimental Design**

  - (B-02) Review and interpret articles from the behavior-analytic literature.

- **Fundamental Elements of Behavior Change**

  - (D-01) Use positive and negative reinforcement.
  - (D-02) Use appropriate parameters and schedules of reinforcement.
  - (D-05) Use shaping.
  - (D-07) Conduct task analyses.
  - (D-21) Use differential reinforcement (e.g., DRO, DRA, DRI, DRL, and DRH).

- **Specific Behavior-Change Procedures**

  - Use instructions and rules.

- **Identification of the Problem**

  - (G-01) Review records and available data at the outset of the case.
  - (G-04) Explain behavioral concepts using nontechnical language.

- **Assessment**

  - (I-05) Organize, analyze, and interpret observed data.
  - (I-06) Make recommendations regarding behaviors that must be established, maintained, increased, or decreased.

- **Intervention**

  - (J-10) When a behavior is to be decreased, select an acceptable alternative behavior to be established or increased.

- **Implementation, Management, and Supervision**

  - (K-03) Design and use competency-based training for persons who are responsible for carrying out behavioral assessment and behavior-change procedures.
  - (K-05) Design and use systems for monitoring procedural integrity.
  - (K-09) Secure the support of others to maintain the client's behavioral repertoires in their natural environments.

KEY TERMS:

- **Differential Reinforcement**

  - Differential reinforcement is a procedure within applied behavior analysis that is used to simultaneously increase desired behaviors while reducing problematic behaviors. This is accomplished by providing reinforcement to only

those behaviors that meet a predetermined criterion, and withholding reinforcement for behaviors that do not meet the criterion (Vladescu and Kodak
2010). For example, increasing a child's in-seat behavior and decreasing his or
her out-of-seat behavior are by only providing reinforcement for in-seat
behavior and withholding reinforcement for out-of-seat behavior.

- **Shaping**
    - Shaping is a technique within applied behavior analysis used to teach new
      behavior. This technique follows a systematic approach to prompt and
      reinforce predetermined successive approximations toward a target behavior
      (Alberto and Troutman 2006).

- **Successive Approximations**
    - Within a shaping program, successive approximations are behaviors that are
      sequential steps toward a terminal behavior, or approximations of the ter-
      minal behavior. Over the course of a shaping program, reinforcement is
      stopped for less accurate approximations of the terminal behavior, and
      reinforcement is provided for more accurate approximations until the ter-
      minal behavior is reached (Cooper et al. 2007).

- **Terminal Behavior**
    - Within a shaping program, the terminal behavior is the desired behavior that
      the program is working toward (Alberto and Troutman 2006), for example,
      gradually prompting and reinforcing the duration of child's sitting behavior
      until the behavior reaches the desired 15-min duration. Sitting for 15 min,
      therefore, is the terminal behavior.

Let's Just Get Moving Along!

"Seriously," the parent said, with quite an upset tone to her voice, "they can't even
be in the room for five minutes together, and they are fighting. And I don't mean
sticking their tongues out or yelling at each other, though we get that, too." She
looked at her partner for confirmation. "But it's rolling around on the ground, hands
around each other's necks. It's kicking over boots in the hallway, and kicking each
other. I just don't get it at all. I didn't act like this as a child. It's just so frustrating!
Everyone told me that having kids close together was a great idea, but it seems like
it just making things worse. We should be able to put them on the same soccer
team, for example, to make our schedules a little easier, but last time we tried that,
we ended up with a bloody nose and an almost-broken arm."

Iris, the behavior therapist nodded, made soothing sounds, took notes, and asked
questions (though she hardly needs to do so). She was well familiar with the
background story of this family. The same-gender parents had a rough yet successful start to parenting, sacrificing time, peace-of-mind, and much of their
combined incomes with the happy addition of two boys to their family, born just
14 months apart.

"Don't get me started on school, either! With Andre following Anton into Kindergarten in a few months, I anticipate disaster! It's not like we have a choice. Our school only has one Kindergarten classroom: I guess that is what happens with life in a small town. I have already warned their teachers, but I don't think they can begin to understand what it's really like for us at home. They think Anton is an angel!"

"It sounds like it's time to try something new," Iris suggested. "Are you willing to make a few changes?"

With support from both parents firmly in place, Iris spent the next few days researching clinical cases in the applied literature. She was aware that, from time to time, the two brothers did engage in cooperative play, both within and outside their sibling dyad. She refreshed her memory about best practices for **shaping** behavior successfully and developed a program using shaping for the boys to teach the remaining essential skills of cooperative play and to gradually increase its duration.

The shaping program started with the level of cooperative play that both the boys could successfully engage in, and this duration was determined by the data that were collected. The data showed that Anton had more cooperative play skills than Andre, and he was able to engage in cooperative play for a longer period of time. Iris noted that this was likely due to being 14 months older and having more experience in the classroom setting. Iris's program broke down each step of cooperative play, and then, reinforcement was delivered. Once the boys were able to demonstrate the next step of play, the therapist or parent would reinforce their behavior. When they went back to a level of play that they had previously mastered, **differential reinforcement** was provided, whereby the lower level was no longer reinforced, but the next step of play was required for the same level of reinforcement.

During a follow-up consultation visit, Iris reviewed a graph, showing the data that have been collected to date from Anton and Andre's parents, the preschool instructors, and the Kindergarten teachers. While their parents could clearly appreciate the progress that was being made, it was pretty clear as well that they were very enthusiastic about the next steps in the shaping program and expressing frustration that even though the graph shows progress, everything seems to be moving slowly. *Let's just get moving along!* was the clear theme of the consultation. Iris left a little frustrated, already trying to work out how to explain to the parents in this situation that behavior change is a process, and that systemic, long-term change takes time and practice, but is well worth it.

The Response: Principles, Processes, Practices, and Reflections

Principles

(Q1) In the situation with Andre and Anton, list two benefits and two limitations of a shaping program?

(Q2) What are three benefits of a reinforcement-based approach, such as the shaping program, as compared to one based solely on extinction or punishment (Reference Ethics Box 5.3, Behavior Analyst Certification Board, 2014)?

Ethics Box 5.3

Professional and Ethical Compliance Code for Behavior Analysts

- 4.08 Considerations Regarding Punishment Procedures.
  (a) Behavior analysts recommend reinforcement rather than punishment whenever possible.
  (b) If punishment procedures are necessary, behavior analysts always include reinforcement procedures for alternative behavior in the behavior-change program.
  (c) Before implementing punishment-based procedures behavior analysts ensure that appropriate steps have been taken to implement reinforcement-based procedures unless the severity of dangerousness of the behavior necessitates immediate use of aversive procedures.
  (d) Behavior analysts ensure that aversive procedures are accompanied by an increased level of training, supervision, and oversight. Behavior analysts must evaluate the effectiveness of aversive procedures in a timely manner and modify the behavior-change program if it is ineffective. Behavior analysts always include a plan to discontinue the use of aversive procedures when no longer needed.
- 4.09 Least Restrictive Procedures
  Behavior analysts review and appraise the restrictiveness of procedures and always recommend the least restrictive procedures likely to be effective.

Processes

(Q3) Below is a sample of ideas that are involved in preschool cooperative play. Write out the task analysis for one aspect of cooperative play for one of the boys (Table 5.2).

(Q4) Based on the task analysis above, outline how you would differentially reinforce each successive approximation of each behavior in your task analysis to get to the terminal behavior. Identify the reinforcer used on the current behavior that has not yet been mastered and the previous behavior that has been mastered.

Table 5.2 Example of behavior involved in preschool-aged cooperative play (Best Start Expert Panel on Early Learning, 2007; Cecchini, 2008)

Types of cooperative play	Examples of cooperative play
• Allow interaction with other children and manipulation of objects between play • Being a part of setting the rules for play and asking others to join in • Playing a game together that involves cooperating with one another to achieve an outcome • Vote: Have a vote with the group to decide which course of action to take	• Set up the setting so that children can engage in different activities where they are facing one another • Have children work together to achieve a task such as cleaning up an area, raking leaves, or building a tower • Think about creating activities and engaging with children to create ideas that promote cooperation

Practice

(Q5) Given your task analysis above, write the shaping program using the attached template (Table 5.3).

Table 5.3 Example skill acquisition template

Skill Acquisition:	
Start Date:	**Mastery Date:**
ABLLS-R Criteria: **VB-MAPP Milestone**:	
Objective:	
Materials:	
Discriminative Stimulus (SD):	
Error Correction:	
Mastery Criteria:	
Data Collection Guidelines:	
General Teaching Procedures and Notes:	
Prompt Hierarchy and Procedure:	
Skill Acquisition Procedure	

(Q6) Given your shaping program, how would you teach the parents how to run the program and what type of data would you have them collect. Describe the training program. Make a data collection sheet for the family.

(Q7) Provide three examples of how you would generalize this skill into other environments. How would you teach this?

Reflection

(Q8) Although sustainable behavior change takes time, Andre and Anton's parents expected a "quick fix" with immediate results. How might you address this? Explain how you might balance the need for a quick reduction in problematic behavior, with a longer-term skill building-based approach to addressing the presenting behavior difficulties?

(Q9) Why might it be important to celebrate small successes with Andre and Anton's parents along the way to their larger goal of sustainable behavior improvements in their children's behavior? How might this be accomplished?

(Q10) Andre and Anton's parents appear to believe that their children should be the focus of Iris's behavior-change program. Would you agree? How might you respond to the assertion that in order to change a child's behavior, behavior change must first occur in adults' behavior?

Additional Web Links
Shaping
http://www.txautism.net/uploads/target/Shaping.pdf
Task Analysis http://www.erinoakkids.ca/getattachment/Resources/Growing-Up/Autism/Applied-Behaviour-Analysis/ABA-for-Families-Task-Analysis.pdf.aspx

CASE: iii-I4

When is "ENOUGH"?
Setting: School   Age-Group: Preschool
LEARNING OBJECTIVE:

- Interpret graphic displays of behavior data and utilize the findings to inform and guide decisions in applied behavior analysis research and practice.

TASK LIST LINKS:

- **Measurement**

    - (A-13) Design and implement discontinuous measurement procedures (e.g., partial and whole interval, and momentary time sampling).

- **Experimental Design**

    - (B-06) Use changing criterion designs.

- **Behavior-Change Considerations**

  - (C-03) State and plan for the possible unwanted effects of extinction.

- **Fundamental Elements of Behavior Change**

  - (D-01) Use positive and negative reinforcement.
  - (D-03) Use prompts and prompt fading
  - (D-18) Use extinction
  - (D-21) Use differential reinforcement (e.g., DRO, DRA, DRI, DRL, and DRH).

- **Behavior-Change Systems**

  - (F-02) Use token economies and other conditioned reinforcement systems.
  - (F-03) Use direct instruction.

- **Measurement**

  - (H-01) Select a measurement system to obtain representative data given the dimensions of the behavior and the logistics of observing and recording.
  - (H-02) Select a schedule of observation and recording periods.
  - (H-03) Select a data display that effectively communicates relevant quantitative relations.
  - (H-04) Evaluate changes in level, trend, and variability.

- **Assessment**

  - (I-01) Define behavior in observable and measurable terms.

KEY TERMS:

- **Data Path**

  - When data points on a line graph are connected with a straight line, a data path is created that highlights the level and trend of the displayed data. In ABA, the data path is a central focus when interpreting and analyzing graphic displays of data (Cooper et al. 2007; Kahng et al. 2010).

- **Graph**

  - A graph is a visual representation of data. In Applied Behavior Analysis (ABA), graphic displays of behavior are used to document and communicate the occurrence of selected target behaviors. Graphs are also used to provide an at-a-glance summary of data collected and to show changes in behavior before, during, and after the introduction of a behavior-change tactic. Graphs are the main process by which behavior analysts communicate the effects of an intervention (Kahng et al. 2010; Dixon et al. 2009).

- **Visual Analysis**
  - Behavior analysts rely on graphic displays of behavior data to summarize, communicate, and interpret measurements of observable behavior. In ABA, the primary method of determining the extent to which meaningful changes in behavior are occurring is by visually analyzing graphic displays of behavior. This involves identifying the level (value on the vertical access where data points converge), trend (overall direction of the data collected), and variability (extent to which multiple measures of behavior produce similar outcomes) of the data displayed before, during, and after a behavior-change program has been introduced (Kahng et al. 2010)

- **X-axis**
  - On a simple line graph, the x-axis is the horizontal axis, also called the abscissa. In ABA, this axis typically represents the passage of time (Cooper et al. 2007).

- **Y-axis**
  - On a simple line graph, the y-axis is the vertical axis, also called the ordinate. In ABA, this axis typically represents a measureable dimension of behavior (Cooper et al. 2007).

When Is "ENOUGH"?

Ms. Lafferty slumped at her cubicle in the staff room, after leaving her new-to-her grade four classroom as soon as the last student exited the school. She lifted her hand to rub her face in despair, and ended up wiping sweat from her brow and neck, even though it was a fairly cool winter day and she had not just been teaching physical education. *It's stress! I am stress sweating!* she concluded, grimacing as she made her way across the staffroom to wash her hands and face with soap and cool water. *Why did I think that taking over this group of 9-year-olds and 10-year-olds within four weeks until the end of the school year was a good idea? I just can't seem to get their attention, and when I do I can't keep it!* Pausing as she exited the washroom, she made a snap decision and turned left instead of her usual right, heading down the hallway to visit the school's behavior consultant. *How lucky we are to have this person on our staff! And how lucky we are again that our principal has an open-door policy with referrals. Good thing I was paying attention at my first (and maybe last) staff meeting.*

She only had to wait about 10 min before the behavior consultant showed up with a smile, clipboards in one hand, her laptop in the other. "Ms. Lafferty!" The consultant—Miss King—called her by name, obviously happy to see her, but of course followed her greeting with an inquiring question, "What's up with you today?" The two educators entered the office and shut the door firmly behind them.

"Remember," said Miss King, "what we talk about here is between you and me, unless there is a safety issue or other serious concern with our school that needs to be referred right away. So let's talk."

Reverting to first names now that they were out of hearing range of any lingering students, Ms. Lafferty began. "As you know, I got here only a few weeks ago. Since then, I have had no luck getting this class on track. The students spend far more time doing nothing than learning anything. They do not listen, they do not follow instructions, they do not complete tasks: they basically do not do anything I ask. It's not just one or two students. It's pretty much everyone! But they do seem to have a really good time chatting it up with one another. I have to say there is lots of laughter in the room. It seems like a really strong community of students who get along together really well. But it's like I am invisible, behind some sort of transparent wall, ineptly waving my arms around and mouthing words that nobody can hear—or nobody chooses to hear. I am like that proverbial fly on the wall: hearing everything but doing nothing that has any effect on what's happening. They just flick me out of the way, metaphorically, of course. And that's my rant. Now, can you help?"

"Of course I can help," replied Miss King. "And today is your lucky day, even though I know it doesn't feel like it right now. We have an ABA student starting tomorrow, and she is a superstar at data collection. She is here to learn about how to collaborate with teachers and to use her skills in the school environment. Since I know that the words 'data collection' aren't everyone's favorite words, I am pretty sure you would be happy to have her help, too. Am I right? We'll start tomorrow, collect some baseline data, and look at implementing a class-wide behavior plan."

The following morning before school began Miss King, Ms. Lafferty and the ABA student collaborated to develop an operational definition for both on-task and off-task behavior, as well as a plan for time sampling of these behaviors every fifteen minutes. The ABA student felt that baseline data were stable after four days and an unexpected field trip, and suggested another meeting with the behavior consultant, Miss King, Ms. Lafferty, and herself to create a plan for change. Together, they make a plan to implement direct instruction to try to increase on-task behavior, and Differential Reinforcement of Other Behavior (DRO), specifically focusing on verbal praise and token reinforcers for on-task behavior in the class-room. By the middle of next week, after only three more days at school, Miss Lafferty found herself back in the consultant's office, looking for an update. As she rounded the doorway, she could see a **graph** projected on the wall over a piece of taped-up chart paper: "Is this it? Is it us?"

"It *is* all of you!" the behaviorists smiled enthusiastically. They began to explain the graph to Ms. Lafferty. "These four days, here is the baseline, that is, when we observed before we made any changes. As you can see, the levels of off-task behavior are quite high, but it is level and stable. Often behavior gets worse before it gets better when a behavior is put on extinction, that is, it is no longer being reinforced. This temporary increase in behavior is called an extinction burst. So basically, the same pattern happened every day. Then, you can see the phase line we drew here, showing that we started the intervention plan. These three days are after we started the intervention...you can see here that the line is way down below the first one, and each of the data points—the small triangles—show how things have changed since then. The first day must have been hard, because you can see that first data point is really high. But the last two days have been much better. You are doing really well! Each day so far, the off-task behavior in your class is decreasing. That's great news and shows us, already, that what you are doing is working!"

Caitlyn interrupted, "Well, to be honest, I don't know about that. I came to see you today because I really feel like nothing has changed. I really feel like it's not working! When can we try something new?"

The Response: Principles, Processes, Practices, and Reflections

Principles

(Q1) Differential Reinforcement of Other Behavior (DRO) involves delivering reinforcement when the target behavior has not occurred for a specific period of time and reinforcing other behaviors with the absence of the target behavior (Mayer et al. 2014). Explain why this approach might be helpful for Ms. Lafferty.

(Q2) Looking at the attached graph of data collected in Caitlin's classroom. Please explain the level, variability, and trend in baseline data and discuss what your next step would be based on the data collected. Would you have continued to collect additional baseline data points or would you have introduced your intervention program as was done in the graph? Explain your decision (Fig. 5.3).

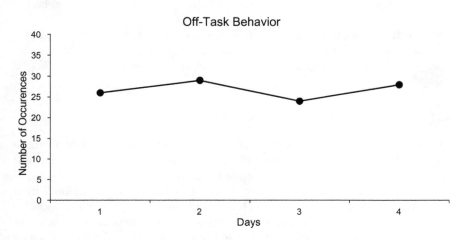

Fig. 5.3 Graph of off-task behavior in Ms. Lafferty's classroom

Processes

(Q3) Draw the graph that was explained in the story above. Please ensure that all of the components of a graph listed below are included and labeled:

- x-axis,
- y-axis,
- condition change lines/phase lines,
- condition labels,
- data points,
- data path, and
- graph title.

(Q4) Outline at least 3 benefits of constructing graphic displays of behavior data (Reference Ethics Box 5.4, Behavior Analyst Certification Board, 2014).

Ethics Box 5.4

Professional and Ethical Compliance Code for Behavior Analysts

- 3.01 Behavior-Analytic Assessment.
  (a) Behavior analysts conduct current assessments prior to making recommendations or developing behavior-change programs. The type of assessment used is determined by client's needs and consent, environmental parameters, and other contextual variables. When behavior analysts are developing a behavior reduction program, they must first conduct a functional assessment.
  (b) Behavior analysts have an obligation to collect and graphically display data, using behavior-analytic conventions, in a manner that allows for decisions and recommendations for behavior-change program development.

Practice

(Q5) Write a DRO program for Ms. Lafferty and outline how you might approach training Ms. Lafferty in the delivery of this program. How might you determine when she has mastered the delivery of the program?

(Q6) Write an operational definition for both off-task and on-task behavior. Why is it important for Ms. Lafferty to have clear definitions of these target behaviors?

(Q7) A token economy involves delivering tokens that are symbolic representations of a reinforcer in response to displays of the target behavior, and then exchanging tokens earned for preferred items, activities, or privileges (Alberto and Troutman 2013). How might a token economy, used in collaboration with a DRO program, be helpful to Ms. Lafferty? Indicate the teaching steps in delivering the token system, so that the tokens become conditioned reinforcers (Fig. 5.4).

Fig. 5.4 The cycle of a token economy

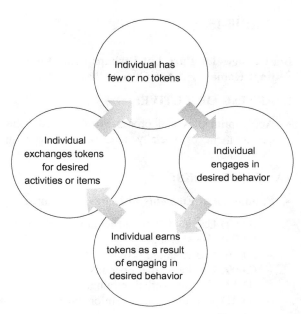

Reflection

(Q8) How would you respond to Ms. Lafferty's concerns? Why might there be a discrepancy between what the data is showing and Mrs. Lafferty's perception of what is happening in the classroom?

(Q9) Time sampling involves measuring the presence or absence of the target behavior within specific time intervals, such as breaking a 30-min behavior observation period into 5-min intervals (Mayer et al. 2014). Examples include momentary time sampling (e.g., recording if the behavior is occurring at the moment each time interval ends), partial-interval time sampling (e.g., recording if the behavior occurred at any time during the interval), and whole-interval time sampling (e.g., recording if the behavior occurred throughout the entire interval). Why might time sampling be a useful approach for Ms. Lafferty? Outline at least one advantage and one limitation of using each method of time sampling listed above as a method for data collection.

(Q10) When planning for this intervention and using a DRO procedure, the unwanted behavior is put on extinction. How would you plan for the side effects of an extinction burst with Ms. Lafferty?

Additional Web Links
Differential reinforcement
http://iris.peabody.vanderbilt.edu/module/bi2/cresource/q4/p05/#content
Time sampling
https://my.vanderbilt.edu/specialeducationinduction/files/2013/07/DC.Time-Sampling.Sample.pdf

CASE: iii-I5

Big Changes for Bart, but Perhaps Little Value
Setting: Home   Age-Group: Preschool

LEARNING OBJECTIVE:

- Apply principles and processes of applied behavior analysis to support the development of socially mediated behavior in a youth with Asperger's Syndrome.

TASK LIST LINKS:

- **Fundamental Elements of Behavior Change**

  – (D-04) Use modeling and imitation training.
  – (D-05) Use shaping.
  – (D-06) Use chaining.
  – (D-09) Use the verbal operants as a basis for language assessment.
  – (D-13) Use intraverbal training.
  – (D-21) Use differential reinforcement (e.g., DRO, DRA, DRI, DRL, and DRH).

- **Specific Behavior-Change Procedures**

  – (E-03) Use instructions and rules.

- **Identification of the Problem**

  – (G-03) Conduct a preliminary assessment of the client in order to identify the referral problem.
  – (G-04) Explain behavioral concepts using nontechnical language.
  – (G-06) Provide behavior-analytic services in collaboration with others who support and/or provide services to one's clients.

- **Measurement**

  – (H-03) Select a data display that effectively communicates relevant quantitative relations.
  – (H-04) Evaluate changes in level, trend, and variability.
  – (H-05) Evaluate temporal relations between observed variables (within and between sessions, and time series).

- **Intervention**

  – (J-02) Identify potential interventions based on assessment results and the best available scientific evidence.
  – (J-11) Program for stimulus and response generalization.

  (J-14) Arrange instructional procedures to promote generative learning (i.e., derived relations).

KEY TERMS:

- **Chaining**

  - Chaining is a procedure within Applied Behavior Analysis (ABA) that can be used to teach a long sequence of behaviors (e.g., making a sandwich). The sequence of behaviors is broken down into smaller discrete behaviors, and each behavior is taught using prompting (to increase the likelihood of occurrence) and reinforcement (to increase the future frequency of the behavior). The discrete behaviors are then put together to form a "chain." When making a sandwich for examples, each step or behavior in the process would be taught (e.g., get a plate from the cupboard, put plate on counter, get the bread, etc...) until all of the steps involved are learned and the "chain" can be independently completed in proper sequence (Granpeesheh et al. 2009).

- **Generalization**

  - One of the defining characteristics of ABA is generality, meaning that a behavior change lasts over time and continues after an intervention has been withdrawn, occurs in environments in which training did not occur, and brings about changes in behaviors not targeted by an intervention (Baer et al. 1968, 1987). In most intervention programs, a behavior change is not considered mastered until evidence of generalization has been documented.

- **Imitation**

  - Imitation is any physical movement that evokes an imitative behavior that immediately follows, resembles, and is controlled by the modeled behavior. For example, a child watching a video and then immediately imitating the same behavior is being modeled in the video (Cooper et al. 2007).

- **Intraverbal Training**

  - An intraverbal occurs when a speaker differentially responds to the verbal behavior of others (Cooper et al. 2007), for example, answering the question "where do you live?" with the response "1234 Avenue Road," or providing a comment (a different comment than the comment that the speaker provides) on an item or an experience in response to hearing another's comments. Intraverbal training focuses on developing reciprocal verbal exchanges (e.g., the foundation of a conversation) by bringing one's verbal responses under the control of another's verbal behavior (e.g., Ingvarsson et al. 2007)

- **Verbal Behavior**

  - Verbal behavior has been defined by Skinner as "behavior that is reinforced through the mediation of another person's behavior" (Skinner 1957 in Sundberg and Michael 2001 p. 701). This can be differentiated from nonverbal behavior that is reinforced through direct contact with the physical environment (Sundberg and Michael, 2001). Within ABA, language is seen as a learned behavior, developed through the same principles and processes as nonlanguage behavior (e.g., reinforcement, punishment...).

Big Changes for Bart, But Perhaps of Little Value?

Eleven-year-old Bartholomew or Bart—or a range of other not-as-complimentary rhyming names used by his peers—was often called a "warrior" by his father. Although Bart's dad used this term in a kindly way, Bart really was a playground warrior, at least up until about midway through grade three, when his peers stopped tormenting him, and started ignoring him, instead, as they were drawn into mutually agreeable conversations about music trends, sports, and television shows, all of which was highly disinteresting to Bart. Over grade three and grade four, and past his eleventh lonely birthday with only his little brother Stewart around for company, Bart seemed to have fewer and fewer social interactions with his peers. His dad noticed this was also becoming true at home and, over the past several months, had been becoming increasingly concerned about Bart's social skills. When Bart got up in the morning, and when he returned home from school, he preferred to engage in solitary activities, with hardly a morose "Hi," before he disappeared into his bedroom to work on his complex engineering tasks. The most conversation he voluntarily elicited with his dad, these past six months or so, was to ask for a ride to the library so he could print his gears, gadgets, and other elements with their free 3D printer.

It was this almost complete lack of social interaction that brought Bart and his dad back to the ABA therapists. After a fruitless search for a business card that had been provided to him years ago when Bart was first diagnosed with an Autism Spectrum Disorder (at the time, called Pervasive Developmental Disorder-Not Otherwise Specified), Bart's dad went online and found the name of the service in the archives of his email. Not wanting to have a complex conversation by email, he picked up the phone, got in touch with the clinical coordinator of *Step-by-Step Disability Services*, and told them his story. By the time another week had passed, Bart and his dad had a late morning appointment to visit the clinic and start to work on his conversational skills. "It's unfortunate that we are only open during the day," said the therapist, "but I think you will find that learning conversational skills will support Bart in his school success, rather than taking away from his learning. It will be worth it! Let's start with appointments twice a week, in the mornings when our adolescent program is taking place, and then go from there. Bart will be back at school by recess time, and he can practice what we have learned together with his peers at school right away." After Bart's therapist completed a thorough assessment of Bart's **verbal behavior** and social skills, Bart's dad and his therapist agreed on the specific details of Bart's ABA program, and began.

After less than six weeks, Bart's dad was back on-site for a follow-up meeting. A little nervous, he waited in the child-sized waiting room until he was called into to meet with the obviously delighted therapist. "I am happy to report," she began, "that Bart has been doing wonderfully well in our sessions. Like you mentioned about his social behavior at home and at school, he was indeed quite quiet at the beginning. I think the best word I could use to describe him would have been "avoider." He was avoiding everything! But from the time that he discovered our electronics cache that we keep meaning to recycle, he has been nonstop talk. It has been quite easy to teach new behaviors using **imitation** and **chaining.** At the same time, we have been able to shape his behavior into not only answering questions within our goal of two sections, but also **intraverbal training** and engaging in three or more conversation turns with both the other therapists and his same age peers in our setting with appropriate amounts of information being shared. Unlike before, he is regularly initiating conversations, too. I have some data and graphs here to show you just how much his skills have improved. It is already time to set new goals." After looking at the visual depictions that Bart's therapist showed to his dad, and discussing and celebrating Bart's progress in the clinical setting, the conversation got a little harder. "What are you hearing about school? And what about home?" asked the therapist?

"In all honesty," replied Bart's dad, "home has been pretty status quo. And so has school. I have actually been pretty worried that you were going to tell me that nothing good has been going on at your sessions, either! So I am quite relieved, really, that you are seeing all sorts of new skills in Bart. I have been asking his teachers to watch him a little more closely when it comes to conversational skills, and they are telling me that he won't say much, even when other people approach him, he won't talk to anyone else first, and sometimes he even turns around and walks off while people are in the process of trying to get his attention. It's pretty frustrating."

This phrase was one that Bart's therapist used later that day, when debriefing with her clinical supervisor. "It's so frustrating!" she began. "I have done quite a few assessments, I have been tracking his skills, his growth, his mastery, and his movement toward independence, but he is only doing it here. Part of it is probably my fault. I thought it was too early to plan for **generalization** to different people and to different settings. I thought we would see some changes everywhere. It is important to pick behaviors so they are important and meaningful in everyday life far beyond the room where we train. So, what's wrong, and what's next? What's the key to success?"

The Response: Principles, Processes, Practices, and Reflections

Principles

(Q1) Use the attached list of specific behaviors identified by Bart's father as skills he would like to see Bart develop. Using the relevance of behavior rule as a guide, select two behaviors as priorities for an intervention program. Explain your selection (Table 5.4).

Table 5.4 List of specific behaviors Bart's dad would like him to acquire

Conversation skills	Initiating conversation
	The give and take of conversation
	Appropriately ending a conversation
	Conversing about things that are not special interests
Conflict resolution	Compromise
	Being open to other ideas (flexibility)
	Controlling emotions
Friendship skills	Nonverbal communication (reciprocating a smile)
	Keeping promises
	Being kind
	Being open to friendship

(Q2) For the behaviors selected in question 1, outline how, once mastered in a treatment setting, you would work to support Bart with the generalization of the behavior. How will you determine when mastery of the behavior has been achieved?

Processes

(Q3) Using the following article as a guide, select one of the training procedures to develop an outline of an intraverbal training program for one of the behaviors chosen for Bart. http://www.ncbi.nlm.nih.gov/pmc/articles/PMC3297336/
(Q4) Outline a systematic and progressive generalization process for the intraverbal program outlined in question #3.

Practice

(Q5) Why might there be differences in reports of Bart's program at home, in the treatment setting, and at school? How could you work with other individuals to promote communication and consistency between home, the treatment setting, and school?
(Q6) Provide a summary of the intraverbal training program, using nontechnical behavioral analytic terms that individuals in other settings can understand and apply with Bart (Fig. 5.5).
(Q7) Why is consistency between home, the treatment setting, and the school important for Bart's short-term and long-term progress? How might this consistency be measured? What indicators would suggest that consistency has been established and maintained over time?

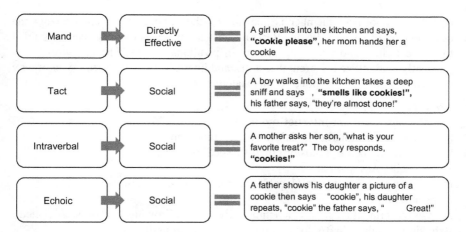

Fig. 5.5 The four verbal operants, the consequences to those operants and an example of each operant

Reflection

(Q8) Bart's father blames himself for some of Bart's difficulties. How might you respond to comments of this nature made by Bart's father?

(Q9) An applied behavior-analytic understanding of language development differs from other theories of language development that might emphasize biological and cognitive aspects before environmental. As a behavior consultant trained in a verbal behavior approach, how might you work collaboratively with others from other disciplines (e.g., speech and language therapist, cognitive psychologist, and developmental psychologist) to develop a single-supportive multidisciplinary team and program for Bart (Reference Ethics Box 5.5, Behavior Analyst Certification Board, 2014)?

Ethics Box 5.5

Professional and Ethical Compliance Code for Behavior Analysts

- 2.03 Consultation.

  (a) Behavior analysts arrange for appropriate consultations and referrals based principally on the best interests of their clients, with appropriate consent, and subject to other relevant considerations, including applicable law and contractual obligations.

  (b) When indicated and professionally appropriate, behavior analysts cooperate with other professionals in a manner that is consistent with the philosophical assumptions and principles of behavior analysis, in order to effectively and appropriately serve their clients.

(Q10) A school staff member is questioning the importance of emphasizing the development of social skills for Bart and, instead, believes that Bart can be guided toward activities and later employment in positions in which he can work independently, and utilize his strengths, skills, and interests. Do you agree? Why or why not? How would you respond to this statement?

Additional Web Links

Social skills—Autism internet modules

http://www.autisminternetmodules.org/user_mod.php

http://www.gov.pe.ca/photos/original/BldSocSkills_11.pdf

Social Skills Assessment

http://www.scaswebsite.com/docs/SST-resource-book-low.pdf

Generalization

http://www.erinoakkids.ca/getattachment/Resources/Growing-Up/Autism/Applied-Behaviour-Analysis/ABA-for-Families-Generalization.pdf.aspx

References

Alberto, P. A., & Troutman, A. C. (2006). *Applied behavior analysis for teachers* (7th ed.). Upper Saddle River, NJ: Pearson Education Inc.

Baer, D. M., Wolf, M. M., & Risley, T. R. (1968). Some current dimensions of applied behavior analysis. *Journal of Applied Behavior Analysis, 1*(1), 91–97. http://doi.org/10.1901/jaba.1968. 1-91

Baer, D. M., Wolf, M. M., & Risley, T. (1987). Some still-current dimensions of applied behavior analysis. *Journal of Applied Behavior Analysis, 20*, 313–327.

Behavior Analyst Certification Board (2014). *Professional and ethical compliance code for behavior analysts*. Retrieved from http://bacb.com/wp-content/uploads/2016/01/160120-compliance-code-english.pdf

Best Start Expert Panel on Early Learning. (2007). *Early learning for every child today: A framework for Ontario early childhood settings*. Retrieved from: https://www.edu.gov.on.ca/childcare/oelf/continuum/continuum.pdf#page=24

Bicard, S. C., Bicard, D. F., & The IRIS Center. (2012). *Measuring behavior*. Retrieved from https://iris.peabody.vanderbilt.edu/wp-content/uploads/pdf_case_studies/ics_measbeh.pdf

Cecchini, M. E. (2008). *Encouraging cooperative play*. Retrieved from http://www.earlychildhoodnews.com/earlychildhood/article_view.aspx?articleid=707

Cooper, J.O., Heron, T.E., & Heward, W.L. (2007). *Applied behavior analysis* (2nd ed.). Upper Saddle River, NJ: Pearson

Davis, A. (n.d.). *4 functions of behaviour*. Retrieved from: http://in1.ccio.co/sB/w2/OC/c0c8d6261e5bcbe325bc445c85518241.jpg

Dixon, M. R., Jackson, J. W., Small, S. L., Horner-King, M. J., Lik, N. M. K., Garcia, Y., et al. (2009). Creating single-subject design graphs in microsoft excel™ 2007. *Journal of Applied Behavior Analysis, 42*(2), 277–293.

Filter, K. J., & Nolan, J. D. (2012). A function-based classroom behavior intervention using non-contingent reinforcement plus response cost. *Education & Treatment of Children, 35*(3), 419+. Retrieved from: http://go.galegroup.com.ezpxy.fanshawec.ca/ps/i.do?id=GALE%7CA301649976&v=2.1&u=ko_acd_fc&it=r&p=AONE&sw=w&asid=9e8573f7e23c3536ef135d7b5b160258

Fryling, M. (2011). The impact of applied behavior analysis on the science of behavior. *Behavior and Social Issues, 19*, 24–31.

Granpeesheh, D., Tarbox, J., & Dixon, D. (2009). Applied behavior analytic interventions for children with autism: A description and review of treatment research. *Annals of Clinical Psychiatry, 21*(3), 162–173.

Ingvarsson, E., Tiger, J., Hanley, G., & Stephenson, K. (2007). An evaluation of intraverbal training to generate socially appropriate responses to novel questions. *Journal of Applied Behavior Analysis, 40*(3), 411–429.

Johnston, J., & Pennypacker, H. (1993). *Strategies and tactics for human behavioral research* (2nd ed.). Hillsdale, NJ: Erlbaum.

Kahng, S. W., Chung, K. M., Gutshall, K., Pitts, S. C., Kao, J., & Girolami, K. (2010). Consistent visual analyses of intrasubject data. *Journal of Applied Behavior Analysis, 43*(1), 35–45.

Kelly, M., Shillingsburg, M., Castro, M., Addison, L., & LaRue, R. (2007). Further evaluation of emerging speech in children with developmental disabilities: Training verbal behavior. *Journal of Applied Behavior Analysis, 40*(3), 431–445.

Mayer, G. R., Sulzer-Azaroff, B., & Wallace, M. (2014). *Behavior analysis for lasting change* (3rd ed.). Cornwall-on-Houston, NY: Sloan Publishing.

Mesibov, G., & Shea, V. (2011). Evidence-based practices and autism. *Autism, 15*(1), 114–133.

Skinner, B. F. (1957). *Verbal behavior*. New York: Appleton-Century-Crofts.

Springer, B., Brown, T., & Duncan, P. (1981). Current measurement in applied behavior analysis. *The Behavior Analyst, 4*(1), 19–31.

Sundberg, M., & Michael, J. (2001). The benefits of Skinner's analysis of verbal behavior for children with Autism. *Behavior Modification, 25*(5), 698–724.

Vladescu, J. C., & Kodak, T. (2010). A review of recent studies on differential reinforcement during skill acquisition in early intervention. *Journal of Applied Behavior Analysis, 43*(2), 351–355.

Chapter 6
Implementation-Based Case Studies from Adolescence to Adulthood

Abstract The current chapter explores the implementation of applied behavior analysis (ABA)-based interventions through the adolescent, adult, and senior stages of life. Throughout this chapter, technical considerations such as the selection of evidence-based behavior-change tactics, objective measurement systems, reliable interobserver agreement methods, and valid procedural integrity checks are highlighted. At the same time, the cases presented prompt readers to reflect on decisions often faced by behavior analysts such as the prioritization of behaviors identified for change, the extent to which programs should balance skill development with behavior reduction tactics, and when and how to utilize punishment procedures within ethical guidelines. This chapter also guides readers to consider the importance of involving adolescents, young adults, adults, and seniors in each stage of the behavior intervention implementation process. The value, benefits, challenges, and limitations of engagement in the planning, implementation, and evaluation stages of behavior programs are critically explored. Further, important ethical and clinical considerations, particularly for individuals with developmental disabilities or cognitive impairments, are highlighted throughout the cases presented. In this chapter, entitled "Implementation-Based Case Studies from Adolescence to Adulthood," technical, professional, and ethical considerations surrounding the implementation of ABA-based behavior-change programs are explored through five case scenarios in home, school, clinical, and community settings.

Keywords Adolescent · Adult · Seniors · Objective measurement systems · Interobserver agreement methods · Procedural identity checks · Skill development · Behavior reduction tactics · Ethical guidelines · Developmental disabilities · Cognitive impairment

CASE: iii-I6

Right, Wrong, or Different?
Setting: School   Age-Group: Adolescence

LEARNING OBJECTIVE:

- Critically assess the quality of behavior measurement.

TASK LIST LINKS:

- **Measurement**

  - (A-01) Measure frequency (i.e., count).
  - (A-06) Measure percent of occurrence.
  - (A-07) Measure trials to criterion.
  - (A-08) Assess and interpret interobserver agreement.
  - (A-09) Evaluate the accuracy and reliability of measurement procedures.
  - (A-10) Design, plot, and interpret data using equal-interval graphs.
  - (A-12) Design and implement continuous measurement procedures (e.g., event recording).

- **Fundamental Elements of Behavior Change**

  - (D-02) Use appropriate parameters and schedules of reinforcement.
  - (D-21) Use differential reinforcement (e.g., DRO, DRA, DRI, DRL, DRH).

- **Measurement**

  - (H-03) Select a data display that effectively communicates relevant quantitative relations.
  - (H-04) Evaluate changes in level, trend, and variability.

- **Intervention**

  - (J-01) State intervention goals in observable and measurable terms.
  - (J-02) Identify potential interventions based on assessment results and the best available scientific evidence.
  - (J-04) Select intervention strategies based on client preferences.
  - (J-10) When a behavior is to be decreased, select an acceptable alternative behavior to be established or increased.

- **Implementation, Management, and Supervision**

  - (K-03) Design and use competency-based training for persons who are responsible for carrying out behavioral assessment and behavior-change procedures.
  - (K-04) Design and use effective performance monitoring and reinforcement systems.
  - (K-05) Design and use systems for monitoring procedural integrity.

- (K-06) Provide supervision for behavior-change agents.
- (K-07) Evaluate the effectiveness of the behavioral program.

KEY TERMS:

- **Differential Reinforcement of Other Behavior**

  - Differential Reinforcement of Other Behavior occurs when reinforcement is delivered when a target behavior does not occur for a specified period of time (Simonsen et al. 2008).

- **Interobserver Agreement**

  - Interobserver agreement or reliability is the extent to which two or more individuals independently report the same values when observing the same behavioral event. In applied behavior analysis research and practice, high rate of agreement between independent observers is an indicator of quality measurement (Mudford et al. 2009).

- **Reinforcer**

  - A reinforcer is a consequence that follows a behavior that increases the future frequency of that behavior (Azrin et al. 2006).

- **Schedule of Reinforcement**

  - A schedule of reinforcement is a protocol that outlines how often reinforcement is delivered in relation to occurrences of target behaviors (Rasmussen and O'Neill 2006).

Right, Wrong, or Different?

The day began with the usual events. From inside the classroom, Mr. Helio could hear the seemingly far-flung sounds of 12-year-old Edgar—Gar—approaching the school's propped-open double doors to the outside. Not only was Gar identifiable by his growling talk and his high-pitched, almost hysterical giggle, but also by his nearly endless stream of profanity. Brief moments later, Gar burst through the classroom door itself, surrounded closely by his usual gang of adolescent boys and girls, tumbling to the floor and laughing as they tossed their knapsack, lunch bags, and boots aside to head to the class's "clubhouse." In the corner of the class sectioned off by two low bookcases and two well-worn couches, Gar's group sat, slouched, and laid out on the floor. As usual, Mr. Helio greeted each student and allowed them their transition time before the bell rang. He did his best to ignore the swearing—totally unacceptable in a school environment—but made sure that he headed over to the general vicinity of the disruptive group when the profanity got too loud, motioning with both of hands in what he thought was a pretty universal hands-down motion. Even though the profanity was just as bad as usual, Mr. Helio felt optimistic about how the day might go, he was hoping for better than usual!

Yesterday, Mr. Helio and the paraprofessional who spends most mornings in his classroom due to the high levels of disruptive behavior (which seemed to swirl in a vortex around Gar) met with the district's behavior consultant. Following a week of observations, a functional behavior assessment, and a meeting with their principal and Gar's foster parents, the consultant had sat them both down and asked them to complete an incredibly detailed list that she called a "preference survey" to figure out things Gar really likes and to rate each one as a potential reinforcer. She had told them both that she understands they know their student well, but that this form would help them to recall any ideas that might otherwise be missed. Next, she had explained to them what "frequency of behavior" meant, and gave them each a data sheet to complete for each period of the day. The definition of the target problem behavior had been defined at the top of the sheet as: "the audible utterance of any words considered to be profanity in the school setting." Mr. Helio and the paraprofessional agreed that they would each count and record the number of incidences of Gar's profanity each morning during each of the four periods of academic classes. "Apart from the actual collection of data," she had further explained "you are going to be implementing Differential Reinforcement of Other Behavior (DRO). Since the function of Gar's problem behavior is socially-mediated attention, your job is to give him lots of attention, praise, and these tokens for extra free time when he is doing anything —except swearing. If you have to give him any attention at all when he swearing—or right after—use as few words as possible, turn your body away, and don't make eye contact. Since he likes attention so much, any attention you give him at that point will actually make him swear more." Following a lengthy but productive discussion, they all departed for home, anticipating the events of the next classroom day.

Mr. Helio smiled widely as the paraprofessional entered the room—happily the same one he met with yesterday—and quickly gathered up their clipboards, data sheets, and pencils. In addition, he taped some pieces of masking tape onto the leg of his pants in order to easily count the frequency of the data quickly and wherever he was in the classroom, and the paraprofessional opened her relevant cell phone app. The cell phone app was the way that the paraprofessional collected data that worked for her! They were ready to go for their first day of data collection—and DRO!

Monday through Thursday (Friday was part of a long weekend) consisted of the two educators busily implementing DRO and collecting frequency data on Gar. Every time Mr. Helio heard profanity from him, he wrote a tally mark on his piece of masking tape on his leg and provided no attention or as little as possible. Each time the paraprofessional heard him swear, she clicked a tally mark on her cell phone app and gave him no attention or as little as possible. Each transferred the total number of tally marks to their separate data collection sheet at some point at the end of the period. The same paraprofessional was available all week, and neither Mr. Helio nor the paraprofessional missed filling in any of the information onto the data collection sheets. At the end of the short week, they were pretty pleased with themselves, scanned, and emailed off their data collection sheets as required by the consultant, and went home early as a special reward.

The following Monday, they met again with the behavioral consultant, with their neat stacks of four carefully penciled data collection sheets in tow. They sat at the behavior consultant's roundtable, anticipating some helpful feedback—and they were not disappointed! However, what she said was a little different than what they expected. On a legal-sized sheet of white paper, she presented a graph to them.

"This section," she said, "is my baseline observations. Remember that week where I was at the back of the classroom, observing every morning? You can see here that the frequency of profanity each morning is quite high, but it is also stable and level: it's about the same every day." "Now, this data path or line, with the triangles, is yours"—she pointed to the paraprofessional—"and the one with the circles is yours"—she pointed to Mr. Helio. "You can see the one line with the triangles is quite high. It's even higher than mine, by quite a bit. You can see that the other one is quite low. It's lower than mine, by quite a bit. It's good that both of them seem to be on a downwards path, which means the behavior is decreasing over time, but it doesn't tell us if our plan is working. What we want to see is what we call interobserver agreement (IOA), where the two of you collect data separately in the same situation, we want that data to tell us the same thing, and then, we will know if the behavior is truly decreasing! But right now, we are not really sure if much change is happening in the direction we want to see."

After another prolonged discussion, it became clear that the paraprofessional was counting each separate swear word as a separate tally mark, and the teacher was counting each time when she could hear Gar swearing as a tally mark, no matter how many times he said swear words together. Together, they rewrote their definition of profanity, and recreated a data plan for next week. Neither of the educators was right—nor wrong—just different.

The Response: Principles, Processes, Practices, and Reflections

Principles

(Q1) Interobserver agreement also has different words to describe the same concept. What other terms are used to describe this concept?

(Q2) From the case study, determine from the graph provided, what may be happening with the DRO procedure with regard to the reinforcement of other behaviors, not taking into the account the difference between educators? How may the behavior data differ if it was DRA or DRI procedures?

Processes

(Q3) Using the graph in Fig. 6.1 that the behavior consultant presented to the team, describe the level, trend, and variability from baseline to intervention.

(Q4) Based on the first-week difference in frequency of behaviors, it was clear that the operational definition of the behavior was not agreed upon to each individual and thus led to differences in the two professionals' count. Write an operational

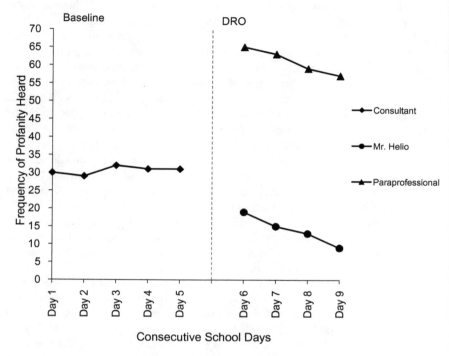

Fig. 6.1 Gar's profanity during his four-period school day

definition of the profanity that is clear for both parties. What else could be done before collecting data in the real environment to ensure both Mr. Helio and the paraprofessional are counting similar behaviors?

Practice

(Q5) Below are the IOA data from the paraprofessional and Mr. Helio. Calculate the percentage of interobserver agreement (Table 6.1).

(Q6) The data sheet for the frequency count for each period throughout the day is below. What else does the data tell you besides the difference in frequency counts across observers (Table 6.2)?

(Q7) Since Gars' behavior is reinforced by social attention, what other reinforcers could be used? What social reinforcers may be naturally occurring in the environment which may act as a confounding variable?

Table 6.1 Frequency data of Gar's profanity during each period of class time for four days during intervention phase by Mr. Helio and the paraprofessional

Day and period	Mr. Helio	Paraprofessional
Monday—Period 1	5	16
Monday—Period 2	6	17
Monday—Period 3	5	14
Monday—Period 4	3	18
Tuesday—Period 1	1	1
Tuesday—Period 2	8	19
Tuesday—Period 3	3	20
Tuesday—Period 4	3	23
Wednesday—Period 1	4	25
Wednesday—Period 2	4	22
Wednesday—Period 3	3	10
Wednesday—Period 4	2	2
Thursday—Period 1	3	21
Thursday—Period 2	0	0
Thursday—Period 3	3	17
Thursday—Period 4	3	19

Table 6.2 Four days of scatterplot data of Gar's use of profanity during class time at school

Half Hour Intervals	Period	Monday	Tuesday	Wednesday	Thursday
8:30 - 9:00 AM	Period 1				
9:00 - 9:30 AM					
9:30 - 10:00 AM					
10:00 - 10:30 AM	Period 2				
10:30 - 11:00 AM					
11:00 - 11:30 AM					
11:30 AM - 12:30 PM		Lunch Break – No teacher observation			
12:30 - 1:00 PM	Period 3				
1:00 - 1:30 PM					
1:30 - 2:00 PM					
2:30 - 3:00 PM	Period 4				
3:00 - 3:30 PM					
3:30 - 4:00 PM					

Reflection

(Q8) What could you have done differently before implementing the procedure to ensure that the two professionals were collecting data on the same behaviors?

(Q9) Do you think the DRO schedule of reinforcement is the most suitable for Gar when his behavior is attention driven? Would you consider using other schedules of reinforcement such as DRI, DRA, or DRL?[1]

---

[1]**see Fig. 3.4 for definitions of each procedure

(Q10) How could you include Gar on this discussion and the design and implementation of his behavior program? What benefits or downfalls do you see with this approach?

Additional Web Links
Differential Reinforcement
http://www.appliedbehavioralstrategies.com/reinforcement-101.html
Interobserver Agreement
http://www.ncbi.nlm.nih.gov/pmc/articles/PMC3357100/
Preference Assessments
http://www.asatonline.org/research-treatment/clinical-corner/conducting-preference-assessments-with-individuals-with-autism/

CASE: iii-I7

He Just Needs to Learn a Lesson
Setting: School Age-Group: Adolescence

LEARNING OBJECTIVE:

- Understand the principles of punishment and overcorrection.

TASK LIST LINKS:

- **Behavior-Change Considerations**

  – (C-02) State and plan for the possible unwanted effects of punishment.

- **Fundamental Elements of Behavior Change**

  – (D-15) Identify punishers.
  – (D-16) Use positive and negative punishment.
  – (D-17) Use appropriate parameters and schedules of punishment.
  – (D-18) Use extinction.
  – (D-19) Use combinations of reinforcement with punishment and extinction.

- **Implementation, Management, and Supervision**

- (K-03) Design and use competency-based training for persons who are responsible for carrying out behavioral assessment and behavior-change procedures.
- (K-05) Design and use systems for monitoring procedural integrity.
- (K-06) Provide supervision for behavior-change agents.
- (K-07) Evaluate the effectiveness of the behavioral program.

KEY TERMS:

- **Overcorrection**
    - Overcorrection is a form of punishment in which, following a display of problem behavior, an individual is asked to engage in behaviors that fix the damage caused by the problem behavior (Anderson and Le 2011).

- **Procedural Drift**
    - Procedural drift occurs when those implementing a behavior-change program, begin to stray from the detailed program instructions (Vollmer et al. 2008).

- **Restitutional Overcorrection**
    - Restitutional overcorrection is a form of punishment in which the individual, following a display of problem behavior, must bring the environment to a state better than it was before the problem behavior occurred (McAdams and Knapp 2013).

Jerry Just Needs to Learn a Lesson

MONDAY

"Seriously? Again?" was the principal's immediate reaction when the on-site police officer approached him first thing in the morning. In fact, the officer was waiting by his door as he entered the school at 7:30 AM. Although this was a fairly common site, her heart fell, as she immediately guessed what it was regarding. Yet again, Jerry, their perpetual grade nine student, had been causing a fuss.

Opening her door and taking off her coat, the principal motioned for the officer to sit with her at her consultation table. "Tell me," she said with a concerned sigh and a downturned mouth.

"One of the neighbors found Jerry around 1:00 AM. He was spray-painting 'School Sucks' on the brick wall around the back entrance. As you probably saw, it's still there, and you know as well as I do that there is going to be quite a fuss about it today when the other students see it. I suspect Jerry—if he is even here—will be getting more than one high-five from the others." The officer stood to take care of his other school responsibilities: "I will leave this with you. We haven't been able to find his parents yet—I think his dad works the night shift. I will see you later today, no doubt."

The principal wrote the main points on the sticky note and sent an email for the itinerant behavior specialist assigned to her school and two other high schools, requesting her to switch up her schedule and head into their school this morning. She tapped a red flag onto the email and sent it on its way. Next, she called the maintenance staff to put in a priority request to have the Jerry's handiwork—no doubt very artistic—scrubbed off the wall. Thirdly, she walked to the back of the school herself to check out the graffiti first-hand, noting happily that which Jerry likes to mistakenly call "street art" was limited (this time) to a small section of the wall.

By the time she was on her way back to the front office area of the school, she was already being paged to meet with the behavior specialist. After a necessarily prolonged conversation, the specialist was dispatched to meet up with Jerry's parents, and the principal was ready to talk to Jerry, who was surprisingly in attendance that day. With the notes for a preliminary program plan in hand, the principal found Jerry outside of an obviously unsuccessful poetry class, leaning against the wall in the school hallway, busily engaged in his handheld game, pretending to ignore her presence. "Jerry," she intoned, "I know you can hear me, I know you can understand me, and I know that you know why I am here." She paused, and Jerry responded with no more than a sarcasm-ridden snort. "I have unfortunately already started our maintenance staff on the thankless job of cleaning up your early-morning mess, but from now on, the agreement is going to be that you clean up whatever mess you make—even if it's here at the school—and in fact you get to clean the whole wall or other area of whatever mess you make. I already have a support from your father in the form of an email that he is in full support of our plans. It would be great if you can keep your vandalism away from the school, or maybe stop it altogether."

She remembers that the behavior specialist spoke about punishment, as that is what the family and the others involved had wanted. She indicated that we would also look at behaviors we wanted to reinforce and increase, besides this behavior we wanted to decrease. She talked about implementing **overcorrection**, since that seemed to be a socially valid approach for the community and was common, especially engaging in **restitutional overcorrection**. Her notes for the behavior specialist were as follows:

TUESDAY
I received a call from home economics class that Jerry drew male genitalia on the cupboards using icing. I asked the teacher to tell Jerry to wash off the icing and also the front of the cupboard.

WEDNESDAY
I received a call from math class that Jerry drew algebraic equations (incorrectly) on the top of his desk with nail polish borrowed from a girl across the aisle. I asked the teacher to tell Jerry to scrape off the nail polish and also clean the inside and outside of the desk with a cloth from the maintenance staff.

THURSDAY
The police officer told me they found more graffiti outside, and they were pretty sure it is Jerry's tag, but nobody caught him doing it. The secretary told me Jerry filled some of staff mailboxes with shredded paper from the recycling bin. I told her to order Jerry to clean it out, also to take the contents of her paper shredder out to the recycling bin and then take the recycling bin out for collection.

FRIDAY
Jerry was absent.

MONDAY
Our music class teacher called me down to the choir room. During class, Jerry snuck into the instrumental music room and snapped all the woodwind reeds in half. I directed Jerry to pick them up and put them in the garbage, and showed him how to fit new ones into the woodwinds. I also showed him how to clean out the mouthpieces from the brass instruments and required him to clean them all before he went back to class.

TUESDAY
Jerry was on a class trip.

WEDNESDAY
I received the news that Jerry spent the whole trip the previous day spreading litter around the environment from his lunch, from garbage bins, from a tissue package in his pocket. When Jerry arrived this morning, I directed him to collect all the classroom and bathroom garbage cans from the whole school and put their contents into the dumpster outside. **NOTE TO SELF:** *Meeting with the behavior specialist, Jerry, and his father tomorrow after school. What are we going to do next? I think he just needs to learn a lesson, but he really doesn't seem to be getting it.*

The behavior therapist received the notes prior to the scheduled meeting and starts to see a pattern. She wonders to herself whether this is a result of **procedural drift**?

The Response: Principles, Processes, Practices, and Reflections

Principles

(Q1) Describe the overcorrection procedures that occurred for each day (Fig. 6.2).
(Q2) In this instance, the behavior specialist implemented punishment procedures. Was this positive or negative punishment? Why?

Processes

(Q3) How would you explain these punishment procedures to the staff that are implementing them? How would you ensure that they are implementing them correctly? What other safeguards do you need to put in place?
(Q4) What other data could be collected to record Jerry's behavior? What information would it provide?

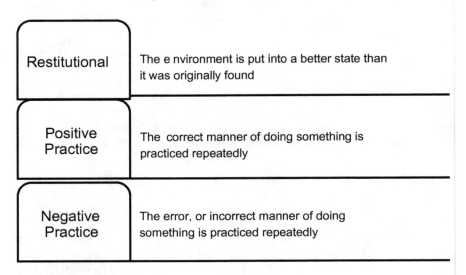

Fig. 6.2 Overcorrection procedures

Practice

(Q5) Using the ABC chart below, indicate the antecedents, behaviors, and consequences for each instance of the behavior that Jerry completed. Tuesday is done for you. What seems to be the possible function(s) of the behavior (Table 6.3)?

(Q6) Culminating the information from the above chart, does the punishment seem to be working? Why or why not?

(Q7) When using a punishment procedure, it is vital to include a reinforcement system. Why is this so? What reinforcement system(s) would you implement with the punishment procedures to ensure that other behaviors are also being increased simultaneously? Why?

Table 6.3 Antecedent–Behavior–Consequence data sheet

Setting	Antecedent	Behavior	Consequence
Home economics	• Jerry had no cake pan • Teacher was supporting another group of students	• Drew male genitalia across a set of cupboards	• Peers laughed and gave him high-fives • Jerry washed the icing off the cupboards and then washed the cupboard doors with soap and water

Reflection

(Q8) Would you have implemented this punishment strategy with Jerry? Do you agree with the behavior analyst? Would you have tried other strategies first? If so, what strategies would you implement?

(Q9) List three potential side effects of punishment and indicate whether you see any of these side effects with Jerry's behavior.

(Q10) Do you see any ethical difficulties with the way that this behavior specialist implemented the punishment procedures according to the Professional and Ethical Compliance Code for Behavior Analysts (2014) (Reference Ethics Box 6.1)?

Ethics Box 6.1

Professional and Ethical Compliance Code for Behavior Analysts

- 4.08 Considerations Regarding Punishment Procedures.

  (a) Behavior analysts recommend reinforcement rather than punishment whenever possible.

  (b) If punishment procedures are necessary, behavior analysts always include reinforcement procedures for alternative behavior in the behavior-change program.

  (c) Before implementing punishment-based procedures, behavior analysts ensure that appropriate steps have been taken to implement reinforcement-based procedures unless the severity of dangerousness of the behavior necessitates immediate use of aversive procedures.

  (d) Behavior analysts ensure that aversive procedures are accompanied by an increased level of training, supervision, and oversight. Behavior analysts must evaluate the effectiveness of aversive procedures in a timely manner and modify the behavior-change program if it is ineffective. Behavior analysts always include a plan to discontinue the use of aversive procedures when no longer needed.

Additional Web Links

Overcorrection and Positive Practice

http://165.139.150.129/intervention/Overcorrection.pdf

Difficulties with Punishment

http://stophurtingkids.com/wp-content/uploads/2013/05/Views-on-the-Efficacy-and-Ethics-of-Punishment-Results-from-a-National-Survey.pdf

Punishment and Extinction

http://www.ncbi.nlm.nih.gov/pmc/articles/PMC1224409/

CASE: iii-I8 Guest Author: Drew MacNamara

"It's just too time-consuming. I'm pretty sure that things are getting better. Is that enough?"

Setting: Community Age-Group: Adult

GUEST CASE: Drew MacNamara

LEARNING OBJECTIVE:

– Implementation of a high-probability request sequence with prompts and a visual schedule.

TASK LIST LINKS:

- **Measurement**

    – (A-01) Measure frequency (i.e., count).
    – (A-02) Measure rate (i.e., count per unit time).
    – (A-03) Measure duration.
    – (A-04) Measure latency.
    – (A-09) Evaluate the accuracy and reliability of measurement procedures.
    – (A-12) Design and implement continuous measurement procedures (e.g., event recording).
    – (A-13) Design and implement discontinuous measurement procedures (e.g., partial and whole interval, and momentary time sampling).

- **Fundamental Elements of Behavior Change**

    – (D-03) Use prompts and prompt fading.
    – (D-07) Conduct task analyses.
    – (D-20) Use response-independent (time-based) schedules of reinforcement (i.e., noncontingent reinforcement).

- **Specific Behavior-Change Procedure**

    – (E-09) Arrange high-probability request sequences.
    – (E-10) Use the Premack principle.

- **Behavior-Change Systems**

    – (F-01) Use self-management strategies.

- **Assessment**

    – (I-07) Design and conduct preference assessments to identify putative reinforcers

KEY TERMS:

- **High-Probability Request Sequence**

  – A behavioral principle based on the concept of momentum, whereby a behavior persists with a change in reinforcement schedule. A series of requests are given that have a high probability of a correct response, followed by a low-probability request to maintain the momentum and increase the likelihood of a correct response to the low-probability request (Houlihan et al. 1994).

- **Premack Principle**

  – The principle that a high-rate behavior can be used to reinforce a low-rate behavior when the reinforcer is contingent upon that behavior. For example, a student may be reinforced for a low-rate behavior of doing homework with an opportunity to go out with friends afterward (Klatt and Morris 2001).

- **Prompt**

  – A cue that guides the learner to engage in expected, or appropriate behavior that is given between the antecedent and discriminative stimulus before the behavior occurs (MacDuff et al. 2001).

- **Reinforcer Survey**

  – A list of potential reinforcers that is given to the individual for self-report or to the caregiver to determine the client's preferences. These preferences are then used as reinforcers. It is well known for its ease and efficiency in administration (Northup 2000).

It's Just Too Time-consuming. I'm Pretty Sure That Things Are Getting Better. Is That Enough?

Friday morning at 7:00 A.M. Tom, a staff person on the day shift, knocks on the door and says," You need to hurry Hadeel. You are going to miss your bus to the college." Hadeel angrily replies, "I know, I know. Stop bugging me." Fifteen minutes goes by and Hadeel still has not appeared to have for breakfast. Tom returns to Hadeel's room and through the door says, "Please hurry Hadeel so you can have your breakfast in time to catch the bus." Hadeel replies, "I'm coming, I'm coming. Just leave me alone!" And so goes another weekday morning.

Hadeel is a 20-year-old woman with an intellectual disability. She is in the process of moving from a supervised residential setting to an assisted living apartment. Hadeel is quite independent with her activities of daily living, and she requires consistent but not intense support to ensure she completes her daily routines. The staff in the residential setting reported that Hadeel is noncompliant to daily requests. Fatima, a behavior consultant, had put in place an intervention to improve compliance by having the staff **prompt** responding and then provide reinforcement when Hadeel does complete the requested tasks. The residential staff are not consistently completing the data collection procedures, saying it is too time-consuming on top of all the other demands that they face each day.

The behavior consultant called a meeting with a group of residential staff. During the meeting, one staff member Amy, who spends the most time with Hadeel, says that she has noticed that when she follows Hadeel's lead and joins her in an activity that she really enjoys, Hadeel is more likely to follow her directions after the activity. Amy goes on to say," it is almost as if she becomes motivated to do what I ask just so that I will keep spending positive time with her."

Based on this latest information, Fatima is *thinking* there is a **high-probability request sequence** occurring. Fatima decides to conduct a new functional behavior assessment. She asks the staff to record the activities that Hadeel completes in response to a staff request, the activities that she does not start completing in response to a staff request within 3 min of the demand, and, most importantly, the activities that Hadeel enjoys completing on her own or with staff. In addition, Fatima asks Amy, who has a good relationship with Hadeel, to assist Hadeel in completing a **reinforcer survey**. To assist with this data collection, Fatima develops a checklist that contains all the tasks that Hadeel is required to complete. Next to the tasks is an area where staff can place a checkmark if completes willingly or with a protest or refusal. Finally, there is an area where staff members are instructed to record Hadeel's preferred activities. With this checklist, the staff can check off everyday tasks and quickly record preferred tasks resulting in a much less time-consuming data collection process. Fatima will also visit the residence for the first three mornings of the week as mornings seem to be most problematic.

Monday evening at 7:00 P.M. Hadeel and Amy are in the kitchen of the residence just finishing the dishes. Amy says, "Hadeel, do you have some time now? I just wanted to ask you some questions about things that you like to do. Could we go to your room and talk about this?" To assist with the process, Amy has put together a list composed of activities that she has done with Hadeel and she has seen Hadeel enjoy on her own. The activities that Hadeel identifies include cooking with Amy, enjoying a cup of coffee with staff, going to the movies, going for a walk to a nearby park, and playing board games with other residents and staff.

Fatima visits on the next three weekday mornings. She notices that there is only one staff present in the mornings to assist residents and it seems that there is no consistency in the schedule of activities. The other three residents of the home seem to be able to manage their routines independently and get to their activities in the community on time. It seems that Hadeel is the only resident who is struggling. Fatima also notices that the staff seem to be able to reliably record the data using the new system.

Fatima meets with the staff on Friday afternoon to review the results of their investigations. The staff report that indeed it was much easier to record the data using a checklist and they began to take better notes of the activities that Hadeel enjoyed. Fatima also shared her observations with the staff. She noted that the other three residents seemed to be able to get themselves up and out the door with minimal assistance. On the other hand, Hadeel seemed to require numerous prompts to help her through her routine. Due to the need for so many prompts, there was a little time or opportunity to engage in reinforcing activities with Hadeel.

Fatima had several suggestions for the staff. First of all, she suggested that they sit down with Hadeel to develop a morning schedule with her. Once this schedule that consisted of words and pictures had been developed, it could be posted in Hadeel's room and in other relevant areas of the house. The schedule would consist of the activities that Hadeel needed to complete in the morning (e.g., get out of bed on time, get dressed, have breakfast) and the completion of these activities would be followed by the opportunity to engage in a special activity (e.g., enjoy a cup of coffee with staff before heading out of the house or onto the daily events). Fatima explained that the visual schedule would be a reminder for Hadeel of the things that she needed to complete in the morning and would utilize the **Premack principle** by the completion of the less preferred activities would be followed by the opportunity to engage in a preferred activity. Further, since Hadeel seemed to enjoy activities with others, completion of other less preferred activities across the day could be followed by any of the preferred activities that Hadeel had identified during the reinforcer survey. Fatima suggested that they begin with the morning routine only and then gradually integrate the intervention into other parts of the day. The staff all agreed with the plan and would put it into action the following week.

Amy agreed to work on the weekend before the plan was to be implemented in order to develop the visual schedule with Hadeel and explain the plan to her. Amy enthusiastically agreed that getting up on time, getting dressed, and having breakfast in time to be ready for the bus were certainly worth the cup of coffee with staff. They selected pictures from one of Hadeel's favorite magazines to represent these tasks, including the coffee time, and together they printed the words on the visual schedule. They posted the schedule in three prevalent areas in house. Amy told Hadeel that she would be in on Monday morning to help start the new routine.

Monday morning at 7:00 A.M. Amy knocked on Hadeel's door, "Hadeel, are you up?" "I'm coming, I'm coming," Hadeel angrily replied. "Don't forget your schedule. I will get the coffee ready," responded Amy. Thirty minutes later Hadeel appeared. She was dressed and ready for breakfast. And together, Hadeel and Amy enjoyed a cup of coffee. The next few mornings went fairly smoothly with only one occurrence of Hadeel missing her bus. By the next week, Hadeel was getting through her morning routine with only the use of the visual schedule. Staff then started to implement the strategy across Hadeel's day. After a month went by, the morning routine was no longer an issue and compliance with other requests has increased significantly.

At a month-end staff meeting, Fatima reviews the progress made. The staff report their concerns about Hadeel's compliance and that she and the other residents and staff are spending a lot of social positive time together. Fatima outlined that the data have been collected much more consistently and praised the staff for the effective implementation of the strategy. The staff commented that the use of a checklist was much more efficient and gave them time to attend to Hadeel and the other residents and to, more importantly, effectively implement the procedure.

The Response: Principles, Processes, Practices, and Reflections

Principles

(Q1) Based on the definition of the Premack principle, indicate these components of Hadeel's program:

– Low-probability event and
– High-probability event.

(Q2) Indicate the types of prompts that were used in the program with Hadeel. Which were stimulus prompts and which were response prompts?

Processes

(Q3) To implement the visual schedule, usually a task analysis of the person's required behavior is needed to determine the schedule. Then, the visual schedule needs to be taught. Write a task analysis for Hadeel's morning routine and indicate the teaching procedures for teaching the visual schedule (Fig. 6.3).

(Q4) Indicate how you would teach the Premack principle to Hadeel. How would you let her know what expectations are required before obtaining the reinforcer? What behaviors are required to gain access and not gain access to the reinforcers?

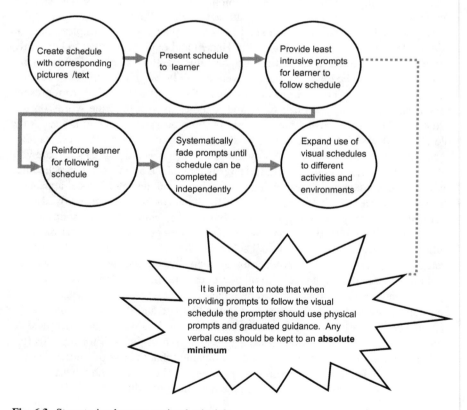

Fig. 6.3 Steps to implemente a visual schedule

Practice

(Q5) Using the checklist below that Hadeel's staff completed, determine how you would graph these data? Why (Table 6.4)?

(Q6) Given the prompts that were used in the scenario, which prompt hierarchy would you use to teach Hadeel—most-to-least or least-to-most. Read the following article before making your decision (Table 6.5):

Table 6.4 Data from first three weeks of Hadeel's morning routine. Each task has seven opportunities to occur independently (without reminders) unless noted. The data below are the sum of each day's occurrences

Task	Number of times completed independently Week 1	Number of times completed independently Week 2	Number of times completed independently Week 3
Gets out of bed	4	6	7
Gets dressed	3	5	6
Gets breakfast	5	5	7
Eats prepared breakfast—alone	0 (2 opportunities)	1 (2 opportunities)	2 (2 opportunities)
Eats prepared breakfast—with others	3 (5 opportunities)	4 (5 opportunities)	5 (5 opportunities)
Brushes teeth	3	4	6
Does hair	2	6	7
Goes to bus stop	1 (5 opportunities)	3 (5 opportunities)	4 (5 opportunities)
Participates in house activity	1 (2 opportunities)	1 (2 opportunities)	2 (2 opportunities)

Table 6.5 Functional assessment summary statement/hypothesis (Maryland State Department of Education, n.d.)

Meets expectations	Partially Meets expectations	Does Not Meet expectations
Good	Fair	Poor
A summary statement is provided, including a hypothesis and all of the following components: • antecedents • behavior • function • setting events	A summary statement is provided, including two of the following components: • antecedents • behavior • function • setting events	A summary statement is provided, including one or none of the following components: • antecedents • behavior • function • setting events Or, a summary statement is not provided

• **Antecedents** are immediate triggers of the behavior.
• The **function** of the behavior is what the student is trying to get/obtain or escape/avoid
• **Setting events** for the behavior are environmental, physical, instructional, or interpersonal factors that may influence how likely it is that the behavior will occur

Strengths	**Needs Improvement**

http://www.ncbi.nlm.nih.gov/pmc/articles/PMC2846579/

(Q7) Based on the case study, what is the function of Hadeel's behavior? Complete the hypothesis statement based on the following guidelines (Table 6.5):

Reflection

(Q8) At first, the staff had difficulties completing the behavior program as determined by the behavior consultant. The data collection sheet was made easier to assist with this. What other factors would you have implemented to assist with staff adherence to the program?

(Q9) The visual schedule has worked nicely for Hadeel to complete her morning routine. List three ways that the staff could generalize this to other parts of Hadeel's life and three ways that the visual prompts of the schedule could be faded.

(Q10) What are two advantages and two disadvantages of implementing a reinforcer survey? What alternatives could have been used?

Additional Web Links
Visual Schedules
http://praacticalaac.org/strategy/ideas-for-teaching-the-use-of-visual-schedules/
Premack Principle
http://study.com/academy/lesson/applying-the-premack-principle-in-the-classroom.html
Task Analyses
http://www.iidc.indiana.edu/pages/Applied-Behavior-Analysis
Least-to-Most Prompting
http://www.autisminternetmodules.org/up_doc/PromptsLeasttoMostSteps.pdf
Instruction Plans
http://mast.ecu.edu/modules/sip/concept/

CASE: iii-I9

It only happens to Sophia when these people are here!
Setting: Community   Age-Group: Adult

LEARNING OBJECTIVE:

- Determine the behaviors under stimulus control.

TASK LIST LINKS

- **Measurement**

  – (A-14) Design and implement choice measures.

- **Fundamental Elements of Behavior Change**

  - (D-14) Use listener training.
  - (D-20) Use response-independent (time-based) schedules of reinforcement (i.e., noncontingent reinforcement).

- **Specific Behavior-Change Procedures**

  - (E-01) Use interventions based on manipulation of antecedents, such as motivating operations and discriminative stimuli.
  - (E-02) Use discrimination training procedures.
  - (E-07) Plan for behavioral contrast effects.

- **Intervention**

  - (J-06) Select intervention strategies based on supporting environments.
  - (J-07) Select intervention strategies based on environmental and resource constraints.
  - (J-08) Select intervention strategies based on the social validity of the intervention.

- **Implementation, Management, and Supervision**

  - (K-01) Provide for ongoing documentation of behavioral services.
  - (K-02) Identify the contingencies governing the behavior of those responsible for carrying out behavior-change procedures and design interventions accordingly.
  - (K-05) Design and use systems for monitoring procedural integrity.
  - (K-06) Provide supervision for behavior-change agents.
  - (K-07) Evaluate the effectiveness of the behavioral program.
  - (K-09) Secure the support of others to maintain the client's behavioral repertoires in their natural environments.

KEY TERMS:

- **Antecedent Stimulus**

  - An antecedent is a stimulus that occurs before a target behavior. Antecedent stimuli cue an individual to display learned behaviors, based on that individual's history of reinforcement in the presence of that stimuli (Travis and Sturmey 2013).

- **Discriminative Stimulus**

  - A discriminative stimulus is a stimulus that signals to a learner that particular behavioral responses are likely to be reinforced (Cooper et al. 2007).

- **Stimulus Control**

  - Stimulus control is when an individual displays certain behaviors in the presence of certain stimuli and not in the absence of those stimuli (Green 2001).

It Only Happens to Sophia When These People Are Here!

The staff at Seven Pines try hard to maintain a family home-like setting in their residential care home. With a five-bedroom rambling ranch home, a beautifully treed outdoor space, and a huge family room for everyone to gather in regularly, it is not hard for the lived environment to be a success for their full-time, live-in adult clients with varied needs. Most importantly, however, is the personal attention they are able to pay to their clients. With an interdisciplinary team at their service on an as-needed basis, and at least two staff members on-site daily, they know their clients well. With a full year's worth of half-day professional development sessions on behavior strategies focused on proactive teaching combined with the prevention of potentially disruptive behaviors, the staff feels ready for almost everything, and enjoy their weekly meetings with the behavior consultant assigned to Seven Pines.

This week, the staff brought a concern about 50-year-old Sophia to the behavior consultant. One staff member started with some very recent history. "Sophia has recently been to a routine medical appointment for her yearly check-up," she began, "and the physician pronounced her with what she called 'prediabetic.'" She did not give her any additional medications but said she is strongly suggesting careful dietary planning, a 25-pound weight loss, and regular exercise. She actually wrote it down on her prescription pad, so I think she was pretty serious. As well, she asked us to monitor Sophia's blood glucose before and after meals and again before bedtime. As Sophia ages, she said, it becomes even more important to take care of her health proactively and to transition her carefully into a new routine respectfully, being sure to account for her Autism Spectrum Disorder. This is just like we talk about with the everyday routines of our group home," she compared. The other staff member continued the conversation. "We have been observing Sophia and collecting data so we have a steady baseline of eating habits, exercise, and weight. As you know, Sophia eats our evening meal with everyone else, and these are carefully monitored by our dietician and typically cooked by the staff along with the residents. Sophia only deviates from this pattern when it comes to takeout food. She chooses, prepares, and cooks her own breakfasts, lunch, and snacks with minimal supervision and has a lot of choice from what we stock in our fridge and pantry. We have sufficient data to show what's happening. What do you suggest we do next?"

The behavior consultant listened, took notes, and examined the data and graphs. "Let's try to structure choice a bit more. How about we cut down on the junk food that is in the pantry. I see that Sophia likes salty treats like potato chips, so let's stock up on healthy alternatives. In other words, decreasing the presence of unhealthy snacks, and increase the presence of healthy ones. Let's meet together next week and see if there is any change in the data, especially snacking patterns and blood glucose levels."

One week later, they gathered together again—this time also including the dietician—to see how things were going with this initial intervention. While they reviewed the data, they noted that a few changes were evident. First, the majority of the time Sophia seemed quite happy to choose from the healthy snacks the dietician had suggested. Her snacking frequency remained the same but her intake was healthier. When they pulled out her blood glucose records, the dietician raised one brow. "What's this?" she inquired. "Here, here, and here, her blood glucose levels have risen quite dramatically after supper. Can you see any patterns in her behavior at that time?" Interestingly, a review of Sophia's eating patterns and the activity notes accompanying them showed that her family members were visiting at these three times—only these three times. It was also noted that Sophia had asked staff members for chips, chocolate, and dessert after her family had left. While her family was visiting on the first occasion, they ate pizza, chicken fingers, and brownies while they gathered together in the kitchen for board games. And that was only one example. The other family visits had similar patterns of food intake.

"This is fascinating," said the one staff member. "We generally give our clients a great deal of privacy with family visits and we have never had a reason to monitor what Sophia was eating or doing at these times. This certainly shows why data—and not assumptions—is important in making programming decisions."

"I agree," the behavior consultant responded. "Since we are all trained here, I can use some behavioral language. It looks like takeout food is acting as the **discriminative stimulus** (S^D) for requesting junk food. Takeout food is leading to junk food, and this behavior is under **stimulus control**. Sophia doesn't seem to request junk food at all if it's not in front of her (or hasn't just been eaten). If it's not in sight, the **antecedent stimulus** is not present, and it seems to be out of mind, speaking more colloquially. A second problem that seems to be in front of us is with **procedural adherence**. If you will remember, when we spoke with Sophia's parents, they were totally on board with the plans for healthy living, as I thought they would be. But either they didn't think this extended to their visits, or they don't think that this kind of eating is detrimental for Sophia. Also, I noticed her brother was here during one of these visits. Did we even talk to extended family—or did we just assume that the parents would do this? We have a bit of work to do, moving forward. Let's try and get everyone fully invested with dietary planning, and then let's talk about starting some daily exercise. We want to make slow and sustainable changes to keep Sophia healthy and even healthier as time passes. She needs everyone's support."

The Response: Principles, Processes, Practices, and Reflections

Principles

(**Q1**) Indicate the behaviors under stimulus control and how they have been reinforced in the past.

(**Q2**) Indicate the SD and the S Delta in the current situation (Fig. 6.4).

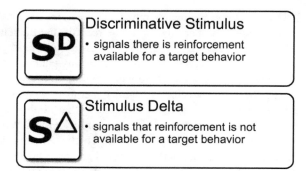

Fig. 6.4 The difference between SD and S Delta

Processes

(Q3) Examining the graph that the behavior consultant examined, what components are missing (Fig. 6.5)?

(Q4) What type of self-management strategy could be used with Sophia? Determine a treatment plan for Sophia to self-monitor her food intake and/or blood glucose level (Reference Ethics Box 6.2, Behavior Analyst Certification Board, 2014).

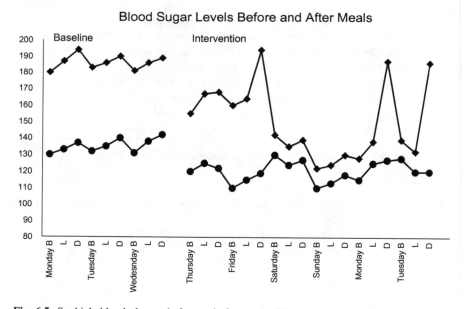

Fig. 6.5 Sophia's blood glucose before and after meals. What elements are missing?

Ethics Box 6.2

Professional and Ethical Compliance Code for Behavior Analysts

- 4.03 Individualized Behavior-Change Programs.
  (a) Behavior analysts must tailor behavior-change programs to the unique behaviors, environmental variables, assessment results, and goals of each client.
  (b) Behavior analysts do not plagiarize other professionals' behavior-change programs.

Practice

(Q5) List all of the potential antecedent stimuli in Sophia's environment? What other antecedent manipulations could you complete in order to help Sophia with her diet and blood glucose levels?

(Q6) It has been demonstrated that also including a differential reinforcement system can help strengthen stimulus control. What differential reinforcement strategies could you implement and how would you design these?

(Q7) Looking at the data below after the family was informed about Sophia's diet changes, what trends and patterns do you see? Is there any additional hypothesis or interventions you would implement to offset these (Fig. 6.6)?

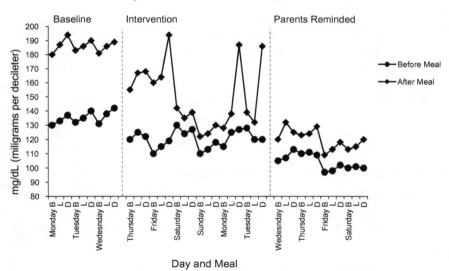

Fig. 6.6 Sophia's blood glucose levels over baseline, intervention, and when her parents were reminded of the importance of her eating habits

Reflection

(Q8) Why may Sophia's parents and other family members have difficulty with adhering to Sophia's diet? What could you do to assist them?

(Q9) When working with adults and behavior programs that involve food, there is sometimes ethical concerns about restricting food since many adults with health concerns do not have their food restricted. How do you feel about restricting Sophia's food in this situation? Are there alternative strategies?

(Q10) How could Sophia be involved in this treatment plan and the decisions regarding her diet and prediabetic condition?

Additional Web Links
SD and S Delta
http://www.educateautism.com/applied-behaviour-analysis/discriminative-stimulus-and-stimulus-delta.html
Self-Management
http://www.iidc.indiana.edu/pages/Dont-Forget-About-Self-Management
Components of Single-Subject Line Graphs
http://www.kipbs.org/new_kipbs/fsi/files/graphingtips.pdf

CASE: iii-I10

I wish Hilde could just tell us!
Setting: Home   Age-Group: Adult

LEARNING OBJECTIVE:

- To design a functional communication method using discrimination training, stimulus equivalence, and an augmentative communication system.

TASK LIST LINKS:

- **Experimental Design**

    - (B-03) Systematically arrange independent variables to demonstrate their effects on dependent variables.
    - (B-04) Use withdrawal/reversal designs.

- **Fundamental Elements of Behavior Change**

    - (D-09) Use the verbal operants as the basis for language assessment.
    - (D-14) Use listener training.
    - (D-21) Use differential reinforcement (e.g., DRO, DRA, DRI, DRL, and DRH).

- **Specific Behavior-Change Procedures**

    - (E-02) Use discrimination training procedures.
    - (E-06) Use stimulus equivalence procedures.

- **Behavior-Change Systems**

  - (F-07) Use functional communication training.
  - (F-08) Use augmentative communication systems.

- **Measurement**

  - (H-05) Evaluate temporal relations between observed variables (within and between sessions, and time series).

- **Assessment**

  - (I-04) Design and implement the full range of functional assessment procedures.

- **Intervention**

  - (J-05) Select intervention strategies based on the client's current repertoires.
  - (J-08) Select intervention strategies based on the social validity of the intervention.
  - (J-10) When a behavior is to be decreased, select an acceptable alternative behavior to be established or increased.
  - (J-11) Program for stimulus and response generalization.
  - (J-12) Program for maintenance.
  - (J-13) Select behavioral cusps as goals for intervention when appropriate.
  - (J-15) Base decision-making on data displayed in various formats.

KEY TERMS:

- **Discrimination Training**

  - Using selective reinforcement and extinction to evoke differential responding between two or more stimuli. For example, when the instructor says, "point to cat," and after the learner responds, the instructor provides reinforcement when the learner points to cat versus the other pictures of dog or fish (those responses are on extinction) (Strand 2007).

- **Functional Communication Training**

  - A method of teaching behaviors that are functionally equivalent to the individual's challenging behavior by using a communication strategy that produces a functionally equivalent response in the environment (Durand and Carr 1991).

- **Stimulus Equivalence**

  - A method of teaching that provides economical and efficient methods to teach complex behavior. Through the use of symmetry, transitivity, and reflexivity, select relations are taught, and then, other relations derive as a result of their relationship to the taught response. This decreases the number of targets that need to be taught (Rose et al. 1996).

- **Tact**

  - A tact is a verbal behavior that occurs when an individual names or identifies objects, actions, or events. A tact occurs when an individual comes into contact with a stimuli, and as a result of that contact, names or identifies that stimuli, such as saying "car" when that individual sees a car (Wallace et al. 2006).

I Wish Hilde Could Just Tell Us!

Hilde was nearing the end of her long life. She was in her early 80 s and placed in a long-term, intensive-care home for the developmentally disabled, where she was finding it increasingly difficulty to make her wants and needs known to the staff. Although she never had a formal method of communication, when she was younger she could say basic things such as "more" or "no," and she would often pointed to things in her environment or led people to what it is she wanted. When her difficulty with verbal language, fine motor skills, and her ability to walk around the house increased, her challenging behavior also increased, and it seemed like her dementia might be more severe. The staff members were seeing her exhibiting new behaviors such as tossing food, cutlery, bedclothes, and items off her bedside table. She was not only tossing them haphazardly, but regularly tossing them at the staff members with impressive accuracy as they went about their daily care tasks.

After a few weeks of this aggressive behavior being present, the staff in the home decided to jot her name down on the weekly meeting agenda. Unfortunately, Hilde's only sister and only relative was elderly herself, had limited mobility, and was unable to attend the planning meeting.

At the large, roundtable where the home's **multidisciplinary team**, consisting of a consulting physician, a consulting behavior consultant, on-site occupational therapist and speech/language therapists, and a family social worker regularly, met the team came to Hilde's name on the agenda and began discussing the current challenges.

The physician began, "It is clear to me that we need to start a trial of medication. Hilde has been very lucky so far that she has rarely needed consistent medication, but to me it would be ridiculous to let this continue. If we give her the right kind of medication, this aggression will likely not continue. I would be so bold to predict that it will reduce quickly within hours."

The behavior consultant, holding onto the notes and data sheets from the staff, added to the conversation, "I think we need to take a functional approach to solving this issue. If we don't know why Hilde is throwing items on the floor and at staff members, we won't be able to provide very effective interventions. We need to know the reason for it: the why, the function. Right now, she has no functional means of communication. If she is trying to get something from the staff—a special food, an activity, a blanket, any sort of request—and she is unable to do so, this is a problem. We need to find a replacement method for Hilde to communicate with us, which will involve some teaching. From the initial data it looks like a functional communication program may be needed. She could use pictures to tell us what she is communicating more effectively than getting upset or throwing things."

"I am not so sure," the speech and language therapist jumped in. "She could be having oral motor issues. I would like to begin a series of exercises to strengthen the motions of her mouth, tongue, and jaws. Perhaps she is unable to form the speech sounds she is used to be able to use. I can only imagine how frustrating that would be!"

"In addition," interjected the social worker, "looking simultaneously at emotional wellness is of highest importance. If she is feeling anxious or stressed, she is probably not functioning at her best. I think we need to be careful to encourage her and to placate her when problems arise. It must be scary for her right now. I could easily start working on a program of stress management that would take some time to change her current behavior patterns, but it would support her emotional domain, which it turn affects everything else."

"Not to start on too many therapies at one time ..." The occupational therapist spoke up during a brief lull in the conversation. "But I think we need to think about activities of daily living. Since Hilde has started with these outbursts, I can see that she has been far less involved than she was a few months ago. She used to be involved with activities happening around here, such as cooking, crafts, and even attending casual activities like games in the recreation room. If she is staying in her bed or in a chair all the time, we are going to start to see other problems."

After a long debate, the behavior analyst tried to bring the team together, "I hear what everyone is saying, and I think we need to see how we can come up with an integrated plan. I want to suggest something to the team. What if I completed a functional assessment to see why the behaviors are occurring, and write up a program for **functional communication training,** particularly **tacts**—to see what communication we can give her to replace the current way she communicates. I think with some simple **discrimination training**, she will be able to differentiate between pictures to communicate to us, what we call an augmentative communication system. Using **stimulus equivalence**, we can plan for her to get the most vocabulary without having to teach each relationship for communication. I will take data as we go, and if we don't see a decrease in challenging behavior within two weeks, then we can start looking at the other options. We can do a **reversal treatment design** where we look at the data phase-by-phase and implement one thing at a time to see the resulting effect on behavior. Then, we can determine how we are going to generalize and maintain these skills across people, situations, and over time."

The team looked at her and smiled. The team agreed that this plan was ideal. The behavior consultant would take the lead and each team member would check in with her each week to see how their strategies could be implemented into the plan as well.

The Response: Principles, Processes, Practices, and Reflections

Principles

(Q1) Discrimination training is often used in Picture Exchange Communication System (PECS) for the client to learn to discriminate between the different pictures when choosing what they would like to communicate. Given the PECS steps below, indicate where the discrimination training occurs (Fig. 6.7).

PECS Phases

Phase I
How to Communicate
- Spontaneous Requesting
- 2-Person Prompt Procedure
- Pick up, reach, release

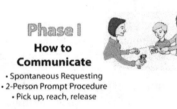

Phase II
Distance and Persistence
- Travel to Communicative Partner
- Carry PECS Book
- Persistence across obstacles

Phase IIIA
Simple Discrimination
- Highly-preferred vs. non-preferred
- 1/2 second rule
- 4-Step Error Correction Procedure

Phase IIIB
Conditional Discrimination
- Correspondence Checks
- 4-Step Error Correction Procedure
- Find pictures in book

Phase IV
Sentence Structure
- Construct and exchange Sentence Strip
- Backstep Error Correction Procedure
- Constant Time Delay to encourage speech

Attributes
Descriptive Vocabulary
- Request specific items
- Size, Color, Shape, etc.
- Action words

Phase V
Answering, "What do you want?"
- Maintain spontaneous requesting
- Progressive Time Delay

Phase VI
Commenting
- Responsive Commenting
- Commenting versus requesting
- Spontaneous Commenting

©2012, Pyramid Educational Consultants   *"FLEX your PECS!"*

www.pecs.com

Fig. 6.7 Phases of the Picture Exchange Communication System (Pyramid Educational Consultants, 2012)

(Q2) Based on the functional assessment data that the behavior consultant continued to collect, she found that the behavior was caused by Hilde wanting to gain access to something tangible. Based on this, what would you teach her within functional communication training to replace this behavior (Fig. 6.8)?

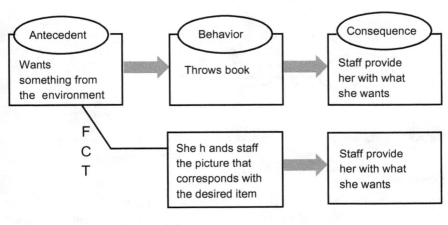

Fill in the empty behavior boxes below.

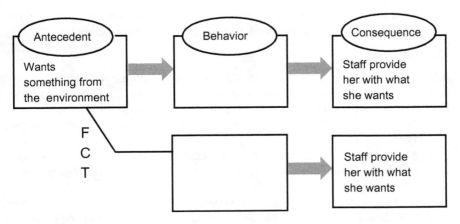

Fig. 6.8 Current behavior contrasted with potential future behavior after functional communication training (FCT)

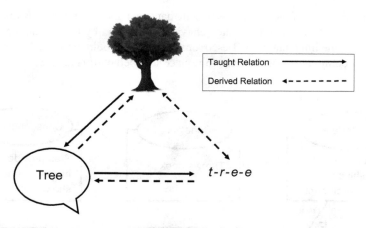

Fig. 6.9 Stimulus equivalence, a depiction of trained relations and derived relations

Processes

(Q3) How would you use stimulus equivalence to ensure that Hilde gets the most out of her vocabulary training without having to teach each everything? See the example below and create your own stimulus equivalence image for Hilde (Fig. 6.9).

(Q4) What other augmentative communication systems could be used with Hilde? What are some advantages and disadvantages of using these systems?

Practice

(Q5) Below are the data for baseline and after implementing the functional communication training. Next, you are going to pair with the occupational therapist to use this communication method to teach daily living skills, and then, you will pair with the social worker to decrease anxiety. Finish the graph by drawing the remaining two phases of the graph (Fig. 6.10).

(Q6) Write out a discrimination training program for Hilde using the template and below. Consider teaching her how to discriminate between requests (mands) in a communication program (Table 6.6).

(Q7) Looking at the final data from the implementation of all different treatment approaches in the graph you completed in Fig. 6.10, describe the temporal relations.

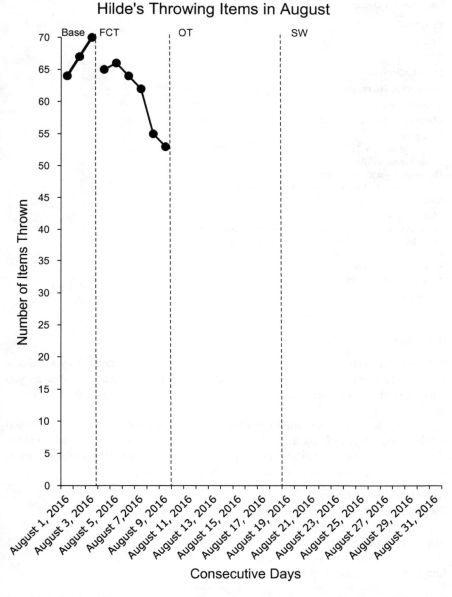

Fig. 6.10 Graph of items thrown by Hilde in the month of August. Baseline and functional communication phases have been done for you. Complete the graph with the occupational therapy (OT) and social worker (SW) phases

Table 6.6 Template to use to make stimulus equivalence program for Hilde

Program	
Trials:	
Sd:	
Data Collection:	
Prompting Hierarchy:	**Materials:**
Teaching Steps:	**Error Correction:**
Mastery Criteria:	**Revision Criteria:**
Generalization: P—**people**—new IT's, school staff, various family members L—**location**—different rooms, away from table, on floor O—**object**—with novel targets P—**placement of object**—have objects out of view S—**SD**—various placement of board, objects, etc.	
Maintenance: **Once mastery is attained at independence for each teaching step,** **complete the following maintenance schedule:** • Weekly: 3 consecutive Y's • Bi-Weekly: 3 consecutive Y's • Monthly: 3 consecutive Y's	
Targets:	

Reflection

(Q8) What do you think about the approach that was implemented? Do you think it was wise to implement it systematically, adding one procedure at a time or do you think it would have been better to work more collaboratively as a team from the start? Why or why not?

(Q9) Implementing a program for functional communication training may be called a behavioral cusp. Do you think this was the case for Hilde? Why or why not?

(Q10) Functional communication training is considered a differential reinforcement strategy. Explain why using information about Hilde.

Additional Web Links
Steps for Implementing Functional Communication Training
http://autismpdc.fpg.unc.edu/sites/autismpdc.fpg.unc.edu/files/FCT_Steps_0.pdf
Stimulus Equivalence
http://journal.frontiersin.org/article/10.3389/fpsyg.2011.00122/full
Single-Subject Research Designs
http://www.winginstitute.org/Graphs/Mindmap/Single-Subject-Design-Examples/

References

Anderson, J., & Le, D. (2011). Abatement of intractable vocal stereotypy using an overcorrection procedure. *Behavioral Interventions, 26*, 134–146.

Azrin, N., Ehle, C., & Beaumont, A. (2006). Physical exercise as a reinforcer to promote calmness of an ADHD child. *Behavior Modification, 30*(5), 564–570.

Behavior Analyst Certification Board (2014). *Professional and ethical compliance code for behavior analysts.* Retrieved from http://bacb.com/wp-content/uploads/2016/01/160120-compliance-code-english.pdf

Cooper, J., Heron, T., & Heward, W. (2007). *Applied behavior analysis* (2nd ed.). New Jersey: Pearson.

Durand, V.M., & Carr, E.G. (1991). Functional communication training to reduce challenging behavior: Maintenance and application in new settings. *Journal of Applied Behavior Analysis, 24*(2), 251–264.

Green, G. (2001). Behavior analytic instruction for learners with Autism: Advances in stimulus control technology. *Focus on Autism and Other Developmental Disabilities, 16*(2), 72–85.

Houlihan, D., Jacobson, L., & Brandon, P. K. (1994). Replication of a high-probability request sequence with varied interprompt times in a preschool setting. *Journal of Applied Behavior Analysis, 27*(4), 737–738.

Klatt, K. P., & Morris, E. K. (2001). The Premack principle, response deprivation, and establishing operations. *The Behavior Analyst, 24*(2), 173.

McAdams, D., & Knapp, V. (2013). Overcorrection. *Encyclopedia of Autism spectrum disorders.* New York: Springer.

MacDuff, G. S., Krantz, P. J., & McClannahan, L. E. (2001). *Prompts and prompt-fading strategies for people with autism* (pp. 37–50). Making a difference: Behavioral intervention for autism.

Maryland State Department of Education. (n.d.). *Discipline of Students with Disabilities.* Retrieved from http://www.marylandpublicschools.org/NR/rdonlyres/5F4F5041-02EE-4F3A-B495-5E4B3C850D3E/22801/DisciplineofStudentswithDisabilities_September2009.pdf

Maryland State Department of Education. (n.d.). *Discipline of students with disabilities.* Retrieved from: http://www.marylandpublicschools.org/NR/rdonlyres/5F4F5041-02EE-4F3A-B4955E4B3C850D3E/22801/DisciplineofStudentswithDisabilities_September2009.pdf

Mudford, O., Taylor, S., & Martin, N. (2009). Continuous recording and interobserver agreement algorithms reported in the Journal of Applied Behavior Analysis. *Journal of Applied Behavior Analysis, 42*(1), 165–169.

Northup, J. (2000). Further evaluation of the accuracy of reinforcer surveys: A systematic replication. *Journal of Applied Behavior Analysis, 33*(3), 335.

Pyramid Educational Consultants. (2012). *PECS phases.* Retrieved from: http://1.bp.blogspot.com/-M5TuLSDMlm8/UeW2mXgKIkI/AAAAAAAADPY/WYJ_nYQQmGo/s1600/Poster+layout-PECS+Phases+copy.jpg

Rasmussen, K., & O'Neill, R. (2006). The effects of fixed-time reinforcement schedules on problem behavior of children with emotional and behavioral disorders in a day treatment classroom setting. *Journal of Applied Behavior Analysis, 39*(4), 453–457.

Rose, J. C., Souza, D. G., & Hanna, E. S. (1996). Teaching reading and spelling: Exclusion and stimulus equivalence. *Journal of Applied Behavior Analysis, 29*(4), 451–469.

Simonsen, B., Fairbanks, S., Briesch, A., & Myers, D. (2008). Evidence-based practices in classroom management: Considerations for research and practice. *Education and Treatment of Children, 31*(3), 351–380.

Strand, P. (2007). Discrimination training. In M. Herson, J. Rosqvist, A. M. Gross, R. S. Drabman, G. Sugai, & R. Horner (Eds.), *Encyclopedia of behavior* doi:10.4135/9781412950534.

Travis, R., & Sturmey, P. (2013). Using behavioral skills training to treat aggression in adults with mild intellectual disability in a forensic setting. *Journal of Applied Research in Intellectual Disabilities, 26*(5), 481–488.

Vollmer, T., Sloman, K., & Pipkin, C. (2008). Practical implications of data reliability and treatment integrity monitoring. *Behavior Analysis in Practice, 1*(2), 4–11.

Wallance, M., Iwata, B., & Hanley, G. (2006). Establishment of mands following tact training as a function of reinforcer strength. *Journal of Applied Behavior Analysis, 39*(1), 17–24.

Part IV
Evaluation

Chapter 7
Evaluation-Centered Case Studies for Preschool to School-Age Children

Abstract The current chapter examines important considerations surrounding the evaluation of applied behavior analysis (ABA)-based programs. The cases prompt learners to consider the perspectives of both ABA researchers and practitioners, while critically exploring strengths and limitations associated with the measurement and evaluation of behavior-change programs. Throughout this chapter, emphasis is placed on the evaluation of behavior changes within a mediator model in applied settings. Within this context, key areas of focus include interpreting and analyzing graphic displays of behavior data, determining the social significance of behavior changes, and weighing the strengths and limitations of various experimental and nonexperimental designs. Learners will be guided to consider indicators of success and determine the extent to which behavior-change programs are responsible for the achievement of meaningful outcomes. In this chapter, entitled "Evaluation-Centred Case Studies for Preschool to School-Aged Children," technical, professional, and ethical considerations surrounding the evaluation of ABA-based research and practice are explored through five case scenarios in home, school, clinical, and community settings.

Keywords Measurement · Evaluation · Preschool · School-age children · Behavior-change programs · Behavior data · Graphic displays · Mediator model · Experimental designs · Nonexperimental designs · Social

CASE: iv-E1 Guest Author: Jocelyn Prosser

GUEST AUTHOR

Jocelyn Prosser
Jocelyn.prosser@tvcc.on.ca

"My teaching strategies are working! Aren't they?"
Setting: Home   Age Group: Preschool

LEARNING OBJECTIVE:

- To interpret and critically analyze graphic displays of behavior data.

© Springer International Publishing AG 2016   229
K. Maich et al., *Applied Behavior Analysis*,
DOI 10.1007/978-3-319-44794-0_7

TASK LIST LINKS:

- **Measurement**

  - (A-06) Measure percent of occurrence.

- **Experimental Design**

  - (B-02) Review and interpret articles from the behavior-analytic literature.
  - (B-03) Systematically arrange independent variables to demonstrate their effects on dependent variables.

- **Fundamental Elements of Behavior Change**

  - (D-03) Use prompts and prompt fading.
  - (D-08) Use discrete-trial and free-operant arrangements.
  - (D-09) Use the verbal operants as a basis for language assessment.
  - (D-14) Use listener training.

- **Measurement**

  - (H-04) Evaluate changes in level, trend, and variability (H-04)
  - (H-05) Evaluate temporal relations between observed variables (within and between sessions and time series)

KEY TERMS:

- **Baseline Phase**

  - The baseline phase is when the practitioner or researcher collects data on the dependent variable prior to any intervention or independent variable being put into place. Data collected during the baseline phase is used to determine any effects of the independent variable (Horner et al. 2005).

- **Intervention Phase**

  - The intervention phase is when the practitioner or researcher introduces the independent variable or intervention, and continues to collect data on the dependent variable (Horner et al. 2005).

- **Least-to-Most Prompt Hierarchy**

  - A "least-to-most prompt hierarchy" involves starting a teaching process using the least intrusive prompt possible to support a learner display a target-desired behavior. If the learner is not successful, the instructor then moves to successively more intrusive prompts. This prompt sequence is typically used when a learner has shown success demonstrating the target behavior in the past (Libby et al. 2008).

- **Receptive Language**

  - Receptive language refers to our ability to understand language that we hear or read. This is often contrasted with expressive language, or how we convey a message to others, or how we express our wants and needs (Thurm et al. 2007).

- **Teaching Targets**
  - Items within a program that are the focus of teaching. For example, the teaching targets could be the different animals in a tacting program. Often multiple trials are run to teach the learner each teaching target (Severtson 2012).

My Teaching Strategies Are Working! Aren't They?

Like many others, I often get asked, "What do you do for a living?" It is a significant challenge to explain this most people, especially to those who are truly interested in a detailed response. I create and supervise individualized programming for children with Autism Spectrum Disorder (ASD). Here is what this looks like on a day-to-day basis ...

One of the first things we behavior therapists focus on is an understanding of spoken language. This might be following an instruction to carry out an action, or following an instruction to select the appropriate item from an array. This is called receptive language and is of utmost importance. Hannah, a behavior therapist for children with ASD, handed me a completed **baseline** graph one morning for three-year-old Jo's—a child in our program—**receptive language** program. Jo's receptive language goal, written below the graph, read: *When presented with 3 familiar foods, Jo will select the correct item upon hearing the corresponding word* (Fig. 7.1).

Fig. 7.1 Graph of Jo's baseline receptive identification data

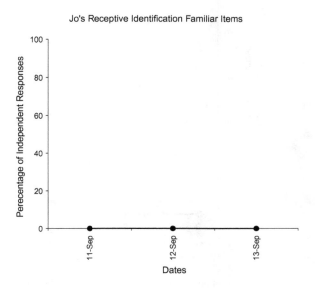

Moving my eyes down the page, I was easily able to make an educated decision on the direction of Jo's program. Letting my eyes move across the graph of "percentage of correct independent responses" for this area of his learning, the visually displayed data show his level at zero percent of these hoped-for correct responses across all three days of data collection so far. My next job, then, was to go to the clinical literature around evidence-based methods to teach receptive language and to use this information to develop a program to help Jo reach this goal through precise instruction around introductory receptive language skills. Ultimately, all of those of us working with Jo and supporting Jo in any of his environments (home, community, and childcare) want to see Jo acquiring reach this one. After I finished researching and writing Jo's current receptive language program, I reviewed it with his parents and his therapist and left it with his therapist to begin immediate implementation during their next morning session.

Five days later, I returned to evaluate the current phase of Jo's program, to see how its implementation was progressing—hoping (and expecting) to see great things from this program that was made just for Jo. Almost as soon as I walked in the door of the children's center, Hannah pulled me aside and quietly exclaimed, "You should see how well he is doing!" She passed me his binder—where we keep all of our programs and data for Jo—and I flipped through a few pages to find his updated implementation graph placed efficiently near the front (Fig. 7.2).

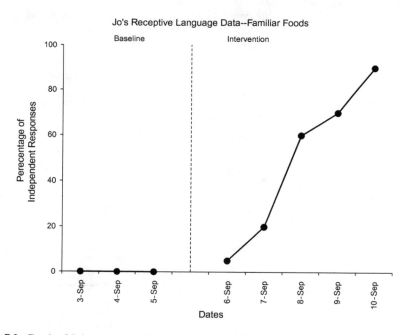

Fig. 7.2 Graph of Jo's progress with first target set–familiar foods

I smiled and nodded as my eyes and mind took in the increasing trend in the **intervention condition.** I could see the graph—flat in the baselines before we started Jo's new program—moving steeply upward in each and every session over the last five days. This positive development showed me that our current teaching strategies were indeed effective—just right—in teaching Jo receptive language with the support of everyone in his environment, including an excellent therapist.

With a tight timeline ahead and an increase in Jo's therapy hours, we decided a prudent next step would be to introduce another receptive language teaching set into Jo's current programming. Since we had such good success with familiar foods— our first focus area—we added, operationalized, and set our next goals around *receptive identification of familiar items.* We even chose to do a **least-to-most prompt hierarchy** to teach it since he had been so successful on the first teaching step. But a week later, Hannah told me that Jo is not doing nearly as well on his second receptive language targets, letting me know by email that his understanding of familiar foods is still going well but asks me to review the second teaching set. I clicked on the attachment to her email (familiar items) and opened the following graph of baseline data for the new **teaching targets,** which looked very different than his intervention for familiar foods (Fig. 7.3).

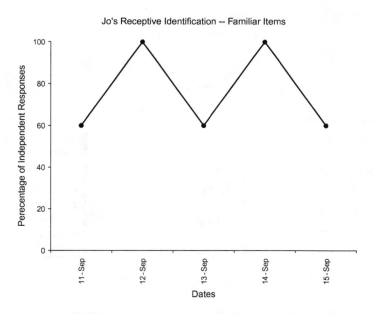

Fig. 7.3 Graph of Jo's progress with second target set—familiar Items

Discouraged, I knew that I needed to figure out what to do next, but I wasn't sure where to start. So I turned to my agenda and began to check over tomorrow's packed agenda, trying to find a time to fit in a visit during Jo's therapy.

And this was only one case—one child—at one of my centers, only over a few days. My job is highly complicated with a matching high level of responsibility; thankfully, a high level of reward comes with it, in the form of helping children and seeing progress on a daily basis.

The Response: Principles, Processes, Practices, and Reflections

Principles

(Q1) What is the purpose of gathering baseline data, and how might it help with the development and implementation of a behavior intervention program?

(Q2) Looking at the baseline data collected for Jo, do you think enough data were collected before introduction of the intervention? Explain your response (Fig. 7.4).

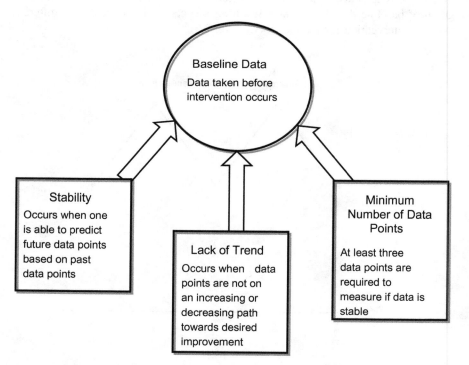

Fig. 7.4 Desirable qualities of baseline data and their definitions (Byiers et al., 2012)

Processes

(Q3) In behavior programs, teaching steps are often introduced to make the program increasingly more difficult as time goes on, in a supportive, stagelike manner. Currently, Jo can receptively identify an array of 3 for familiar foods. What would your next teaching step be (Fig. 7.5)?

(Q4) Explain how the therapists would have collected the data during the receptive language trials. Why did they convert it to percentage of opportunity data? How would they have calculated this?

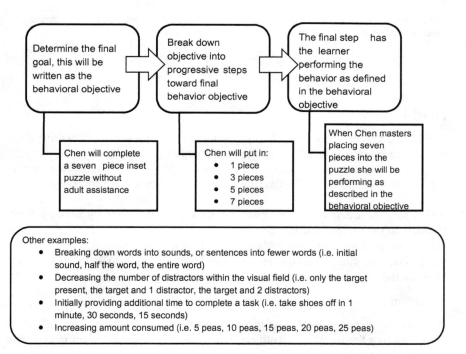

Fig. 7.5 Breaking a behavior objective down into teaching steps

Table 7.1 Common issues and potential solutions during receptive language training (Grow and LeBlanc, 2013)

Issue	Potential solution
The learner chooses one side consistently over another	• Continually mix-up position of materials • Use a larger array • Add an extra-stimulus or within-stimulus prompts to fade later
The learner watches the instructor for prompts	• Use video recording for the instructor to self-identify behavior changes to make • Model correct behavior • Identify and coach instructor on behavioral changes to make
When targets are similar, the learner does not discriminate reliably between them	• Put the similar targets into two separate learning sets • Introduce distinctly different targets to intermix with targets

Practice

(Q5) If the mastery criteria for Jo's program were 80 % over 3 consecutive days, would you say Jo mastered the familiar food targets?

(Q6) What may be some reasons that Jo is not as highly successful on the receptive identification program for *familiar item* targets as compared to the *familiar food* targets (Table. 7.1)?

(Q7) Using the article below as a guide, which prompting hierarchy would you use to teach Jo the receptive language program?
http://www.ncbi.nlm.nih.gov/pmc/articles/PMC2846579/

(Q8) What are some potential intermediate teaching steps to help Jo transition between the targets of *familiar foods* to *familiar items*?

Reflection

(Q9) As the therapist overseeing the case, what might you have done differently before starting the receptive identification programs to assist the team in choosing and teaching targets to Jo?

(Q10) Before implementing the program modification for Jo's receptive language program, who needs to approve the changes (Reference Ethics Box 7.1, Behavior Analyst Certification Board, 2014)?

Ethics Box 7.1

> **Professional and Ethical Compliance Code for Behavior Analysts**
>
> Behavior analysts are required to gain consent from the client in a number of situations regarding behavior-change programs and procedures:
> - 3.03 Behavior-Analytic Assessment Consent
>   (a) Prior to conducting an assessment, behavior analysts must explain to the client the procedures(s) to be used, who will participate, and how the resulting information will be used.
>   (b) Behavior analysts must obtain the client's written approval of the assessment procedures before implementing them.
> - 4.02 Involving Clients in Planning and Consent.
>   Behavior analysts involve the client in the planning of and consent for behavior-change programs
> - 4.04 Approving Behavior-Change Programs.
>   Behavior analysts must obtain the client's written approval of the behavior-change program before implementation or making significant modifications (e.g., change in goals and use of new procedures).

Additional Web Links
Determining Baseline and Interpreting Data
http://pisp.ca/strategies/documents/BaselineDataCollection.pdf
Visual Analysis of ABA Data
http://www.educateautism.com/applied-behaviour-analysis/visual-analysis-of-aba-data.html
Teaching Receptive Identification in Discrete Trials or Natural Methods
http://www.ncbi.nlm.nih.gov/pmc/articles/PMC3592489/

CASE: iv-E2

It's Working for Tito ... Right?
Setting: Home   Age Group: Preschool

LEARNING OBJECTIVE:

- To critically evaluate behavior changes within a mediator model.

TASK LIST LINKS:

- **Experimental Design**
  - (B-01) Use the dimensions of applied behavior analysis to evaluate whether interventions are behavior analytic in nature.
  - (B-03) Systematically arrange independent variables to demonstrate their effects on dependent variables.

- **Identification of the Problem**

  - (G-06)Provide behavior-analytic services in collaboration with others who support and/or provide services to one's clients.

- **Implementation, Management, and Supervision**

  - (K-02) Identify the contingencies governing the behavior of those responsible for carrying out behavior-change procedures and design interventions accordingly.
  - (K-06) Provide supervision for behavior-change agents.
  - (K-09) Secure the support of others to maintain the client's behavioral repertoires in their natural environments.

- **Intervention**

  - (J-09) Identify and address practical and ethical considerations when using experimental designs to demonstrate treatment effectiveness.

KEY TERMS:

- **AB Design**

  - An AB design involves two phases: the "A" phase, or the baseline phase, during which the target behavior or dependent variable is measured before the intervention is introduced, and the "B" phase, or the intervention phase, during which the independent variable or intervention is introduced and the target behavior continues to be measured (Odom et al. 2003).

- **Level**

  - When visually analyzing a graph displaying behavior data, level of the data refers to the position of the data on the y-axis. Do most of the data points seem to be at a "high" level on the graph (e.g., fall between approximately 70 and 100 %), a moderate level (e.g., fall between approximately 40 and 70 %), or a low level (e.g., fall between 0 % and approximately 40 %) (Kratochwill et al. 2010)?

- **Reversal/Withdrawal Treatment Design**

  - A single-subject research design whereby the intervention is implemented and then withdrawn and reimplemented to investigate whether there is a functional relationship between the intervention and the behavior targeted for change. Although an ABAB design is the most common, other treatments can be implemented as well to make it an ABC… ABCD… etc., design (Engel and Russell 2012).

- **Trend**

  - When visually analyzing a graph displaying behavior data, trend refers to the direction that the data points seem to be going. For example, are the data points going up, or showing an increasing trend? Are the data points going down, or showing a decreasing trend? Are the data points not showing either an increasing or a decreasing trend, but rather a "zero" trend, remaining level? (Kratochwill et al. 2010).

- **Variability**
  - When visually analyzing a graph displaying behavior data, variability refers to how different each data point is from one another or the extent to which multiple measures of behavior result in different findings (Kratochwill et al. 2010).

It's Working for Tito … Right?

The grade one teacher began, "His classmates sometimes call him 'Tito the Turtle' because it seems to take him FOREVER to do anything. I don't know if he's not paying attention, or if he just doesn't care, or he doesn't have the skills, maybe at times? It's just not clear to me. Yesterday was a routine after-school set of events. We finished up class, the bell rang, and all the other grade one students rushed to get ready for theirs parents to pick them up, to meet with their older sibling to walk home, or to get to their buses on time. Tito, has a developmental disability but our class is very inclusive and caring, we have all sorts of diverse children here. Anyhow … yesterday, everyone else was gone—everyone—and Tito was still around. He had his boots on the wrong feet, and his coat on upside down, and he was very unconcerned about what was happening next. He was happy—but definitely disengaged. This is the same way he is with class work. If he has to write his name on a paper, he does everything BUT write it. He seems happy enough, but is looking around, or laughing, or chewing his pencil, or getting up to go to the bathroom. Really, he does everything EXCEPT what he is supposed to be doing. I know we are only in the second week of school, but this off-task behavior is just not going to work."

The school's behavior consultant replied to the grade one teacher: "It sounds like you are saying that off-task behavior is the issue with Tito. Remember last year with your student who was hiding under her desk, we will start in the same manner, we will begin with collaborating with Tito's parents, operationalizing the behavior, creating a data sheet, and then collecting baseline data until we see a stable pattern. Since we need to know how much time Tito is off-task, it would probably make sense to use momentary time sampling. And you are in luck, because I have a student starting with us next week who is learning the clinical work of behavior analysis, and I can get him to help you with this data collection. Agreed?"

The teacher and the behavior student started collecting data the week after next, on a Monday. The student carefully graphed the off-task data each day and took the additional step of graphing the behavior of two typically developing peers to see the comparison in the inclusive classroom. "It's important," she explained to the grade one teacher, "to not only know details regarding Tito's off-task behavior, but also to know if this behavior is any different from that of his peers, and if it is to what extent."

Predictably, the grade one teacher laughed and responded with, "I don't need any data sheet or graph to tell me that!" However, she let the student move on with his work. Five days later, the school's behavior consultant, the classroom teacher, the resource teacher, and the student studying ABA reviewed the graph together using visual analysis. Together, they concluded that Tito's **level** of off-task behavior is stable; the **trend** is increasing (far higher than that of his peers); and the **variability** is low. According to the collected data, there was no difference in academic tasks when compared to tasks of everyday living, such as reading and taking off his outdoor shoes in the morning. It was apparent that Tito was on-task during anything that involved technology. Together with the functional behavior analysis that they would be completing in the coming weeks, they had a plan for intervention.

Over the next week, the behavior student's data collection continued, while the teacher put a number of her self-created interventions in place. On Monday, she placed visual schedules around the class, including one about how to get dressed for home, and showed Tito—and the rest of the class—how to use them. On Tuesday, she took the class to the computer laboratory for an hour in the morning and again at the end of the day. On Wednesday, she borrowed the cart of iPads and used them in her two learning centers through the day. On Thursday, there was a substitute teacher. On Friday, a parent volunteer came in and spent most of the day with Tito, prompting him to help with his on-task behavior.

When the behavior consultant dropped by on Friday after school, the grade one teacher excitedly said to the ABA student, "Show her!" She then reported to the behavior consultant, "See? The plan working … right? I am so happy. The student showed me this week's graph and how much better it is and we are both celebrating. Tito's doing great!" They told the behavior consultant the activities of their week and the variety interventions and activities that had happened each day.

Not sure what to say next—and wanting to be supportive rather than the cynic of the team—a number of fleeting thoughts and concerns ran though the behavior consultant's head.

- *An **AB design** does not tell us much. At the best of times, it cannot tell us whether a change was caused by the intervention.*
- *Even if it could, how do we know what was making a change happen? Every day was a different intervention!*
- *Did Tito learn new skills that will be maintained so quickly? Is he even attending to the visual schedules put in place?*
- *Does it appear that he is more on-task simply because there are more electronics in the environment this week?*

She tried to be very gentle: "You are quite right that the graph is looking better, far better. But at this point, we really can't be quite sure if—or what—is related to this increase in Tito's on-task behavior. We have to do things a little bit differently, in order to tell what is causing the increase in on-task behavior we need to try one intervention or change at a time. So we don't know, yet, if it's working, but with some slight alterations we will keep going until it does!" She thought to herself about the importance of using an experimental design such as a **reversal or withdrawal design** to be sure that it was the intervention that was causing the change, but also had to think through the ethical implications of this in the setting.

The Response: Principles, Processes, Practices, and Reflections

Principles

(Q1) Why is it important to compare Tito's problematic behavior to those of his same age peers?

(Q2) Often in clinical work, an AB design is used to see the difference from baseline to intervention, as was done in this case. What type of design would be most appropriate when the teacher wants to try numerous different interventions?

(Q3) When doing a number of interventions together, this is called a comprehensive treatment model. What are pros and cons of this approach (Fig. 7.6)?

Comprehensive Treatment Models	Focused Intervention Packages
Comprehensive treatment models (CTMs) consist of a set of practices designed to achieve a broad learning or developmental impact on the core deficits of ASD. In their review of education programs for children with autism, the National Academy of Science Co mmittee on Educational Interventions for Children with Autism (National Research Council, 2001) identified 10 CTMs. Examples included the UCLA Young Autism Program by Lovaas and colleagues (Smith, Groen, & Winn, 2000), the TEACCH program developed by Schop ler and colleagues (Marcus, Schopler, & Lord, 2000), the LEAP model (Strain & Hoyson, 2000), and the Denver model designed by Rogers and colleagues (Rogers, Hall, Osaki, Reaven, & Herbison, 2000). In a follow -up to the National Academy review, Odom, Boyd, Hall, and Hume (2010) identified 30 CTM programs operating within the U.S. These programs were characterized by organization (i.e., around a conceptual framework), operationalization (i.e., procedures manualized), intensity (i.e., substantial number of hou rs per week), longevity (i.e., occur across one or more years), and breadth of outcome focus (i.e., multiple outcomes such as communication, behavior, social competence targeted) (Odom, Boyd, Hall, & Hume, in press).	In contrast, focused intervention pract ices are designed to address a single skill or goal of a student with ASD (Odom et al., 2010). These practices are operationally defined, address specific learner outcomes, and tend to occur over a shorter time period than CTMs (i.e., until the individual goal is achieved). Examples include discrete trial teaching, pivotal response training, prompting, and video modeling. Focused intervention practices could be considered the building blocks of educational programs for children and youth with ASD, and they are highly salient features of the CTMs just described. For example, peer-mediated instruction and intervention (Sperry, Neitzel, & Engelhardt-Wells, 2010), is a key feature of the LEAP model (Strain & Bovey, 2011).

Fig. 7.6 Comprehensive treatment models versus focused intervention packages (Wong et al., 2013, p. 3)

Processes

(Q4) Given that there are multiple interventions in place for Tito, what type of alternating treatment design would you use and how would you set up the different interventions (Table 7.2)?

Table 7.2 Different types of multiple treatment designs in single-subject research

Design	Details
1. Alternating treatment design with no baseline 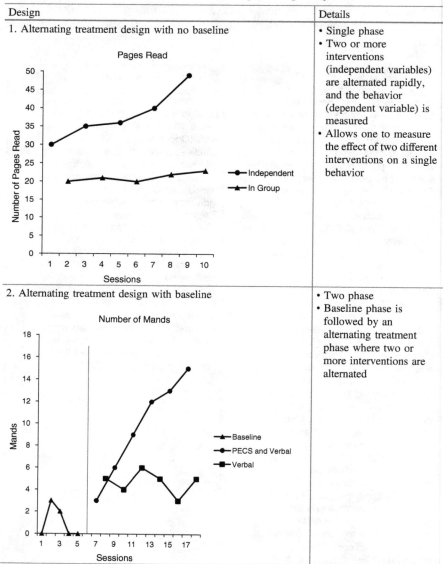	• Single phase • Two or more interventions (independent variables) are alternated rapidly, and the behavior (dependent variable) is measured • Allows one to measure the effect of two different interventions on a single behavior
2. Alternating treatment design with baseline	• Two phase • Baseline phase is followed by an alternating treatment phase where two or more interventions are alternated

(continued)

Table 7.2 (continued)

Design	Details
3. Alternating treatment design—three phase with final phase most effective treatment implemented	• Three phases are used • Baseline is followed by the alternating treatments; then finally, the best treatment is used in the final phase

Pinching at School

| 4. Alternating treatment with no treatment control condition | • Single phase
• Multiple independent variables are alternated; one independent variable is the "no treatment" or control
• Useful for visualizing functional behavior analysis data |

Frequency of Toy Dumping

(Q5) What are the strengths and limitations of an AB design? How could the limitations be addressed?

Practice

(Q6) The behavior that has been identified to increase is "on-task behavior." Create an operational definition of this behavior the team could use.

(Q7) Taking two of the interventions that the teacher utilized, use either an alternating treatments or changing criterion design to determine which intervention is more effective.

(Q8) How might a behavior analyst balance the need for an objective, scientifically based approach to analyzing changes in behavior with the establishment and maintenance of a positive and supportive relationship with mediators implementing a behavior-change program?

Reflection

(Q9) Do you agree with the behavior consultant's response when shown the graph illustrating positive changes in Tito's behavior? Why or why not?

(Q10) It turns out that the ABA student is also Tito's next door neighbor and occasionally watches Tito for a few hours on the weekend. Discuss whether the role the student has at school with Tito is appropriate or not.

Additional Web Links
Defining Normal Behavior
http://www.healthyplace.com/parenting/challenge-of-difficult-children/how-kids-grow-defining-normal-behavior/
Hypothesis Development
http://challengingbehavior.fmhi.usf.edu/explore/pbs/step4.htm

CASE: iv-E3

It's just not happening with Owen!
Setting: Home   Age Group: Preschool

LEARNING OBJECTIVE:
To critically evaluate behavior measurement procedures.

TASK LIST LINKS:

* **Measurement**

    – (A-09) Evaluate the accuracy and reliability of measurement procedures.

* **Experimental Design**

    – (B-02) Review and interpret articles from the behavior-analytic literature.

- **Fundamental Elements of Behavior Change**

  - (D-21) Use differential reinforcement.

- **Behavior-Change Systems**

  - (F-01) Use self-management strategies.

- **Intervention**

  - (J-09) Identify and address practical and ethical considerations when using experimental designs to demonstrate treatment effectiveness

- **Implementation, Management, and Supervision**

  - (K-03) Design and use competency-based training for persons who are responsible for carrying out behavioral assessment and behavior-change procedures.

KEY TERMS:

- **Dependent variable**

  - In ABA research, the dependent variable is the target behavior that is identified for change (Horner et al. 2005).

- **Independent variable**

  - In applied behavior analysis research, the independent variable is the intervention that is put into place to increase or decrease a target behavior (Horner et al. 2005).

- **Treatment Fidelity**

  - The degree in which an intervention was implemented as designed, which ensures reliability in the data (Vermilyea et al. 1984).

It's Just Not Happening with Owen!

"Owen! Stop! You have to stop that, please! O, come on! You know better! Let's just go and talk. Owen, hands down! Hands to yourself!" These were the commonly heard phrases echoing around the Towering Spruce outdoor activity day camp. Parents of campers at Towering Spruce could sign up for any number of weeks, or even the whole summer! Owen was signed up for every week of the summer—what looked like were going to be eight very long, exhausting weeks for the camp staff—and even the first two weeks had been pretty tough to take. Two weeks into summer camp, Owen had already been in four physical fights, filled with yelling, pushing, and punching. *Clearly,* though the head camp counselor, *this is not a personality conflict, as the fights have been with four other children. I can't say I have been enjoying all of the phone calls I have had to make to hysterical parents, and all of the incident reports I have had to complete.*

Each week at the camp had a theme, and week two was "arctic week." Though it was pretty warm outside, 10-year-old Owen's favorite activity for the week was dressing up in the full-body polar bear costume. The costume itself, though made of fairly light material that let in the breeze, had a heavy rubber head and long, black rubberized claws attached to the bear's four paws. Life around camp was quite calm while Owen was getting in and out of the polar bear costume, a stark contrast with life around camp while Owen donned the costume.

Perhaps predictably, Owen enjoyed leaping off of the Styrofoam icebergs when other campers were near, typically scaring them so that they startled and as a result yelled, then they yelled at him. He also enjoyed chasing others with the costume again and growling, with his front paws and claws outstretched. He seemed to do this quite a bit around girls, who often screamed and giggled while they chastised him in a friendly way. Finally, he would roll on his back and pretend to eat the plastic seals as his lunch, hitting anyone near him who dared to interrupt his polar bear "meal."

When the majority of the camp staff had engaged in one or a number of the following, chasing Owen around to get in-between him and the other campers, physically pulling Owen off others, calming Owen, or talking to Owen over and over, the camp director decided next steps had to be taken. *I can't have all my staff quitting on me after week two*, she thought, *as she searched for the right number to call. I am sure I have a number, somewhere, for an agency that will come out and help with problem behaviors and provide some 1:1 support, too, I think.* After easily securing parental consent and finally locating the number to the local behavior support agency, the director made the call. The director gave a brief overview of the situation at hand and arranged an emergency meeting the next morning with Owen's parents, the behavior agency, herself, and the head counselor who had been for many of Owen's exhibitions and who was responsible for debriefing the counselors at the end of the day meetings. The behavior agency explained that they would be bringing along a support counselor to provide extra time and attention for Owen during the planning meeting.

After introductions, the camp director explained to everyone in a quiet, calm voice: "All of the camp staff are struggling with how to support Owen. While we are very relieved that so far no one has been seriously hurt, we are worried that if we don't make a serious change, things will get worse over the next six weeks of camp. We have tried talking, scolding, time outs, and giving him extra jobs to do around the camp's kitchen area. But it's just not happening for us. So we have now brought a behavior consultant on board, who will work with the camp team to develop a behavior intervention program and provide training all of our staff to implement it. While the behavior consultant works out the intervention plan, her and I have discussed that the best route to take right now is assigning someone every half-day to spend that time just with Owen, and that person that person will focus on giving Owen praise and rewards for anything that is **not** physical aggression." Everyone agreed that this was the best possible route to take, and the behavior consultant stuck around for a few more hours to talk with Owen's parents, directly observe, generally start working on Owen's behavioral assessment, and to write up the details of this short-term intervention with the camp team. She began by describing that she wanted to approach this from a scientific perspective, as they do in research, *thinking* about Owen's behavior as the **dependent variable** and the intervention program that they will be developing as the **independent variable,** and the goal being to demonstrate a relationship between these two variables. As part of the intervention, she explained that a **self-monitoring** program might be effective for Owen. Everyone quickly agreed and almost in unison said: "Whatever will help, we are fully on-board. Just tell us what to do!"

Before the behavior consultant had a chance to come up with a data-supported hypothesis, however, she received a frantic phone call from the camp saying that the intervention is not working—it is just not happening—and if the behavior has not improved by the end of the week, Owen will not be able to stay in camp at all— even with 1:1 support. The child's parents, who received the same message, work full time over the summer, are very concerned, and are not sure what they will do if he is not allowed to stay at the camp. After much discussion, the camp staff agreed to continue but allow the behavior consultant to stay on the camp site for a longer period of time to observe the child at camp for a few days. After two days, the consultant has a good idea about why the intervention is not working. *Given the number of different camp staff that interact Owen each day,* she wrote in her notes, *as he moves from activity to activity throughout the day, it is clear that the procedure of attention for everything except the problem behaviors was not consistently implemented in the way it was explained. For example, when Owen was fishing, his 1:1 counselor was off at the tuck shop having ice cream, and the counselor in charge of the fishing activity was giving Owen all sorts of attention for his problem behaviors. Some of the counselors provided lots of praise and positive reinforcement for camp-appropriate behaviors, and others told me that they were not doing it, because he didn't deserve it. This problem with everyone not implementing the program as planned, called **treatment fidelity**, is providing confusing messages to Owen. I think we need to have another emergency meeting with the camp staff and begin to explain the importance of treatment fidelity as well as avoiding treatment drift; that how they are implementing this intervention is the issue, and not in the intervention itself. THIS is why it's "just not happening."*

The Response: Principles, Processes, Practices, and Reflections

Principles

(Q1) Why is procedural fidelity a critical component of any behavior intervention program?

(Q2) What procedure did the behavior consultant implement when she asked them to provide attention to everything except the problem behavior?

Processes

(Q2) Given the graph collected of Owen's behavior below, how may treatment drift have been missed? What other interpretations may be possible (Fig. 7.7)?

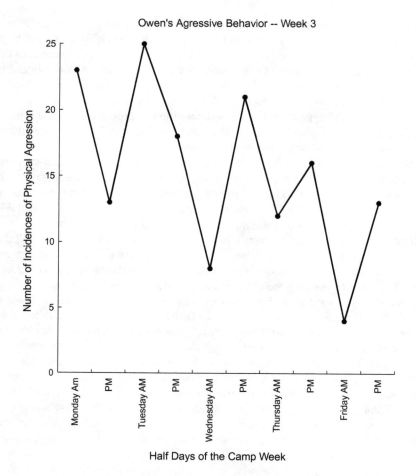

Fig. 7.7 Graph of data collected by camp staff regarding the total frequency of Owen's physical aggression toward others during week 3 of camp

(Q3) In the case of Owen, does the behavior consultant have enough evidence to support the conclusion that treatment drift is the reason that the intervention program is not working?

(Q4) What types of information would be essential to determine that treatment drift is causing the inconsistencies in Owen's behavior? What data sheet would be ideal to collect this information?

Practice

(Q5) Develop a treatment fidelity checklist for Owen's staff using the sample below as a guide (Fig. 7.8).

		M	Tu	W	Th	F
Treatment Fidelity Checklist						
Early Learner's ABA Program						

Learner: **Instructor:**

Week of: **Session Length:**

Instructions: Complete after session and file in binder under "TFC" tab. Circle Y for each component that was completed or implemented; each component that was not completed or implemented circle N.

	M	Tu	W	Th	F
1. Preference assessment completed at start of session	Y N	Y N	Y N	Y N	Y N
2. Mand training completed for at least 50% of session	Y N	Y N	Y N	Y N	Y N
3. Maintenance checks completed	Y N	Y N	Y N	Y N	Y N
4. Data taken as soon as possible after behavior occurred	Y N	Y N	Y N	Y N	Y N
5. Correct response varied position in visual array (left, middle, right positions)	Y N	Y N	Y N	Y N	Y N
6. Transferred data from hand tallies to data sheet at end of session	Y N	Y N	Y N	Y N	Y N
7. Daily mands graphed	Y N	Y N	Y N	Y N	Y N
8. Paired tangible reinforcers with social praise	Y N	Y N	Y N	Y N	Y N
9. Wrote in communication book including: effective reinforcers, overall affect of the learner, and any information relayed to you from parents	Y N	Y N	Y N	Y N	Y N
10. Instructor control program run at least 5 times throughout session	Y N	Y N	Y N	Y N	Y N

Fig. 7.8 Sample treatment fidelity checklist (Wilkinson, 2007)

(**Q6**) Do you agree with the consultant having the staff give Owen praise and rewards for anything that is not physical aggression? Looking at the literature, was this an evidence-based decision? Why or why not?

(**Q7**) Using the chart below, how could treatment drift be avoided when starting to implement a new intervention (Table 7.3)?

Table 7.3 Treatment fidelity assessment grid (UCDHSC Center for Nursing Research, 2006)

Type of fidelity	Steps taken to ensure fidelity	How was fidelity assessed?
Fidelity to theory (*did the intervention include the relevant "active ingredients" based on theory?*)	• Review by experts • Ensure adequate "dose" of treatment is received • Ensure equivalent dose of treatment across conditions (if applicable)	• Documentation of review, comments, suggestions • Statistics on number, frequency, length of contact • Show no difference in number, frequency, length, and type of content
Provider training (*were the treatment providers capable of delivering the intervention as designed?*)	• Initial training of interventionists • Test of provider skills • Ongoing supervision of interventionists • Periodic retraining to prevent "drift"	• Training protocols and standardized materials • Results on post-training test • Forms used to document supervision • Schedule and protocols for retraining
Treatment implementation (*did the treatment providers actually implement the intervention as it was designed?*)	• Standardized intervention protocol • Provider monitoring (e.g., video, audio, in-person) • Participant rating of treatments' credibility • Minimize treatment contamination	• Treatment manual or other standard delivery materials • Individual or aggregate results of monitoring • Survey of participants' perceptions of treatment • Methods used to prevent contamination (e.g., separate sites, patient exit interviews, checklist of *non*allowed provider behaviors)
Treatment receipt (*did the participant receive the relevant "active ingredients" as intended?*)	• Check of participants' understanding • Measure of change in participants' knowledge • Review of homework completion • Self-report or diary to measure use of new skills	• Results from participant measures {note: this section may be "N/A" if the participant is not expected to learn something from the intervention—e.g., in behavioral interventions with cognitively impaired patients}
Treatment enactment (*did the participant put new skills or behaviors into practice? Were all necessary steps completed?*)	• Success in implementing new behaviors • Level of skill in performing new behaviors (e.g., using an inhaler correctly)	• Laboratory assessment of actual participant skills/behaviors • Self-report or home visit to assess actual skills/behaviors {note: This may be N/A in some but not all cases, when behavior is the outcome variable}

Reflection

(Q8) After reading the case of Owen, who is it that may need to change? Owen, the camp staff, or both? Please explain.

(Q9) Within a mediator model, the behavior consultant is focused both on the behavior of the individual displaying the problematic behavior and on the behavior of those charged with implementing the intervention program. Where should a behavior consultant place the emphasis of his or her work? Why (Fig. 7.9)?

(Q10) With emphasis placed on the behavior of Owen as the source of the problem, how might the behavior consultant begin to shift emphasis toward the behavior of the staff while still maintaining positive rapport with the team?

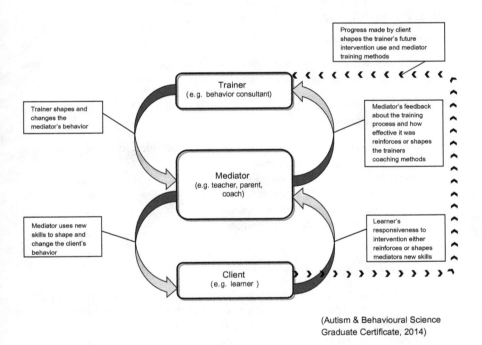

(Autism & Behavioural Science
Graduate Certificate, 2014)

Fig. 7.9 Triadic mediator model of interaction (Autism and Behavioral Science Graduate Certificate, 2014)

Additional Web Links
Helping Children Learn to Manage their own Behavior
http://csefel.vanderbilt.edu/briefs/wwb7.pdf
Acknowledging Children's Positive Behaviors
http://csefel.vanderbilt.edu/briefs/wwb_22.pdf
Differential Reinforcement
http://165.139.150.129/intervention/Differential.pdf

CASE: iv-E4

As long as Molly's improving, nothing else matters
Setting: Home   Age Group: Preschool

LEARNING OBJECTIVE:

- To critically weigh the strengths and limitations with the use of single-subject experimental designs in natural settings.

TASK LIST LINKS:

- **Experimental Design**

    - (B-03) Systematically arrange independent variables to demonstrate their effects on dependent variables.
    - (B-04) Use withdrawal/reversal designs.
    - (B-05) Use alternating treatment designs.
    - (B-06) Use changing criterion designs.
    - (B-07) Use multiple baseline designs.

KEY TERMS:

- **Alternating Treatment Design**

    - The alternating treatment design is a type of single-subject research design that allows for the effects of two or more treatments on a target behavior to be compared. In this design, two or more treatments are presented to an individual in rapidly alternating succession, such as on alternating days or even alternating sessions on the same day, in order to determine whether one intervention is more effective than the other (Cooper et al. 2007; Kratochwill et al. 2010).

- **Changing Criterion Design**

    - A changing criterion design is a type of single-subject research design that involves gradually changing criteria for reinforcement or punishment following a baseline phase. Throughout the changing criteria, the target behavior is measured and the extent to which changes in the behavior correspond to changes in the criteria is documented (Cooper et al. 2007; Kratochwill et al. 2010).

- **Multiple Baseline Design**

  - Multiple baseline designs are a type of single-subject research design that allows for measurement of the effects of an independent variable (e.g., intervention program) on a dependent variable (e.g., target behavior) across individuals or settings, or even across several behaviors displayed by the same individual. For example, when measuring the effects of an intervention program on a problem behavior being exhibited by three individuals, baseline data collection would begin at the same time for all three individuals. The intervention program would then be systematically introduced in a staggered manner across the individuals—the first individual would begin the treatment phase, while the others remain in the baseline phase; then, the second would begin the treatment phase, while the third remains in baseline; then, the third would begin the treatment phase. This staggered introduction of the intervention program allows for any effects on the target behavior to be observed in one individual at a time, so as to establish a functional relationship between changes in the target behavior and the introduction of the intervention (Cooper et al. 2007; Kratochwill et al. 2010).

As Long as Molly's Improving, Nothing Else Matters

Every report card Molly brought home from school in Kindergarten, Grade 1, Grade 2, and now the first term of Grade 3 said the same thing in different words that Molly had hardly any friends. Following Molly's diagnosis of Asperger's disorder in preschool, her parents had watched her carefully. She seemed to get along okay. "Who needs a lot of friends as long as you have one good one?" they asked one another. But when they received this most recent report card, even with all of the encouragement they had given Molly, the meetings with her teacher, the peer sensitivity training in her classroom, and all the community activities that they had enrolled her in, it finally became clear to them. This was not going to "go away" without some sort of systematic intervention.

"Maybe it was my fault?" said Molly's mom. "Maybe I shouldn't have gone back to work so soon and I could have taken her to more moms and tots lessons. But we needed the money."

"Well, maybe it was mine. I took those two years off when she was a toddler because we moved and I couldn't find work. Maybe we should have put in her childcare so she could have had more socialization at an even younger age," countered Molly's dad. "But it doesn't matter any longer. Remember that the psychologist told us that she was going to struggle with social skills. So as much as we didn't want this to happen, it's happening. Let's just move forward."

"Okay, let's do it." Molly's mom, who tended to organize the household affairs now that Molly was in school, sent an email to the agency she had found online that was recommended by Molly's skating coach. Only hours later, she received a reply and set up a time for a behavior analyst to come and work with Molly and their family.

"Tell me about your biggest concerns with Molly when it comes to her social skills" was one of the questions the behavior analyst asked.

"That's easy," replied Molly's dad, eager to contribute to this conversation. "Molly has never had very many friends, but we told ourselves that it's okay. After all, we don't have a ton of friends either, but we do have some really good friends—other parents—that we hang out with as a couple. And that's enough for us! But even when she is with other children regularly, she doesn't really seem to interact much, or really want to make friends. It almost seems like she is withdrawing; like she doesn't want to make friends at all."

"And we have told her this over and over," chimed in Molly's mother. "We have modeled it for her at the playground, during her lessons and activities. She can tell us the steps to making a friend, but she doesn't seem to DO it or even try just one little bit. At school where, obviously, there are tons of other kids, it still doesn't happen. We thought, for a long time, until now, really, that she would 'catch up.' People keep telling us that young children learn skills at their own pace. But it's really past that point now, we think. We are really getting worried and I have big knot in my stomach right now just talking about it." She reached for Molly's dad, and they held hands tightly while the conversation continued. "It might sound silly, but we are feeling almost desperate. We are just really frightened for Molly."

Later, as the conversation concluded, the behavior analyst went back to her office, her desk, and her computer to work out a plan for completing a full assessment and then putting a plan into place. She began to think about how she might be able to determine whether the intervention program that she will be designing is responsible for any behavior changes they might observe. She wondered about the strengths and limitations of a **multiple baseline design**, a **changing criterion design**, a reversal design, and an **alternating treatment design**. *Could I even ethically use any of these experimental designs in this context? Social skills are so complex*, she pondered. *And it looks like, at least for some of Molly's skills, that we are seeing problems with performance of skills that she knows. I think that since Molly has a number of components in her repertoire of social skills that will likely need support, I could plan a multiple baseline across behaviors design, or maybe a multiple baseline across home, school, and community settings design, when we are ready to start working on the actual intervention.*

For the next three months, Molly, her parents, and the behavior analyst worked together on a range of social skills, including approaching other children, initiating conversations, and reciprocal turn-taking in conversation. Each of these interventions began at various times, so that the behavior analyst could easily pinpoint which parts of the interventions were successful—if any. The behavior analyst was quite impressed with the graph he created throughout this period of time, gathering data at home, school, and community settings to see whether the frequency in which Molly demonstrated these new skills was increasing.

At their next meeting, the analyst reported as he displayed the graphs, "I am really thrilled to see that Molly is making so many positive changes. She is really showing her skills in every setting, and I see a strong upward trend in the frequency in which she uses these skills, especially in the last month or so."

Molly's parents nodded, but made very little eye contact. They did not appear to share in the enthusiasm that the behavior analyst was exhibiting. She finally asked, "Is something wrong?"

"Not wrong, no. But we are a bit embarrassed," they began. "We actually started Molly on some new medication for social anxiety suggested by her pediatrician and her child psychiatrist. This was about a month ago, too. Although they told us that we shouldn't tell anyone so the use of the medication could be what they called 'blinded.' But it feels really wrong to us and I think we should have told you."

Molly's behavior analyst hesitated to process this new information and then said, "I think that the intervention, though, is what is making the difference, based on the data we have collected."

Molly's dad interrupted with, "But does it really matter? In the end, as long as Molly is improving, she wins, you win: we all win. Am I right?"

The Response: Principles, Processes, Practices, and Reflections

Principles

(Q1) What is the term used when it is unsure whether another variable is influencing the results that are being seen?

(Q2) Does an ethical dilemma result at all, from the behavior therapist, if she is not sure whether her intervention is effective (Reference Ethics Box 7.2, Behavior Analyst Certification Board, 2014)?

Ethics Box 7.2

Professional and Ethical Compliance Code for Behavior Analysts

- 4.07 Environmental Conditions that Interfere with Implementation.

  (a) If environmental conditions prevent implementation of a behavior-change program, behavior analysts recommend that other professional assistance (e.g., assessment, consultation, or therapeutic intervention by other professionals) be sought

  (b) If environmental conditions hinder implementation of the behavior-change program, behavior analysts seek to eliminate the environmental constraints or identify in writing the obstacles to doing so.

Processes

(Q3) What are the strengths and limitations of a multiple baseline design, reversal design, changing criterion design, and alternating treatment design (Table 7.4)?

(Q4) In this case, which research design would allow the therapist to evaluate whether the medication or the social skills intervention was causing the change?

Table 7.4 Descriptions of reversal, changing criterion, multiple baseline, and alternating treatment single-subject research designs

Design	Description
Reversal (A–B)	Baseline data are taken and then an intervention (A phase) is introduced for a predetermined amount of time. After this time has passed, the intervention is removed (B phase). This can be repeated a number of times in order to determine whether a functional relationship exists between the independent variable (the intervention) and the dependent variable (the behavior)
Changing criterion	This design is appropriate when the target behavior has the potential to change in gradual stages. Baseline data on the behavior are taken first. After baseline data are collected, a criterion level is determined for each phase. The final phase criterion level should match the behavior and terminal goal initially determined. The intervention is then introduced, and the criterion level that had been predetermined is used to control reinforcement (or punishment). Each time the criterion level is met, the next phase is introduced, and this continues until the terminal goal is met
Multiple baseline	A multiple baseline design is similar to the reversal design but is used when there is more than one dependent variable, such as setting, people, or functionally equivalent behaviors. Baseline data are taken on all dependent variables. After the baseline phase, the independent variable, or intervention, is introduced for the first dependent variable, while maintaining baseline for the other dependent variables. Upon reaching predetermined criteria for the first dependent variable, the following dependent variable may enter the intervention phase. This pattern would continue until all dependent variables enter into the intervention phase
Alternating treatment	An alternating treatment design is used when one is interested in the effect of more than one intervention on a dependent variable. The interventions are rotated in a counterbalanced manner to decrease the possibility of treatment effects carrying over from one intervention phase to subsequent phases. Baseline data are not necessary when using this design, though should be included when it is possible. The first independent variable is introduced; data are taken. At the next opportunity, a different independent variable is used. This continues until it is determined whether one independent variable is more effective than another

Richards et al. (2013)

Practice

(**Q5**) Set up a multiple baseline design to determine whether the social skills training is effective. Which type of multiple baseline would you use and why? Would a multiple baseline or a reversal design be more effective?

(**Q6**) Another way to evaluate if change has been achieved is by completing a criterion-based skills assessment. An example from the VB-MAPP is provided below. What are advantages and disadvantages to using this approach (Fig. 7.10)?

(**Q7**) Using the figure below, determine how the changing criterion design would work with Molly? How would self-management play a role with this design? Do you think the medication influenced her performance given the results (Fig. 7.11)?

	ASSESSMENT			
	1ST	2ND	3RD	4TH
TOTAL SCORE				

DOES THE CHILD SPONTANEOUSLY PARTICPATE IN ACTIVITIES WITH OTHER CHILDREN AND SPONTANEOUSLY VERBALLY INTERAC T WITH THEM?

1ST	2ND	3RD	4TH	
1ST	2ND	3RD	4TH	6. Initiates a physical interaction with a peer 2 times (e.g., a push in a wagon, hand holding, Ring around the Rosy) **(TO: 30 min.)**
1ST	2ND	3RD	4TH	7. Spontaneously mands to peers 5 times (e.g., *My turn. Push me. Look! Come on.*) **(TO: 60 min.)**
1ST	2ND	3RD	4TH	8. Engages in sustained social play with peers for 3 minutes without adult prompts or reinforcement (e.g., cooperatively setting up a play set, water play) **(TO: 30 min.)**
1ST	2ND	3RD	4TH	9. Spontaneous responds to the mands from peers 5 times (e.g., *Pull me in the wagon. I want the train.*) **(E)**
1ST	2ND	3RD	4TH	10. Spontaneously mands to peers to participate in games, social play, etc. 2 times. (e.g., *Come on you guys. Let's dig a hole.*) **(TO: 60 min.)**

Fig. 7.10 VB-MAPP milestones, level 2, social behavior, and social play (Sundberg 2008, p. 13)

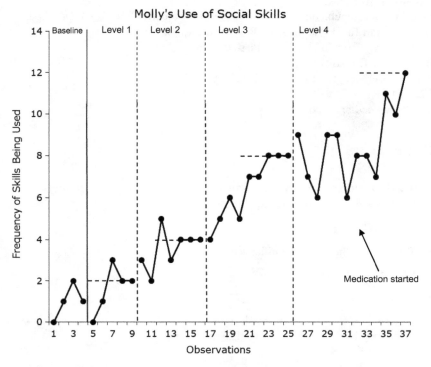

Fig. 7.11 Changing criterion graph showing the number of times Molly engaged in one of the social skills being worked on while behavior analyst was observing

Reflection

(Q8) Can medication be a useful part of a behavior intervention program? If so, in what way? If not, why not?

(Q9) What was the behavior consultant required to discuss with the family with regard to implementing the treatment? Did this change at all since she implemented a multiple baseline design (Reference Ethics Box 7.3, Behavior Analyst Certification Board, 2014)?

Ethics Box 7.3

Professional and Ethical Compliance Code for Behavior Analysts

- 4.04 Approving Behavior-Change Programs.
  Behavior analysts must obtain the client's written approval of the behavior-change program before implementation or making significant modifications (e.g., change in goals, use of new procedures).

(Q10) Were Molly's parents wrong to withhold information about the introduction of medication? Why or why not?

Additional Web Links
Single-Subject Design
http://www.sagepub.com/sites/default/files/upm-binaries/25657_Chapter7.pdf
Introduction to Single-Subject Research Design
https://www.msu.edu/user/sw/ssd/issd10.htm#a
Behavioral Consulting
http://files.eric.ed.gov/fulltext/EJ801232.pdf
VB-MAPP
http://www.avbpress.com

CASE: iv-E5

How is it a success for Ramsey, when WE aren't seeing any change?
Setting: Home   Age Group: Preschool

LEARNING OBJECTIVE:

- To evaluate the social significance of behavior change.

TASK LIST LINKS:

- **Experimental Design**

    - (B-08) Use multiple probe designs.
    - (B-09) Use combinations of design elements.

- (B-10) Conduct a component analysis to determine the effective components of an intervention package.

- **Identification of the Problem**

  - (G-02) Consider biological/medical variables that may be affecting the client.
  - (G-06) Provide behavior-analytic services in collaboration with others who support and/or provide services to one's clients.

- **Intervention**

  - (J-11) Program for stimulus and response generalization.

KEY TERMS:

- **Scatterplot**

  - In applied behavior analysis, a scatter plot is a tool used to discover patterns between the occurrence of certain behaviors within certain times over the course of a day or week. A scatter plot is often used as part of the behavior assessment process to determine when, for example each day, problematic behaviors are occurring, and is often collected within a data sheet (Maas et al. 2009).

- **Self-injurious behavior**

  - Self-injurious behaviors can be described as behaviors that one engages in that harm one's own body. There are many forms of self-injurious behaviors that may include head-banging, hand-biting, and scratching one's self (Matson and LoVullo 2008).

- **Socially significant**

  - In applied behavior analysis, behaviors are selected for change based on their social significance, that is, the extent to which the behavior change will improve the person's quality of life (Bosch and Faqua 2001).

How Is It a Success for Ramsey, When WE Aren't Seeing Any Change?

"Ramsey has really been struggling with **self-injurious behavior** this year at school so far," noted one of the school support team members, Mr. Avro, at their weekly team meeting. "It is quite different from what we saw last year. Last year, he was having trouble with physically aggressive behaviors, mostly around his peers. He kept taking those airplanes that he loves—the ones he carries in his pockets—and hitting his peers with them. Remember? We did a great job working with the school staff and with Ramsey to decrease this particular behavior. But since he was off for the summer months, he has come to school with a whole new one and we have been focusing on that important **socially significant** behavior issue since then. Ms. Lancaster, could you describe your observations around Ramsey?"

"Certainly," Ms. Lancaster—another school support member–responded with confidence. "As you will all remember, Ramsey does not use verbal communication, he has an Autism Spectrum Disorder diagnosis, he just turned 11 a few weeks ago, and is in sixth grade at this school. He has been displaying what we would call self-injurious behaviors: he has been banging his head against the wall and banging his head, at times, with his fists. This has persisted for over two months, and we have full parental support to put changes in place as they see this as both a socially important goal, but also safety concern. Although there is not a great deal of force behind any of the blows Ramsey self-delivers, is it obviously concerning to the school staff, Ramsey's parents, and importantly, Ramsey himself. It is really making his peers shy away from interacting with him: they clearly do not know what to think or to do as they likely wouldn't have seen this type of behavior before. When Ramey was re-referred to use about seven weeks ago, of course we began with requesting that his parents take him for a full medical evaluation. No issues emerged from his check-up. We updated his Functional Behavior Analysis (FBA), which showed a complex combination of sensory and socially mediated attention functions. Our **scatterplot** showed a distinct pattern of occurrence during the periods where Ramsey is included with all the students in his grade level, which typically happen in the afternoon hours before the students leave for the day. He often wants to interact with them, but gets frustrated when they don't interact with him or when he cannot communicate his message. In addition, it was found that the overwhelming nature of the situation was difficult for him when there were many peers and the noise was loud. As you will recall, we planned and implemented a package of interventions here at school: noncontingent attention from peers, teachers, and paraprofessionals; the addition of sensory and other acceptable tools around the school (bongo drums, gel-filled squeezable items); a button coded with phrases to get the attention of peers; learning to ask for a break with a 'break card'; and response blocking if necessary."

Mr. Avro picked up the summary again. "Excellent. That's quite right. We have, of course, been collecting and evaluating data to see if this intervention package has had any effect on the incidence of self-injurious behaviors, as operationalized, and we have seen impressive success so far. In fact, the level of self-injurious behaviors is at a very low level—almost zero and seems quite stable at this point! This is very good news and I think our goals here are pretty much achieved. So, as you know, I have invited Ramsey three parents, his Mom, Dad and Step-Mom, into school today to share this progress. I think they are going to be very happy, as this behavior was noted as particularly concerning in both school and home environments." He glanced at the wall clock and stood up. "I think they should be here by now. I will go and see if they are waiting for us at the office."

Momentarily, Mr. Avro returned with Ramsey's three greatest resources: his parental figures from his two homes. With earnest pleasure, the team greeted Ramsey's parents and excitedly explained—and showed—the tremendously decreased rates of self-injurious behavior happening during the school days. All three listened with avid interest, nodding and smiling as they heard the positive news. Ramey's father began, "We were talking together in the office before you came to get us for this meeting. We wanted to make sure that you know we are thrilled with the positive news that you have been informing us about regularly in Ramsey's communication book and phone calls. It's really good to hear that you have been having so much success, just like you did last year. However, unlike last year, we are still really struggling with something at both of Ramsey's homes, and we haven't really been sure how to approach this. But here goes. We are still having all sorts of problems with these self-injurious behaviors at home. All three of us agree that we want to ask you for help at home, too. Is that possible?"

The members of the school support program awkwardly made eye contact, and Ms. Lancaster responded "Unfortunately, not for us, no. We are privately contracted with this school board in a partnership. It would be a conflict of interest and directly against the boundaries set out in our memorandum of understanding to work in the homes of our students. Even if it wasn't, our job is here, and if we are not busy with Ramsey, we have many other students on our caseloads that occupy our work hours."

"That makes me so angry!" Ramsey's mother blurted, with his father and stepmother nodding in unison. "I mean, you are clearly very skilled professionals, people who are hard to find, but I wonder how meaningful all of these so-called great changes are if they happening only in one place? How are they really meaningful changes?"

"I can understand your frustrations," added Mr. Avro, "but unfortunately our hands are tied with respect to looking at other environments. But I can make a list for you of names and contact information for other community support services that might work for you outside of the school environment. That's the best we can do for Ramsey and all of you right now."

The Response: Principles, Processes, Practices, and Reflections

Principles

(Q1) What would the component of the intervention that focused on noncontingent attention from peers look like?

(Q2) Using the table below, has the principles of generality been achieved in the case of Ramsey? Why or why not (Fig. 7.12)?

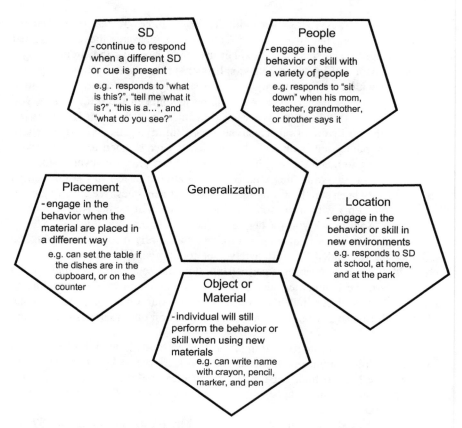

Fig. 7.12 Types of generalization

Processes

(Q3) How could the school personnel have planned for the generalization of Ramsey's behavioral improvements outside of the school environment?

(Q4) What ethical boundaries are in place that prevent the school team from working with Ramsey's parents at home? How might the school personnel have included Ramsey's parents in the process while staying within the scope and boundaries of their roles (Reference Ethics Box 7.4, Behavior Analyst Certification Board, 2014)?

Ethics Box 7.4

Professional and Ethical Compliance Code for Behavior Analysts

- 2.04 Third-Party Involvement in Services.

  (a) When behavior analysts agree to provide services to a person or entity at the request of a third party, behavior analysts clarify, to the extent feasible and at the outset of the service, the nature of the relationship with each party and any potential conflicts. This clarification includes the role of the behavior analyst (such as therapist, organizational consultant, or expert witness), the probable uses of the services provided or the information obtained, and the fact that there may be limits to confidentiality.

  (b) If there is a foreseeable risk of behavior analysts being called upon to perform conflicting roles because of the involvement of a third party, behavior analysts clarify the nature and direction of their responsibilities, keep all parties appropriately informed as matters develop, and resolve the situation in accordance with the code.

  (c) When providing services to a minor or individual who is a member of a protected population at the request of a third party, behavior analysts ensure that the parent or client-surrogate of the ultimate recipient of services is informed of the nature and scope of services to be provided, as well as their right to all service records and data.

  (d) Behavior analysts put the client's care above all others, and should the third party makes requirements for services that are contradicted by the behavior analyst's recommendations, behavior analysts are obligated to resolve such conflicts in the best interest of the client. If said conflict cannot be resolved, that behavior analyst's services to the client may be discontinued following appropriate transition.

Practice

(Q5) Using the competing behavior path diagram below, indicate the current behavior path for the socially mediated component of the behavior and indicate how the intervention has been implemented to teach replacement behaviors (Fig. 7.13).

(Q6) Using the functional analysis data shown in the link (pg. 5), describe the functions that are maintaining the self-injurious behaviors at home.

http://www.pent.ca.gov/frm/functobserv.pdf

(Q7) Given the information provided, what initial hypothesis may you draw as to why the self-injurious behavior is occurring at home? What additional information do you need to confirm this? How and from whom might you obtain this additional information?

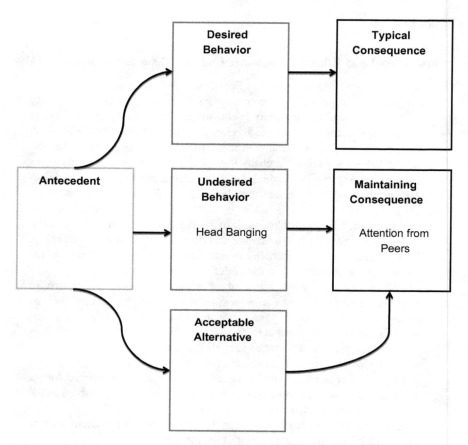

Fig. 7.13 Competing behavior pathway for Ramsey's self-injurious behavior

Reflection

(Q8) Why was a medical examination conducted before Ramsey's self-injurious behaviors were addressed through a behavioral intervention (Reference Ethics Box 7.5, Behavior Analyst Certification Board, 2014)?

Ethics Box 7.5

Professional and Ethical Compliance Code for Behavior Analysts

- 3.02 Medical Consultation.
  Behavior analysts recommend seeking a medical consultation if there is any reasonable possibility that a referred behavior is influenced by medical or biological variables.

(Q9) By still maintaining appropriate ethical guidelines, could the consultants work with the family through a parent coaching or mediator model?

(Q10) How meaningful are the changes in the success that the school has seen in the reduction of Ramsey's self-injurious behaviors if they have not generalized (Reference Ethics Box 7.6, Behavior Analyst Certification Board, 2014)?

Ethics Box 7.6

Professional and Ethical Compliance Code for Behavior Analysts

- 4.03 Individualized Behavior-Change Programs.
  (a) Behavior analysts must tailor behavior-change programs to the unique behaviors, environmental variables, assessment results, and goals for each client.
  (b) Behavior analysts do not plagiarize other professionals' behavior-change programs.
- 4.06 Describing Conditions for Behavior-Change Program Success.
  Behavior analysts describe to the client the environmental conditions that are necessary for the behavior-change program to be effective.

Additional Web Links

Promoting Generalization of Positive Behavior Change: Practical Tips for Parents and Professionals

http://www.centerforautism.com/Data/Sites/1/media/GeneralizationForParents
AndProfessionalsJan06DLS.pdf

Generalization

http://www.kcbehavioranalysts.com/aba-toolbox/generalization

ABA: A Focus on Outcomes

http://www.iidc.indiana.edu/pages/Applied-Behavior-Analysis-A-Focus-on-Outcomes

Self-Injurious Behaviors

http://www.autism.com/symptoms_self-injury

References

Autism & Behavioural Science Graduate Certificate (2014). *Triadic Mediator Model of Interaction*. Toronto, ON: Queen's Printer.

Behavior Analyst Certification Board (2014). *Professional and ethical compliance code for behavior analysts*. Retrieved from http://bacb.com/wp-content/uploads/2016/01/160120-compliance-code-english.pdf

Bosch, S., & Fuqua, W. (2001). Behavioral cusps: A model for selecting target behaviors. *Journal of Applied Behavior Analysis, 34*, 123–125.

Byiers, B. J., Reichle, J., & Symons, F. J. (2012). Single-subject experimental design for evidence-based practice. *American Journal of Speech-Language Pathology, 21*, 397–414.

Cooper, J., Heron, T., & Heward, W. (2007). *Applied behavior analysis* (2nd ed.). New Jersey: Pearson.

Grow, L., & LeBlanc, L. (2013). Teaching receptive language skills: Recommendations for instructors. *Behavior analysis in practice, 6*(1), 56.

Horner, R., Carr, E., Halle, J., McGee, G., Odom, S., & Wolery, M. (2005). The use of single subject research to identify evidence-based practice in special education. *Exceptional Children, 72*(2), 165–179.

Kratochwill, T. R., Hitchcock, J., Horner, R. H., Levin, J. R., Odom, S. L., Rindskopf, D. M., et al. (2010). *Single-case designs technical documentation*. Retrieved from What Works Clearinghouse website: http://ies.ed.gov/ncee/wwc/pdf/wwc_scd.pdf.

Libby, M., Weiss, J., Bancroft, S., & Ahearn, W. (2008). A comparison of most-to-least and least-to-most prompting on the acquisition of solitary play skills. *Behavior Analysis in Practice, 1*(1), 37–43.

Maas, A., Didden, R., Bouts, L., Smits, M., & Curfs, L. (2009). Scatter plot analysis of excessive daytime sleepiness and severe disruptive behavior in adults with Prader-Willi syndrome: A pilot study. *Research in Developmental Disabilities, 30*(3), 529–537.

Matson, J., & LoVullo, S. (2008). A review of behavioral treatments for self-injurious behaviors of persons with autism spectrum disorders. *Behaviour Modification, 32*(1), 61–76.

Odom, S., Brown, W., Frey, T., Karasu, N., Smith-Canter, L., & Strain, P. (2003). Evidence-based practices for young children with autism: Contributions for single subject design research. *Focus on Autism and Other Developmental Disabilities, 18*(3), 166–175.

Richards, S. B., Taylor, R., & Ramasamy, R. (2013). *Single Subject Research: Applications in Educational and Clinical Settings*. Nelson Education.

Severtson, J. M., & Carr, J. E. (2012). Training novice instructors to implement errorless discrete-trial teaching: A sequential analysis. *Behavior Analysis in Practice, 5*(2), 13–23.

Sundberg, M. L. (2008). *Verbal behavior milestones assessment and placement program (VB-MAPP)*. Concord, CA: AVB Press.

Thurm, A., Lord, C., Lee, L., & Newschaffer, C. (2007). Predictors of language acquisition in preschool children with autism spectrum disorders. *Journal of Autism and Developmental Disorders, 37*(9), 1721–1734.

UCDHSC Center for Nursing Research. (2006). *Treatment fidelity assessment grid*. Retrieved from http://www.ucdenver.edu/academics/colleges/nursing/Documents/PDF/TreatmentFidelityChecklist.doc

Vermilyea, B. B., Barlow, D. H., & O'Brien, G. T. (1984). The importance of assessing treatment integrity: An example in the anxiety disorders. *Journal of Behavioral Assessment, 6*, 1–11.

Wilkinson, L. A. (2007). Assessing treatment integrity in behavioral consultation. *International Journal of Behavioral Consultation and Therapy, 3*(3), 420–432. doi:10.1037/h0100816.

Wong, C., Odom, S. L., Hume, K. A, Cox, A. W., Fettig, A., Kucharczyk, S., et al. (2013). *Evidence-based practices for children, youth, and young adults with autism spectrum disorder: A comprehensive review*. Retrieved from http://fpg.unc.edu/sites/fpg.unc.edu/files/resources/reports-and-policy-briefs/2014-EBP-Report.pdf

Chapter 8
Evaluation-Centered Case Studies from Adolescence to Adulthood

Abstract In this chapter, the evaluation of behavior-change programs is explored through a series of case scenarios with adolescents, adults, and seniors. While the reduction and elimination of problematic behaviors are usually key outcomes for behavior-change programs, in these stages of life increased emphasis is often placed on the development and mastery of skills that will lead to independent living and working, and successful engagement in social and recreational activities. Throughout this chapter, learners will evaluate the efficacy and effectiveness of behavioral interventions and determine the extent to which outcomes are being achieved that are meaningful and socially significant for the adolescent adult stages of life. Further, learners will be guided to use a logic model to support the development and implementation of a program evaluation framework, while considering the importance of viewing both positive and negative evaluation outcomes as critical to the success of a behavior-change program. In this chapter, entitled "Evaluation-Centered Case Studies from Adolescence to Adulthood," the strengths and limitations of various direct and indirect measures of behavior are critically examined within a bio-psychosocial framework through five case scenarios in home, school, work, and community settings.

Keywords Adolescents · Adults · Seniors · Measurement · Evaluation · Problematic behaviors · Independent living · Engagement · Social activities · Efficacy of behavioral interventions · Program evaluation framework · Implementation

CASE: iv-E6

I Think it is fair to say that this is Working!
Setting: Community   Age Group: Adolescence—Adulthood

LEARNING OBJECTIVE:

- Construct an evaluation to demonstrate an intervention program's efficacy and effectiveness.

© Springer International Publishing AG 2016   267
K. Maich et al., *Applied Behavior Analysis*,
DOI 10.1007/978-3-319-44794-0_8

TASK LIST LINKS:

- **Measurement**

  - (A-11) Design, plot, and interpret data using a cumulative record to display data.

- **Behavior-Change Systems**

  - (F-06) Use incidental teaching.

- **Implementation, Management, and Supervision**

  - (K-02) Identify the contingencies governing the behavior of those responsible for carrying out behavior-change procedures and design interventions accordingly,
  - (K-06) Provide supervision for behavior-change agents,
  - (K-07) Evaluate the effectiveness of a behavioral program,
  - (K-10) Arrange for the orderly termination of services when they are no longer required.

KEY TERMS:

- **Cumulative Record**

  - A method of data collection whereby the rate of the response is added to the previous data collection and the display is organized such that the steeper the response, the more rapid the responses (Mayer et al. 2014).

- **Effectiveness**

  - Effectiveness refers to whether a treatment improves outcomes when delivered with typical clients in real-world settings, outside of rigorous research or clinical trial conditions (Marchand et al. 2011; Wells 1999).

- **Efficacy**

  - Efficacy refers to whether a treatment improves outcomes under highly controlled conditions, such as in rigorous clinical trials or research that use experimental designs (Marchand et al. 2011; Wells 1999).

- **Program Evaluation**

  - Evaluations are conducted to determine the extent to which programs are achieving their intended purpose. An evaluation may involve an assessment of a program's processes, procedures, or outcomes (Hogan 2007). The Ontario Centre of Excellence for Child and Youth Mental Health (2016) describes program evaluation as gathering information systematically to use results for making decisions and future program improvement.

I Think It Is Fair To Say That This Is Working!

It was the end of another busy, yet successful, day at the center. Checking his watch, Tom, the supervisor of a social skills program at a local treatment center for children and adolescents with autism spectrum disorder (ASD), was happy to see that he had thirty minutes to debrief with the staff and clean up from the day's program. His group of eight adolescents had just been picked up by their parents a few minutes ago, and he was eager to hear from each of the staff about how they thought the session went.

Tom was hired four weeks ago to support the launch of a new program at the treatment center: a social skills program for adolescents between the ages of 10 and 12 with a diagnosis of ASD. The center had received some new funding to try out and evaluate this new program in the hopes that it would be found to be effective. Everyone hoped that, after this trial period, the center would receive permanent funding to expand this social skills program so that more adolescents could participate, and the center could add it to their list of programs offered year-round to the community.

After working together with his staff to quickly put activities and supplies away, disinfect the tables and chairs, sweep the floors, and take the garbage out, Tom asked the staff to meet in the staff room for a quick meeting before they all left for the day. As they settled into the staff room, making themselves comfortable on the couches, Tom began to share with the staff the conversation he had had earlier that morning with the Center Director Sherrie. Sherrie had told Tom that next month, she had to report back to the funders about the progress of the new social skills program and complete a new funding application. "We have to do a small **program evaluation**," Sherrie said. "The funders are interested in both the **effectiveness** and the **efficacy** of our program." Sherrie went on to tell Tom that the future of the program could be dependent upon whether it was seen to be successful and reminded Tom and the rest of the staff that the current funding was just intended for a short, three-month pilot program. At the end of the conversation, Sherrie asked Tom to meet with her next month for an update so that she could complete her report to the funders. As Tom continued to speak with the staff about this upcoming meeting, his mind started to wander.

He remembered how he felt walking away from Sherrie that morning after their conversation about the program's future, as he was reminiscing he felt a wave of anxiety come over him. *I just started*, he thought, *and I really like it here. My staff are great, the youth seem to be enjoying the program, and parents keep thanking me and my team for the work we are doing. What will happen if the funding is cut and the program ends? What will this mean for the youth? For my staff? And what about me?*

As he looked around the room at his five staff members, he could see that they were listening closely to every word he was saying. "But I like it here. I think we are a great team and working with all of you and in this program is a lot of fun," said Tracey, a twenty-year-old post-secondary student working part-time with the program. "And I need this job to help pay for school," Tracey went on to explain.

Tom interrupted the clearly rising anxiety around him and said, "Let's begin by having a quick look at the data you have all been collecting. This should help to explain our case to the funders." One at a time, each staff member held up the graphs they had been constructing over the last four weeks and provided a very brief summary of the progress the youth were making. The thing that struck Tom was the fact that all of the graphs were so different since they were measuring such different social skills for each adolescent. He did not know how he was going to summarize all of this information to ensure that he could demonstrate success across all of the participants, especially since they are using incidental teaching and turning tasks that each youth enjoys into "teachable moments." He thought about it and suggested a **cumulative record**. When asked what it was by the staff, they discussed that they would be able to track the number of different social skills each person exhibited across all of the sessions. This way, if there were some social skills that were dependent on others or what was happening that day, it would not influence the data.

As the staff listened, they became more and more excited, and the anxiety became a thing of the past. One of the staff members could not contain himself any longer and blurted, "This is fantastic! It has given me a great idea! Let us put together a cumulative graph showing the progress of each youth, and then, we can attach each of the individual graphs to a summary across all youth. We can then give this package to Sherrie to show her that our program is indeed successful."

Matt, a 22-year-old part-time staff member and also a full-time student at the local college, looked at Tracey and shared a somewhat concerned look. "But Tom, while it is great that youth in our program are showing the target social skills more often, how can we tell if it is actually because of our program?" asked Matt. "And what about those who we have been able to systematically fade our involvement with? Do we know if our ability to fade our prompts and supports has anything to do with our program? What about other possible explanations?"

"I agree," said Tracey, "I mean, we know that some have been taking medication, some of been receiving other interventions at the same time, and some have not even attended every session. Can we really just put all the data together and say that we are the reason for the changes in behavior? And is this really what Sherrie is looking for?"

But Tom was not listening to the thoughtful input of his team. His mind was back on all of the ways he could put the data together to not only help with planning the next steps for each student, but also show Sherrie how great the social skills program is doing. He thought that *I could save the program!* Tom looked at his staff, thanked them for all of the great work they are doing, and told them to have a great night. He knew what to do, and he wanted to get started right away.

The Response: Principles, Processes, Practices, and Reflections

Principles

(Q1) Describe the similarities and differences between evaluation and research. What considerations will be important for Tom to ensure that he is conducting an evaluation of the social skills program, and not research?

(Q2) When determining whether or not to implement an intervention in an applied setting, would the efficacy or effectiveness of that intervention be of greater importance? Why? Should Tom be concerned about demonstrating the efficacy or the effectiveness of the social skills program?

Processes

(Q3) What would be involved in teaching social skills through incidental teaching? What would be some benefits and drawbacks of the approach from an evaluation standpoint (Fig. 8.1)?

(Q4) What are the strengths and limitations of conducting visual analysis of graphed behavior data? How might you address any limitations in the current study with the cumulative record (Fig. 8.2)?

Fig. 8.1 Steps in incidental teaching (Ryan 2011)

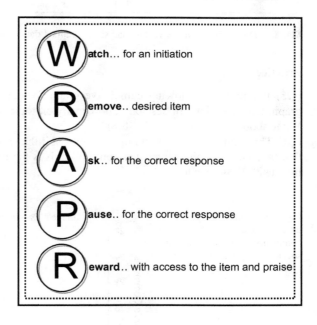

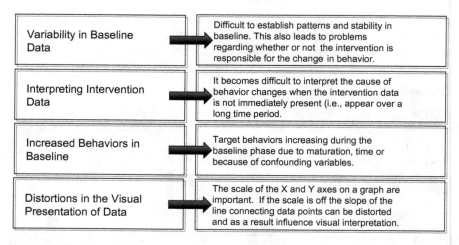

Fig. 8.2 Difficulties with the visual analysis of graphed data (Alnahdi 2015)

Practice

(Q5) Interpret the following cumulative graph for one of the youth. What is the graph demonstrating? In Session 9, how many on-topic comments did Jaako make? What about in Session 13 (Fig. 8.3)?

(Q6) This cumulative graph in Fig. 8.4 looks at if the youth says "Hi" each morning that he comes into the center. Do you think this is the most effective way to graph this data? Why or why not?

Fig. 8.3 Cumulative graph depicting Jaako's on-topic comments to his peers during social skills program sessions

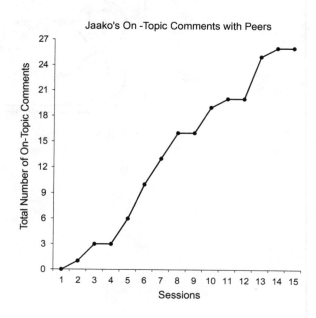

Fig. 8.4 Cumulative graph of one youth in the program's greeting staff each morning at the center

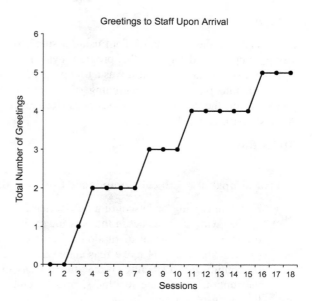

(Q7) Comparing the cumulative graph in Fig. 8.3 to the line graph below, which graph better depicts the frequency of social greetings each day. What is the pros and cons of using each graph (Fig. 8.5)?

(Q8) What confounding variables might pose challenges for Tom? For each confounding variable listed, please outline how you might address the issue.

Fig. 8.5 Line graph depicting one youth in the program's greeting staff each morning at the center

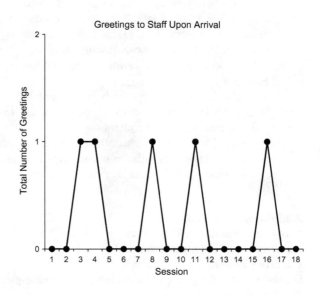

Reflection

(Q9) What are the benefits of Tom using a single-subject design as opposed to a group-comparison design for this program evaluation?

(Q10) Knowing that this project was a trial project, what considerations would need to be put into place at the beginning of the program to ensure that clients are prepared for the termination of services (Reference Ethics Box 8.1, Behavior Analyst Certification Board, 2014)?

Ethics Box 8.1

Professional and Ethical Compliance Code for Behavior Analysts

- 2.15 Interrupting or Discontinuing Services.

  (a) Behavior analysts act in the best interests of the client and supervisee to avoid interruption or disruption of service.

  (b) Behavior analysts make reasonable and timely efforts for facilitating the continuation of behavior-analytic services in the event of unplanned interruptions (e.g., due to illness, impairment, unavailability, relocation, disruption of funding, disaster).

  (c) When entering into employment or contractual relationships, behavior analysts provide for orderly and appropriate resolution of responsibility for services in the event that the employment or contractual relationship ends, with paramount consideration given to the welfare of the ultimate beneficiary of services.

  (d) Discontinuation only occurs after efforts to transition have been made. Behavior analysts discontinue a professional relationship in a timely manner when the client: (1) no longer needs the service, (2) is not benefiting from the service, (3) is being harmed by continued service, or (4) when the client requests discontinuation.

- 4.11 Discontinuing Behavior-Change Programs and Behavior-Analytic Services.

  (a) Behavior analysts establish understandable and objective (i.e., measurable) criteria for the discontinuation of the behavior-change program and describe them to the client

  (b) Behavior analysts discontinue services with the client when the established criteria for discontinuation are attained, as in when a series of agreed-upon goals have been met.

Additional Web Links

Program Evaluation Resources

http://www.cdc.gov/eval/resources/

Planning Evaluation

http://www.excellenceforchildandyouth.ca/evaluation-module-1-planning-evaluation

Incidental Teaching

http://www.special-learning.com/article/incidental_teaching

CASE: iv-E7

Does it matter WHAT worked?
Setting: School   Age Group: Adolescent—Adulthood

LEARNING OBJECTIVE:

- Design and evaluate a school-wide positive behavior support program.

TASK LIST LINKS:

- **Experimental Design**

  - (B-02) Review and interpret articles from the behavior-analytic literature.
  - (B-03) Systematically arrange independent variables to demonstrate their effects on dependent variables.
  - (B-11) Conduct a parametric analysis to determine the effective values of an independent variable.

- **Behavior-Change Systems**

  - (F-02) Use token economies and other conditioned reinforcement systems.

- **Measurement**

  - (H-01) Select a measurement system to obtain representative data given the dimensions of the behavior and the logistics of observing and recording
  - (H-03) Select a data display that effectively communicates relevant quantitative relations

- **Implementation, Management, and Supervision**

  - (K-06) Provide supervision for behavior-change agents
  - (K-07) Evaluate the effectiveness of the behavioral program

KEY TERMS:

- **Positive Behavior Support**

  - Positive Behavior Support (PBS) is an application of behavior analysis. Often described as a system, PBS begins with understanding the function of problematic behaviors, and then focuses on replacing the problematic behavior with functionally equivalent, yet more socially appropriate skills. This reduces the potential that intrusive or aversive interventions will be needed. Additional components of PBS may include lifestyle changes, person-centered values, a life span perspective, ecological and social validity of interventions, and a focus on prevention and empirical validation of behavior-change procedures (Carr et al. 2002).

- **Component Analysis**

  - Intervention programs, either to reduce problematic behaviors or increase pro-social behaviors, are often made up of various components, or parts. For example, a parent training program might be made up of (a) increasing positive parent–child interactions, (b) using time-out, (c) communication skills, and d) parental consistency. A component analysis is an attempt to determine which components, or parts, of the intervention program, either alone or in combination, are associated with larger or smaller effects on the target behaviors (Kaminski et al. 2008; Ward-Horner and Sturmey 2010).

- **Experimental Design**

  - Single-subject research is one of the most commonly used approaches to research in applied behavior analysis. Single-subject research focuses on the measurement of changes within each participant taking part in a study, where the participant acts as their own control, rather than average changes in groups of participants, as is often the focus of group design studies. A single-subject experimental design, such as an ABAB withdrawal design (A = baseline phase, B = treatment phase), or a multiple baseline design, attempts to document causal or functional relationships between the manipulation of the independent variable, such as the introduction and withdrawal of the treatment, and changes in the dependent variable, such as decreases or increases in behavior (Horner et al. 2005).

- **Parametric Analysis**

  - Statistical practices whereby it relies on the assumption that the shape of the distribution is a normal distribution from the sample it is derived from and that there are parameters (means and standard deviations) in this assumed distribution (Hoskin n.d.).

Does It Matter WHAT Worked?

Jennifer, the principal of Sunnyview High School, just left yet another administrative meeting feeling uneasy about the future of her students, her staff, and her school. The meeting that she had attended was chaired by the superintendent of schools in her district. In attendance were most of the principals from schools across the wide and long geographic area in which her school resided. The focus most of the day was on addressing decreasing behavioral difficulties and poor achievement among some of the schools: including Sunnyview. Sunnyview was recognized earlier in the school year (and the last school year, and the one before that) as one of the schools experiencing such challenges, and Jennifer—like her colleagues in similar situations—had been asked to provide an update to her colleagues. After her update, the superintendent said that she would like to send a few school administrators to a workshop being held next week on *s*chool-wide **Positive Behavior Support**. She identified Jennifer, along with four other principals, as individuals she would like to see participate in this workshop. The Superintendent went on to say that at the next meeting of this group–eight weeks away–she would like the five principals, including Jennifer, to share how they have put PBS into practice, and to share the progress they are making in turning their schools around.

As Jennifer started her car and began to drive slowly back to her school, she kept asking herself questions: *How am I going to lead this change in my school? Can I really do this? And in just eight weeks?* Jennifer began to feel her stress build as she thought about where she might even begin—much less end.

After her return from the series of PBS-intensive professional development activities, Jennifer called a meeting of her school administrative, senior teaching staff members, and her heads of guidance and special education. After welcoming everyone to the meeting, Jennifer began to share with her team her experience at the administrative meeting and the expectations of the superintendent. Jennifer went on to say, "We will have to report back in only about seven weeks. That does not give us a lot of time. But I am confident that if we support each other and draw on each other —our knowledge, our experiences, our expertise—we can bring about some of the changes we want to see in our students, and our school. Let us begin by identifying the challenging behaviors you are experiencing. Who would like to begin?"

One at a time, the teachers each shared with Jennifer the challenging behaviors they were experiencing with students in their classrooms. Jennifer listened carefully and worked hard not to interrupt, even as she was shocked at some of this new-to-her information. As she absorbed the ongoing commentary, the school's secretary busily took minutes on her notepad, and she took some additional notes, trying hard to capture what each teacher shared. After all twelve of the teachers finished describing the challenging behaviors they were experiencing, Jennifer took a deep breath and looked back at the notes, then at her staff, for what seemed like several very long minutes.

Without saying a word, Jennifer stood up and began to write on the large white-board behind her. On the left side of the board, she began to list all of the challenging behaviors described by the teachers. As she listed the behaviors, she noticed from the corner of her eye some of the teachers nodding as they saw their concerns reflected. After listing all of the behaviors on the left side of the board, Jennifer wrote three headings on the right side of the board: (1) school-wide/classroom-wide preventive practices; (2) specialized group programs; and (3) specialized intensive individualized programs. She then began to organize the behaviors listed under each heading.

Jennifer then turned around, faced her staff, and said: "I would like to propose a way for us to work together as a team to support our students and turn our school around. Last week, I attended a workshop on school-wide Positive Behavior Support and I think, based on the challenging behaviors you have been facing, it might work well here. Some of the challenging behaviors that you shared, like disrespectful behavior, could be a focus school-wide, with each of us modeling and reinforcing respectful behavior in all parts of the school throughout the whole day. We may want to think of a school-wide reinforcement system. Other challenging behaviors you listed, like social skill difficulties between students in your classrooms, could be a focus for specialized instructions for small groups of students. Still other challenging behaviors, like specific behavioral difficulties experienced by only a select few students—for example, non-compliance to teacher requests and aggressive outbursts toward peers—can become the focus of specialized intensive individualized programs. We have funding for all of it and a promise of its renewal if we get results. We just need, at this point, the initiative and enthusiasm to put it into place."

The teachers in the room were silent as they took in what Jennifer had explained. One by one, the teachers began to nod in agreement. "I like it. I really like how we can all work together to make this happen," said Frank, a senior teacher with more than thirty years of experience. "Me too. I can see the potential in this plan," said Fareed, another senior teacher with twenty-five years of experience. After hearing that the most senior teachers were in support, the other teachers in the room began to express their support for this idea.

Jennifer, in turn, was getting excited: "It is great that you are all in support of this idea. I will contact a behavior analyst to work with us over the next seven weeks to design and implement the intervention programs and help us measure our progress."

"But Jennifer," interrupted Fareed, with a background in applied behavior analysis himself, "with so many parts to this idea for a really complex intervention program, how will we know which part is contributing to which change? How will we know if we are making a difference? Will the behavior analyst do a **component analysis**? Should we start all of the interventions at the same time or maybe stagger the start of each part, maybe as part of some sort of **experimental design**, to help us see which is making a difference?" Jennifer, *thinking* that these were excellent questions but not quite knowing how to respond and feeling the pressure of having to provide an update to her colleagues and the Superintendent in just seven weeks, quickly replied, "As long as we are seeing improvement, does it really matter which part is making a difference?" She thought back to her university days and wondered if she would need to complete **parametric analyses** or if using a single-subject design would suffice. With that, Jennifer thanked the teachers for attending the meeting and said that a behavior analyst will be in touch with each of them to get started over the next week.

The Response: Principles, Processes, Practices, and Reflections

Principles

(Q1) In their article "Positive Behavior Support: Evolution of an Applied Science" (Carr et al. 2002), the authors assert: "Were it not for the past 35 years of research in applied behavior analysis, PBS could not have come into existence" (p. 5). Do you agree or disagree with this statement? Please explain your response (Table 8.1). **(Q2)** Determining the function of behavior is a key component of positive behavior support. What is the difference between a functional analysis and a functional behavior assessment? When would you do one over the other for specific students (Fig. 8.6)?

Table 8.1 Data collection in social skills teaching

Data collection method	How could this data be used to evaluate the social skills group?
Frequency	
Rate	
Duration	
Latency	
Interresponse time	
Percent of occurrence	
Trials to criterion	

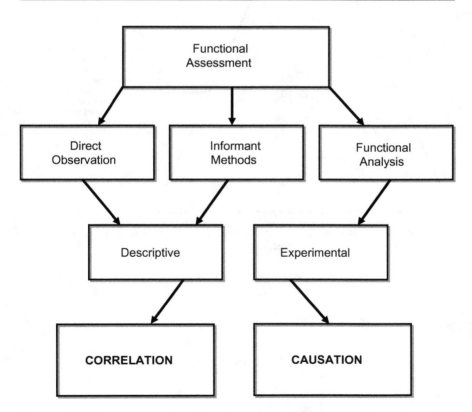

Fig. 8.6 Correlation versus causation within a functional behavior assessment (Educate Autism 2016)

Processes

(Q3) Jennifer outlines a tiered approach to supporting students throughout her school. This approach includes school-wide strategies for all students, specialized instructions for small groups of students, and specialized intensive individualized programs for a small number of students. How might you prepare both staff and students for the implementation of this tiered approach (Fig. 8.7)?

(Q4) An important component of positive behavior support is person-centered planning. What does this mean, and how might it apply to Jennifer's situation (Fig. 8.8)?

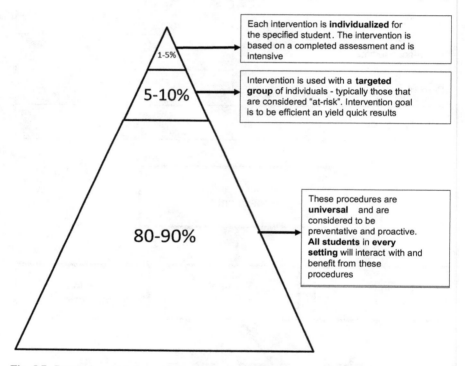

Fig. 8.7 Pyramid model for school-wide positive behavior supports can be used for both academic and behavior systems (Elsbree, n.d.)

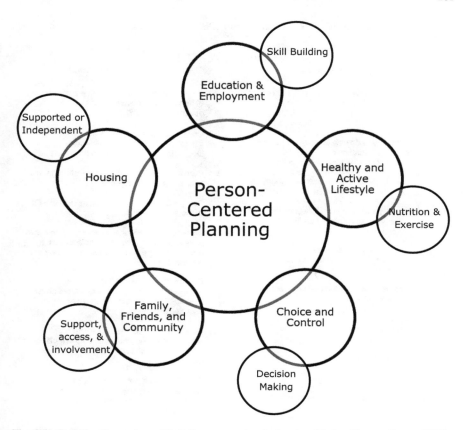

Fig. 8.8 Considerations when utilizing person-centered planning (Caring Homes Group, 2016)

Practice

(**Q5**) As principal, Jennifer's role requires that she not only focus on the behavior of students, but also determine how she will encourage and support her teachers and staff throughout the implementation of this school-wide behavior-change initiative. How might Jennifer apply the principles of applied behavior analysis to encourage engagement and program adherence in her teachers?

(**Q6**) When implementing the primary prevention for 80 % of students in the PBS program, the main focus is on clearly identifying expectations, teaching expectations and behaviors, and reinforcing the targeted behaviors. Often conditioned reinforcement systems and token economies are used school-wide to reinforce these behaviors. Design a school-wide reinforcement system and indicate how you will use it to track data of skill increases within the school.

(**Q7**) Using the school-wide PBS evaluation questionnaire below, what type of data will this produce? Will this information be able to be evaluated with parametric analyses? Why or why not (Table. 8.2)?

Table 8.2 Positive behavior intervention support (PBS) evaluation questionnaire (Todd et al., 2012)

SET MATCHING EXERCISE

Interview Questions	*Evaluation Questions*

What information do you use for collecting office disciplines referrals?
   a) What data are collected?
   b) Who collects those data?
_____
	B2. Do 90% of the staff asked state that teaching of behavioral expectations to students has occurred this year?

What do you do with the office discipline referral information?
   c) Who looks at those data?
   d) How often do you share them with other staff and whom do you share them with?
_____
	B3. Do 90% of team members asked state that the school wide program has been taught/reviewed with staff on an annual basis?

	B4. Can at least 70% of 15 or more students state 67% of the school rules?
What type of problems do/would you refer to the office rather than handling in the classroom? _____	B5. Can 90% or more of the staff asked list 67% of the school rules?
What is the procedure for handling extreme emergencies in the building (i.e. stranger with a gun? _____	C2. Do 50% or more students asked indicate they have received a reward (other than verbal praise) for expected behaviors over the past two months?
What are the school rules/motto and what are they called? _____	C3. Do 90% of staff asked indicate they have delivered a reward (other than verbal praise) to students for expected behavior over the past two months?
Have you received/given a "gotcha" (positive referral) in the past 2 months? _____	
Has the school-wide team taught/reviewed the school wide program to staff this year? _____	D2. Do 90% of staff asked agree with administration on what problems are office-managed and what problems are classroom–managed?
How often does the (PBIS) team meet? _____	D4. Do 90% of staff asked agree with administration on the procedure for handling extreme emergencies (stranger in building with a weapon)?
Do you (administrator) attend team meetings consistently? _____	E2. Can the administrator clearly define a system for collecting & summarizing discipline referrals (computer software, data entry time)?
Does the (PBIS) team provide faculty updates on activities & data summaries? _____	E3. Does the administrator report that the team provides discipline data summary reports to the staff at least three times/year?
Do you have an out-of-school liaison in the state or district to support you on positive behavior support systems development? _____	F1. Does the school improvement plan list improving behavior support systems as one of the top 3 school improvement plan goals?
Have you taught the school rules/behavior expectations to your students this year? _____	F5. Is the administrator an active member of the school-wide behavior support team?
What are your school improvement goals? _____	F6. Does the administrator report that team meetings occur at least monthly?
	G2. Can the administrator identify an out-of-school liaison in the district or state?

Reflection

(Q8) How would you respond to Jennifer's statement: "as long as the behavior challenges are improving, does it matter which part of the intervention program is making a difference?" Please explain your response.

(Q9) *Thinking* about the many ethical considerations that surround the implementation of all applied behavior analysis-based intervention programs is consent required from all students in the school and/or their parents before Jennifer can implement any aspects of this school-wide intervention? Would this vary for different students in the different groups of interventions(Reference Ethics Box 8.2, Behavior Analyst Certification Board, 2014)? Why or why not?

Ethics Box 8.2

Professional and Ethical Compliance Code for Behavior Analysts

- 4.02 Involving Clients in Planning and Consent.
  Behavior analysts involve the client in the planning of and consent for behavior-change programs

(Q10) Given the complexity of the PBS model and the short time frame that the school is working with, which components of the PBS model would be the most effective in making the largest changes?

Additional Web Links
Positive Behavior Support
http://www.nasponline.org/resources-and-publications/resources/mental-health/positive-behavior
Association for Positive Behavior Support
http://www.apbs.org/
The Six Steps of PBS
http://challengingbehavior.fmhi.usf.edu/explore/pbs/process.htm
What is School-wide PBIS?
https://www.pbis.org/school

CASE: iv-E8

We cannot Evaluate our Program!
Setting: Community   Age Group: Adult

LEARNING OBJECTIVE:

- Employ a logic model to support preparations for program evaluation.

TASK LIST LINKS:

- **Measurement**

  - (A-09) Evaluate the accuracy and reliability of measurement procedures.

- **Experimental Design**

  - (B-03) Systematically arrange independent variables to demonstrate their effects on dependent variables.

- **Measurement**

  - (H-01) Select a measurement system to obtain representative data given the dimensions of the behavior and the logistics of observing and recording.

- **Implementation, Management, and Supervision**

  - (K-07) Evaluate the effectiveness of the behavioral program.

KEY TERMS:

- **Logic Model**

  - A logic model is a tool used as part of the program evaluation process that describes linkages between program resources, components, activities, outputs, and outcomes and helps to describe program effectiveness (Bellini and Pratt 2011).

- **Output Measures**

  - Output measures refer to the products of a program's activities. These are often reported as the number of units such as the number of clients served or the number of hours of service delivered (Carman 2007).

- **Outcome Measures**

  - Outcome measures refer to the impact of a program's activities. Examples include an increase in knowledge or skills or improvements in behavior (Carman, 2007).

We Cannot Evaluate Our Program!

Gian, the supervisor of a skills training program for teenagers with developmental disabilities, was preparing the agenda for an upcoming meeting with this staff. Three months ago, he had received a letter from the government department that had long-funded the program. In the embossed letter that came to his mailbox—and not his email inbox—Gian was told that a review of programs funded by this department would be conducted and the skills training program that Gian supervises may be one of the programs carefully examined to see whether future funding would continue. The letter went on to describe that the department is planning to review how available funds are invested, seeking evidence from programs to inform decisions that will be made about future funding allocations in the next six months and beyond.

Up to now, he thought, *the staff have been keeping great notes summarizing how each session has gone, how many participants attended, any questions or concerns raised, and have been completing the checklists confirming that the curriculum we have planned is covered in each session. Participants have also been sending in short feedback surveys comprised of open-ended questions and yes/no questions, and the large majority are positive. Would this be enough to demonstrate the value of the program? Is this the "evidence" that the Ministry would want?* Gian was not sure.

Today, three months after receiving the initial letter, he had not received any further correspondence about this evaluation plan, and he was still not sure what next steps to take. *Maybe we should just hope that this program would not be part the review after all,* he thought. As he thought about this further and with more maturity, Gian felt that he should try to get ahead of any potentially imposed evaluations, and to do more to engage his team in evaluating the program on their own.

After *thinking* about this for several more minutes, Gian doodled "Program Evaluation" at the top of his notepad as the first agenda item to be discussed at his team meeting later that week. He then placed a call to a colleague, Angela, who worked in the research and evaluation branch of his organization. *Maybe she can help,* he silently hoped. And—he was right.

During the team meeting, Angela, a Board Certified Behavior Analyst, began their group discussion by asking each staff member to take out a piece of paper and write out what the skills training program does and how the training happens. After several minutes, when everyone has stopped writing, Angela asked each staff person, one at a time, to read their ideas out loud. Gian was quite surprised at what he heard, listening and taking notes while taking a back seat to the actual events of the day. While his staff each provided valid, truthful statements about the program, they each offered quite different descriptions of the program's day-to-day happenings.

After much deliberation, discussion, consultation, and collaboration, Angela suggested that what is needed is a **logic model**, a tool to help develop a single, agreed-upon description of the program, its purpose and components, and its **output** and **outcome measures.** She went on to explain that, "In order to determine if the program is meeting its goals, we will need to first agree on a single description of the program. Once we agree on how we will describe the program, we can then —and only then—determine well how we will measure it." Gian's staff looked a little concerned. They had been used to collecting frequency, percent of occurrence, duration, and latency data—all which they thought would prove the effectiveness of the program.

Angela set up meetings with the team once every two weeks to continue to develop the logic model together. After several months of work, the team produced a single agreed-upon description of what the program does, how it does it, and what it hopes to achieve.

Angela, who by then had arranged for some of her workday to be spent with this team for at least the next six months, spoke with the team about the importance of moving toward a more objective approach to measuring their program. She stressed the importance of building on the subjective accounts of client progress they had already collected by introducing more objective behavioral data on the progress of each participant.

Angela then asked the staff if they had any questions at this point. After several beats of silence, Marcus, a senior staff member tentatively asked, "I don't really get why we are doing this evaluation in the first place. Am I being evaluated?" Several other staff members joined Mark in expressing their concerns out loud for the first time since this process began.

"I don't understand why we are doing this either. What is wrong with what we have been doing, exactly?" questioned Bruno.

"And how will this information be used?" requested Amber, with stress and concern reflected in her cadence and tone. "I am not sure I am comfortable with all this. I mean, what will happen if it turns out that we are not meeting all of these goals? Will we be penalized? Will I? And who will be looking at this data?"

The room erupted in questions. Angela and Gian looked at each other with concern. *What have I done?* thought Gian to himself. *Why don't they see the importance of this and how this will help us? What are they afraid of? What are they worried about? Don't they get that it is not about us; that it is about our clients?*

The Response: Principles, Processes, Practices, and Reflections

Principles

(Q1) Describe the difference between measurement, evaluation, and research in applied behavior analysis.

(Q2) How might visual representation of a program through the construction of a logic model be helpful to Gian, Angela, and the team?

Processes

(Q3) Explain the role of a logic model in the program evaluation process.

(Q4) What would a logic model provide that other data may not provide (i.e., frequency, rate, trial to criterion).

Practice

(Q5) Completing the figure below, what other ABA data collection measures could be used to evaluate the program?

(Q6) Task list link, K-10, states that the behavior analyst should prepare for the orderly termination of behavior services (BACB, 2012). How would a program evaluation address this principle?

Reflection

(Q8) Is there something that Gian could have done to help prevent these concerns for occurring? If so, what actions could he have taken?

(Q9) Why is it important to include both quantitative and qualitative data in the program evaluation?

(Q10) How might Gian create a climate in which evaluation is seen as safe and a driver of continuous improvement?

Additional Web Links
Recommended Practices: Being an Evidence-Based Practitioner
http://challengingbehavior.fmhi.usf.edu/do/resources/documents/rph_practitioner.pdf
Program Evaluation Checklist
http://www.actcommunity.ca/rasp/information-for-families/program-evaluation-checklist/
Logic Model
http://www.uwex.edu/ces/pdande/evaluation/evallogicmodel.html

CASE: iv-E9

"It worked for them; it will work for us."
Setting: Employment   Age Group: Adult

LEARNING OBJECTIVE:

- To recognize opportunities and limitations associated with generalizing research to practice.

TASK LIST LINKS:

- **Experimental Design**

  - (B-02) Review and interpret articles from the behavior-analytic literature.

- **Behavior-Change Systems**

  - (F-04) Use precision teaching.

KEY TERMS:

- **Direct Replication**

  - Direct replication refers to an experiment that attempts to precisely duplicate a previous study (Barlow 2009).

- **External Validity**

  - External validity refers to the extent that the findings of a study can be generalized to other individuals, settings, or target behaviors (Horner et al. 2005).

- **Replication**

  - Replication refers to repeating a previous study in an attempt to determine the extent to which the findings will hold true. Further, within single-subject research, replication may also refer to repeating a certain condition within an experiment to determine the extent to which the findings of previous conditions will hold true (Horner et al. 2005).

- **Systematic Replication**

  - Systematic replication refers to an experiment that attempts to duplicate a previous study, but varies one or more aspects of the earlier study (Barlow 2009).

It Worked for Them; It Will Work for Us

Raymundo, the manager of a local department store, arrived for work early, looking forward to getting a head start on his long "to-do" list. As he settled into his office at the back of the store, he noticed the message light flashing on his desk phone. It was a message from Stephanie, the behavior consultant from the community support service down the street. Stephanie was calling to see how Vicky was doing.

Three months ago, Vicky began working part-time at the department store. Raymundo still remembers the first phone call he received from Stephanie asking him if he had any part-time positions available. During that call, Stephanie explained that her program supports adults with developmental disabilities in their independent living, and, as with many of the individuals she supports, this often involves supporting individuals to acquire employment within their local community. Raymundo recalls listening especially carefully to Stephanie during that initial call, as she explained that she was calling on behalf of Vicky, a 45 years old with a developmental disability. At that time, Stephanie had also explained that she had consent from both Vicky and her family to contact him in order to explore the possibility of employment for Vicky. Although he had been a little nervous at the time, as he did not have any experience supporting individuals with developmental disabilities at work, as a life-long volunteer in his town and neighborhood, Raymundo remembers being happy with the possibility that his store might be able to help to make an important difference in someone's everyday life.

That was three months ago, thought Raymundo, as he wrote down Stephanie's updated contact information. *Things had started off so well, then.* Lately, however, his floor supervisors had become concerned. According to the reports he had been receiving, Vicky seems to be doing very well following instructions and completing tasks such as placing items on the shelves, sorting returned items, placing price stickers on items, and keeping the sections she is working in neat and clean and up to standard. His supervisors, however, have had to respond to several customer complaints about Vicky over the past few weeks. Customers have complained, for example, that Vicky asks too many questions, speaks too loudly and, at times, is abrupt and rude (according to their perceptions).

Most recently, a customer reported that after being greeted in a friendly manner by Vicky, Vicky became overly interested in a tablet computer that the customer was holding. Vicky asked the customer if she could see it and even use it. After several minutes of showing Vicky the tablet, the customer—who was in a rush and wanting to proceed with her shopping—told Vicky that she was on a tight schedule and had to get her shopping done. Vicky became upset when the customer took her tablet away, followed the customer down several aisles and, in a very loud voice, continuously asked the customer to stop and show her the tablet. The customer eventually went to the customer service desk for assistance.

I am not sure what has changed, thought Raymundo. *Hopefully, Stephanie can turn this around. I am not sure how many more incidents we can take. While the team are very supportive, everyone is concerned about the increase in complaints recently.* Raymundo picked up the phone, called Stephanie, and scheduled a meeting with her later that week.

In preparation for the meeting, Raymundo searched online for examples of how others have supported employment for adults with developmental disabilities. After reading several articles, Raymundo was becoming concerned. Although there were no shortage of examples of interventions that others have used in employment settings to address challenging behaviors, the interventions seemed very complex and way too time-consuming. *I can't add even more to my staff members' work-load, and this certainly would not be in their current job description,* he thought. *And the training that would be involved would be far too extensive—way beyond what I was imagining.* After about a half hour of very detailed searching, Raymundo came across a case in a different environment which a teacher in an elementary classroom used a method called **Differential Reinforcement of Other Behavior** to reduce inappropriate social skill behaviors in children with autism spectrum disorder. Though the terminology and its clinical implications were far beyond his areas of interest and ability, he still recognized that he had found a good thing. *This is it,* thought Raymundo. *I think that we could do something like this.*

As he sat down to meet with Stephanie, as planned, Raymundo was excited to share what he had found. *If this worked for them, it should work for us,* he thought. With that, he began to outline his plan to Stephanie. As she listed, Stephanie became concerned and her mind became consumed with clinical care. *Was there enough **external validity** to support the use of this approach for what Vicky is struggling with? Is there any evidence to support the efficacy and effectiveness of this approach for Vicky's situation? Has this approach been **replicated**, either through a **direct replication** or a **systematic replication**? And did these replications result in enough evidence to support the use of this intervention with Vicky in this setting?* Stephanie was, of course, concerned and did not want to rush into an intervention plan without quite a bit more research into processes and procedures.

As she listened to Raymundo explain what he had found and how he was going to implement this in his store to support Vicky, she tried to determine how she would engage Raymundo in a critical review of this intervention while acknowledging the work he has done and being supportive of the steps he has taken. *I don't want to discourage him*, she thought, *and we have developed a very positive rapport that I don't want to damage.*

"Well," said Raymundo looking up at her from where had been excitedly reading and gesturing, "What do you think?"

The Response: Principles, Processes, Practices, and Reflections

Principles

(Q1) What is meant by evidence-informed practice in applied behavior analysis?
(Q2) What types of evidence can inform the practice of behavior analysts?

Processes

(Q3) Should Stephanie focus on efficacy or effectiveness of research studies when looking for evidence to inform the types of supports provided to Vicky? Please explain your response.
(Q4) What components of a research study should behavior analysts focus on when attempting to generalize from research to their practice (Table 8.3)?

Table 8.3 Efficacy versus effectiveness (Gartlehner et al., 2006)

Efficacy	Effectiveness
Tests whether an intervention produces the desired results under ideal circumstances (i.e., clinical lab, etc.)	Determines whether an intervention produces the desired results in the natural setting (i.e., classroom)

Practice

(Q5) How might Raymundo determine the external validity of the studies he is reviewing (Table 8.4)?

(Q6) When seeking research to inform your practice, would a direct replication study or a systematic replication study be of greater value? Why?

(Q7) How could you determine if an intervention was evidence based? What does it mean for something to be evidence based (Table 8.5)?

Table 8.4 Types of validity (University of Calgary, 2005)

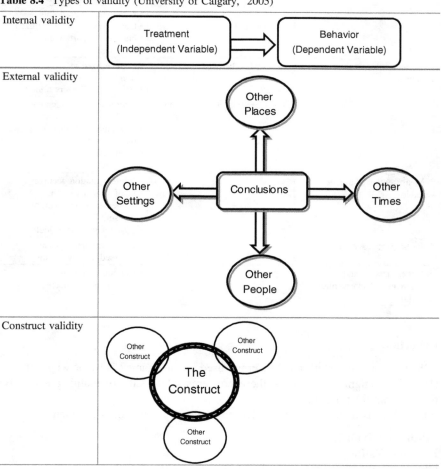

Table 8.5 Scientific merit rating scale (SMRS) when determining if an intervention is evidence based (National Autism Project 2015)

Variables in SMRS		Sample variables considered to give number rating from 1–5
1. Research design	Group design	• Number of groups • Size of groups (N) • Design (i.e., random) • Data loss
	Single-subject designs (not including alternating Treatment)	• Number data points • Number of reversals • Number of Participants • Data loss
	Single-subject designs (alternating Treatment	• Number of data points • Carryover effects minimized • Number of participants • Data loss
2. Measurement of dependent variables	Test, scale, checklist, etc.	• Standardized vs. non-standardized • Are data collectors blind?
	Direct behavioral observation	• Interobserver Agreement (IOA) • Continuous vs. discontinuous data collection • % of sessions where IOA collected
3. Measurement of independent variable		• Implementation accuracy • % of sessions where implementation accuracy measured • IOA for treatment fidelity
4. Participants ascertainment		• How participants were assessed and by whom
5. Generalization and maintenance of intervention effect(s)		• Generalization and maintenance collected

Reflection

(Q8) Do you agree with the concerns raised by Stephanie? Why or why not?

(Q9) How might you address these concerns while still maintaining a positive professional relationship?

(Q10) Why is maintaining a positive professional relationship important?

Additional Web Links
External Validity
http://www.socialresearchmethods.net/kb/external.php
Planning and Conducting Program Evaluation
https://www.fraserhealth.ca/media/2009-05-11-A-Guide-to-Planning-and-Conducting-Program-Evaluation-v2.pdf
Evidence-Based Practices for ASD
http://autismpdc.fpg.unc.edu/evidence-based-practices

CASE: iv-E10 Guest Authors: Sharon Jimson and Renee Carriere

GUEST AUTHORS

Sharon Jimson, MADS, BCBA
Community Consultants
sjimson@wgh.on.ca
Renee Carriere, MADS, BCBA
Regional Support Associates
rcarriere@wgh.on.ca
Raja's Decreasing Disruptive Behavior
Setting: Home   Age Group: Adolescence to Adulthood

LEARNING OBJECTIVE:

- To describe the strengths and limitations of direct and indirect measures of behavior.

TASK LIST LINKS:

- **Measurement**

    - (A-06) Measure percent of occurrence.
    - (A-09) Evaluate the accuracy and reliability of measurement procedures
    - (A-14) Design and implement choice measures.

- **Experimental Design**

    - (B-01) Use the dimensions of applied behavior analysis (Baer et al. 1968) to evaluate whether interventions are behavior analytic in nature.

- **Fundamental Elements of Behavior Change**

    - (D-21) Use differential reinforcement (e.g., DRO, DRA, DRI, DRL, DRH).

- **Identification of the Problem**

    - (G-02) Consider biological/medical variables that may be affecting the client.

- **Measurement**

    - (H-01) Select a measurement system to obtain representative data given the dimensions of the behavior and the logistics of observing and recording.

- **Assessment**

    - (I-03) Design and implement individualized behavioral assessment procedures.
    - (I-05) Organize, analyze, and interpret observed data.
    - (I-06) Make recommendations regarding behaviors that must be established, maintained, increased, or decreased.

- **Intervention**

  - (J-13) Select behavioral cusps as goals for intervention when appropriate.

- **Implementation, Management, and Supervision**

  - (K-10) Arrange for the orderly termination of services when they are no longer required.

Professional and Ethical Compliance Code for Behavior Analysts:

- Avoiding Harmful Reinforcers (4.10)

KEY TERMS:

- **Direct measurement**

  - Direct measurement of behavior involves actually observing episodes of the target behavior under study (Cooper et al. 2007).

- **Indirect measurement**

  - Indirect measurement of behavior involves gathering secondhand information about the target behavior under study. Examples include interviews with parents, teachers, or professionals who may be able to provide insights into the target behavior under study (Cooper et al. 2007).

- **Intellectual disability**

  - An intellectual disability refers to limitations in both intellectual functioning (i.e., IQ) and adaptive behaviors such as social skills and daily living skills (Crocker et al. 2006).

Raja's Decreasing Disruptive Behavior

Raja is a thirty-six-year-old woman who has been assessed by a psychologist to be functioning within the moderate range of **intellectual disability**. She has been residing in a group home with the same two house-mates since she moved into the residence eight years ago. The home is fully supported with two full-time staff members during all waking hours, and one staff member who remains awake during the night shift. Prior to this placement, Raja lived with her mother in their small suburban home. She was placed with the current residential agency when her maladaptive behaviors became too difficult for her mother to manage in the home. Raja began engaging in minor property destruction in the form of ripping and tearing household furnishings (curtains and linens), as well as breaking small household items by pulling out cords or snapping them in pieces.

Prior to Raja moving in, a planning meeting was held between the new team and Raja's mother, as a result of the planning meeting a number of environmental modifications were made to help support her. As such, the home used frosted glass windows in lieu of curtains, all kitchen appliances were kept out of sight in a cabinet until needed for use, and living room electronics were stored in cabinets with Plexiglas fronts to ensure the cords were inaccessible. At that time they decided to limit Raja's smoking too, since it may be a danger to the environment if she did not put it out properly and her health. Since moving into the new residential setting, Raja's maladaptive behavior has escalated to include ripping the clothing off herself and others. She has also begun to target minor items in the home such as books, bills, data collection sheets, or other papers left within sight.

Last year, the agency placed a referral for clinical support from their local behavior support provider. At that time, a behavior analyst was assigned and conducted a full functional assessment of behavior including biopsychosocial variables. A meeting was held with Raja, her mother, and the agency where a full health review screen was completed. The family noted a history of seasonal allergies, and a broken wrist as a child which has since healed. Otherwise, Raja was reported to be in good overall physical health. She has a family doctor whom she sees regularly as he monitors her use of birth control to regulate her menses, as well as lorazepam (Ativan) to help manage anxiety. Raja's staff team are diligent at administering her prescribed medication, and Raja typically takes them when prompted.

After the behavior analyst explained some of the key components of a behavioral program—that it must address behaviors of social importance, that it must focus on observable and measureable behaviors, and that it requires objective measurement and evaluation, a combination of **direct measurement** and **indirect measurement** of Raja's behavior was then completed. The Psychological Assessment Screen for Adults with Developmental Disabilities (PAS-ADD) was conducted and one of the contributing psychological factors was found to be generalized anxiety, which is managed with medication. It was also reported that Raja's father abused alcohol prior to being asked to leave the family home when Raja was sixteen years old. The psychological report obtained by the assessing psychologist determined that Raja functioned in the moderate range of intellectual disability. She is described as nonverbal, however, reportedly demonstrated good receptive language skills. She could reliably follow simple one-step instructions when the assessor used 3–5 word sentences.

The Questions about Behavior Function (QABF) questionnaire was completed by Raja's primary support staff in her residential setting, and focused on the target behavior of minor property destruction. She often engaged in this behavior in the absence of demands, regardless of who was present. Results indicated that Raja's ripping or breaking of items was likely maintained by an automatic/sensory function as evidenced by the high score in the nonsocial section and relatively low scores in the physical, escape, attention, and tangible sections.

Raja currently follows a structured routine in which she attends a day program on Tuesdays, Wednesdays, and Thursdays and participates in scheduled activities with her staff team, housemates, or family when not in attendance. While at the program she follows a visual daily schedule in which she is guided through social activities such as games and karaoke to enhance cooperation and help build a social network with the support of her one-to-one staff member. Friday evenings after dinner, Raja's mother comes to visit her at the group home for approximately one hour. Typical visits include a snack brought by her mother and quiet activities such as reading, listening to music in low light, or receiving back and head massages.

Raja's maladaptive behaviors present themselves across all settings and with everyone in her circle of care. Behavioral incidents were tracked through the use of A-B-C (antecedent-behavior-consequence) narrative data by the staff teams at both her home- and day-program settings. While the behavior was present in all settings, the frequency of minor property destruction varied across those settings. The highest frequency was consistently associated with the home environment, followed by the day program. Data analysis further indicated that the minor property destruction occurred most frequently during unstructured times throughout the day, and during non-preferred activities. For example, when Raja was left alone without an activity to engage in, the frequency of minor property destruction would increase. Her staff team often attempted to interrupt this behavior by offering alternative activities and/or direction to stop with little success. Once the item that Raja had targeted for minor property destruction was completely ripped, this signaled the end of the behavioral incident.

This data were collected for a period of three weeks, and it was forwarded to Raja's behavior analyst on a weekly basis for baseline analysis. In addition, the behavior analyst would visit the group home a minimum of once per week to complete one-hour observation periods in which she collected interobserver agreement (IOA) data. Based on data analysis, it was noted that visits with Raja's mother that commenced with a snack tended to result in increased positive interactions such as smiling and reciprocation; however, if the anticipated snack was withheld or not provided at the onset of the visit, Raja would often engage in minor property destruction such as ripping her mother's jewelry or clothing. When this behavior occurred, her mom would typically provide access to the snack in order to interrupt the behavior in an effort to continue with the scheduled visit. However, upon finishing the snack, Raja was typically ready to end the interaction. She demonstrated this by walking away from her mother. Should her mother choose to remain in her living space, minor property destruction would resume. It was noted that Raja's mother also provided her with cigarettes when she came. Based on the data collected and direct observation, the behavior consultant determined that the behavior was maintained by automatic reinforcement.

Through the analysis of the data obtained in the functional behavior assessment as outlined above, a treatment plan was designed. This support plan was created to help reduce the frequency of Raja's minor property destruction through the use of discrimination training to teach ripping of appropriate materials in order to meet her sensory requirements. Other positive behavioral strategies introduced in the home setting were the use of a choice board to request activities/items including the materials designated for ripping, as well as the use of a visual schedule similar to the one currently being used successfully in the day program. It was suggested that cigarettes also be used as a reinforcement, as they had proven an extremely high reinforcer in the past.

Ethics Box 8.3

Professional and Ethical Compliance Code for Behavior Analysts

4.10 Avoiding Harmful Reinforcers.

Behavior analysts minimize the use of items as potential reinforcers that may be harmful to the health and development of the client or that may require excessive motivating operations to be effective.

Discrimination training began by introducing a response interruption and redirection (RIRD) program in order to block access to the inappropriate materials once minor property destruction was initiated by Raja, followed by immediate redirection to the appropriate materials. These materials are to be kept on a small table in the living room for easy access at all times. In addition, a differential reinforcement of alternative behavior (DRA) schedule was introduced to reinforce any demonstration of the alternative behavior (ripping designated materials).

The visual schedule was to be set up each morning and represent daily activities or expectations in one-hour increments, in an effort to increase predictability and independence. The schedule is designed to mix preferred, non-preferred, or neutral tasks such as daily living skills. During the independent time slots, Raja is provided with a choice board to assist in choosing which activity she would like to engage in. She was taught to use her choice board by pairing preferred activities with their associated pictures. The designated materials in which Raja can utilize for ripping were always provided as an option on the choice board.

Data were collected by the staff team to indicate each time RIRD was used in response to the minor property destruction. Each time Raja initiated an attempt to engage in the target behavior it was indicated on the data sheet, along with her response to the staff member's use of the RIRD program. If Raja was successfully redirected to the alternative designated materials, a check mark would be used, and if she was unsuccessful an "X" would be used. At the end of each day, the percentage of opportunities would be calculated by dividing the total number of checks by the total number of redirection efforts. Raja's independent engagement with the designated materials was also tracked on a separate data sheet to establish any gains in independent initiations of the alternative behavior. A total frequency count was calculated at the end of each day. Both data sheets were retrieved by the behavior analyst on a weekly basis during her scheduled visits, which she would then graph to allow for visual analysis.

Evaluation of the data indicated that Raja responded well to the treatment, as evidenced by an overall increasing trend in the behavior for increase (engagement with the designated materials), and a corresponding decrease in the number of redirection efforts required. The overall frequency of minor property destruction decreased from an average of six times daily (42 times weekly) during the baseline condition, to three to five times weekly during treatment. These treatment gains were maintained at a one-month follow-up with minor property destruction occurring an average of three times per week.

Raja's family and her support team find these gains have had a meaningful impact on her overall quality of life. Since the decrease in property destruction, the staff team have been slowly reintegrating items into her living space including books and magazines as well as small games for her to engage with. The designated ripping materials remain available, and the staff team report that she continues to engage with them periodically. The behavior analyst has asked that the staff team continue to collect data to continue monitoring progress of the treatment program and has began to fade herself out and provide a follow-up plan for her departure on the team.

The Response: Principles, Processes, Practices, and Reflections

Principles

(Q1) Explain the process of discrimination training. Why is it important to teach?
(Q2) What is the response interruption and redirection (RIRD) program? How would it be taught to Raja?

Processes

(Q3) Describe the strengths and limitations of direct and indirect measures of behavior.
(Q4) Using the table and figure below, how might direct and indirect measures of behavior be combined to provide comprehensive insights into behavior and the evaluation of the information collected (Fig. 8.9, Table 8.6)?

Practice

(Q5) Looking at the data below, calculate the percentage of opportunity data (Table 8.7).
(Q6) Use the following checklist to determine whether the following behavior program uses the dimensions of applied behavior analysis listed by Baer et al. 1968 (Table 8.8)?
(Q7) What skills were taught to Raja that would be considered behavioral cusps? Why are behavioral cusps so important?

Sarah's results of the Questions About Behavior Function Questionnaire

Attention	Escape	Non-Social	Physical	Tangible
3	3	15	0	2

Fig. 8.9 Sarah's results of the questions about behavior function questionnaire

Table 8.6 Three days of antecedent-behavior-consequence (A-B-C) data for Sara's property destruction behavior in the group home

Date/time/observer/setting	Antecedent	Behavior	Consequence
September 15/11:30 A. M./Jamal/Living room	• Sara alone in living room	• Use hands and teeth to rip sleeve of shirt	• Interrupt physically • Turned on TV show
September 15/2:30 P. M/Mom/Kitchen	• Sara and Mom in kitchen at table • Mom talking to Sara about her week	• Sara grabbed Mom's bracelet and pulled it off	• Mom got snack off counter and brought it to table
September 15/9:30 P. M/Yasmin/Bedroom	• Sara in her room • I (Yasmin) left briefly to assist other client, directed Sara to put pajamas on	• Sara had ripped the lace off the sleeves of her pajama shirt	• I (Yasmin) came back into room • Directed her to pick up lace and give to me, then get new pajamas
September 16/9 A.M./ Jamal/Kitchen	• Sara at kitchen table with housemates having breakfast	• Used hands to rip up napkin	• Directed to put in garbage and continue eating
September 16/1:30 P.M./ Jamal/Car	• Sitting in backseat • On the way to afternoon program (swimming)	• Used hands to pull off housemate to the left's necklace	• Housemate exclaimed "no! that is mine" and grabbed it back
September 16/Yasmin/8:30 P.M./ Living room	• Sara sitting alone in living room	• Used hands to rip up magazine	• I (Yasmin) asked her if she wanted me to read with her • Read a chapter of the book we are reading
September 17/Jamal/10:30 A.M./ Bedroom	• Sara alone in her bedroom	• Found her ripping papers (not sure where from?)	• Asked her to clean up papers • Asked her to come downstairs with me to join housemates in painting
September 17/Jamal/10:45 A. M/Kitchen	• Sara joined in painting with housemates	• Ripped up paper	• Gave her new paper and prompted her to use paint brush to paint

Table 8.7 Data to calculate the percentage of opportunity

Opportunity	Data								
		Sept 15 1 pm	Sept 15 2:20 pm	Sept 15 8:20 pm	Sept 16 9:00 am	Sept 16 9:30 am	Sept 16 9 pm	Sept 16 10:20 pm	Sept 17 6:20 pm	Sept 17 10:20 pm
Redirection offered to Raja										
Successful redirection		✓	✓	✗	✗	✗	✓	✓	✓	✗

Table 8.8 Mark Sundberg's (2015) ABA program evaluation form: quick assessment

	None	Poor	Fair	Good
(1) **Applied** : Socially significant behaviors	0	1	2	3
Skill assessments completed: language social, academic, play, functional skills, etc.				
Behavioral deficits assessments completed: barriers, FBAs				
IEP goals appropriate and consistent with assessments				
Daily curriculum is consistent with assessments and IEP goals				
Behavior intervention program consistent with FBA				
Structured and intensive ABA style teaching sessions in place				
(2) **Behavioral** : Data system				
Data collection system in place				
Targets are based on the assessment results				
Targets are definable, observable, and measurable				
Uses appropriate measurement procedure for each target				
ABC recordin g system in place for problem behaviors				
Binder system in place				
(3) **Analytic** : Prediction and control				
Demonstrates prediction and control of skills and problem behaviors				
Demonstrates that skill acquisition is a function of the teachi ng procedures and intervention program				
The sources of control for barriers that impair language, social and learning skills are identified and ameliorated				
(4) **Technological** : Standard behavioral procedures are used				
Staff demonstrate corr ect use of basic ABA methodology				
Reinforcers identified and delivered effectively				
Staff have established clear instructional control				
Discrete trial structured teaching (DTT/EIBI) format used				
Natural environment teaching (NET) format used				
Negative behaviors appropriately prevented and/or consequated				
	None	Poor	Fair	Good
(5) **Conceptual Systems** : Procedures are relevant to principles	0	1	2	3
Staff can identify the relevant concepts and principles that underlie teaching proce dures				
Staff use the concepts and principles of behavior analysis to guide the intervention				
Staff use behavioral terminology				
(6) **Effective** : Large enough effects for practical value				
The students are acquiring appropriate and meaningful skills				
Negative behavior is significantly decreasing				
IEP benchmarks and goals are consistently being met				
(7) **Generality** : The skills are durable and generalize				
Daily programming for generalization occurs (different settings, peop le, time, materials, etc.)				
Systematic stimulus and response generalization after acquisition is in place				
Parent training program in place				
Score	None	Poor	Fair	Good
	0	1	2	3
Total tallies				
Sub -total scores (multiple number of tallies times point value)				
Final quick assessment score	/90 possible points			

Reflection

(Q8) Often, for adults with developmental disabilities, teaching them functional skills to keep them engaged is important and can decrease behaviors. Using the following figure as a guide, what self-help skills would you identify as critical to her independence and quality of life, and what self-care skills could increase her functional activities in a day (Fig. 8.10)?

SELF–CARE CHECKLISTS
The focus of the VB-MAPP is primarily on communication and social skills. However, self-care skills are an important part of the child's growing independence. The following self-care checklists can be used for assessment and skills tracking. The list can be downloaded and printed as needed to complete your child's program. As always, the procedures derived from applied behavior analysis provide the best way to teach these skills (Sunberg, n.d)

DRESSING – BY ABOUT 18 MONTHS	
Pulls a hat off	
Pulls socks off	
Pulls mittens off	
Pulls shoes off (may need help with laces, buckles and Velcro straps)	
Pulls coat off (may need assistance unbuttoning and unzipping)	
Pulls pants down (may need assistance unbuttoning and unzipping)	
Pulls pants up (but may need help getting pants over a diaper, and with buttoning, snapping and zipping)	

DRESSING – BY ABOUT 30 MONTHS	
Unties shoe laces	
Unbuttons front buttons	
Unsnaps	
Fastens and unfastens Velcro	
Unzips front zippers (smaller zippers may be difficult)	
Removes shirt (tight shirts may require assistance)	
Removes pants or skirts (may need help unzipping and unbuttoning)	
Puts on shoes (needs help discriminating right from left and tying)	
Puts on pants (may need help zipping and buttoning up)	
Adjusts clothing	
Matches own socks	
Matches own shoes	
Puts dirty clothes in a hamper	

Fig. 8.10 Functional activities in a day

DRESSING – BY ABOUT 48 MONTHS	
Undresses (but may need help with tight pullover clothes)	
Dresses (may need help with back buttons and zippers such as on a dress)	
Puts on coat	
Puts on socks	
Puts on pants	
Buckles and unbuckles most buckles (some may be more difficult)	
Zips and unzips front zippers	
Buttons and unbuttons front buttons	
Snaps and unsnaps front snaps	
Identifies which clothes to wear for various weather conditions	
Attempts to lace shoes	
Puts on shoes (discriminating right from left with a prompt)	
Attempts to tie shoes	
Hangs up own clothes on a hook	
Hangs up own clothes on a hanger (with assistance)	
Folds own clothes (with assistance)	
Puts clothes in drawer	

BATHING AND GROOMING – BY ABOUT 18 MONTHS	
Wipes nose with a tissue (with assistance)	
Washes hands (with assistance)	
Dries hands (with assistance)	
Attempts tooth-brushing (with assistance)	

BATHING AND GROOMING – BY ABOUT 30 MONTHS	
Attempts to use a washcloth and soap while bathing (with assistance)	
Brushes teeth (with assistance)	
Washes face (with assistance)	
Dries face	
Attempts to wash hands independently	
Dries hands	
Attempts to brush hair (with assistance)	

Fig. 8.10 (continued)

BATHING AND GROOMING – BY ABOUT 48 MONTHS	
Wipes nose with a tissue and puts it in the trash	
Gets in and out of a bath tub with minimal assistance	
Uses a washcloth and soap when bathing	
Washes hair (with assistance, especially for longer hair)	
Dries self after a bath or shower	
Brushes teeth	
Flosses teeth (with assistance)	
Washes hands	
Washes face	
Dries both face and hands	
Hangs up towel after washing	
Brushes hair (with assistance, especially for longer hair)	

FEEDING – BY ABOUT 18 MONTHS	
Eats finger foods	
Drinks from a cup by self	
Uses a spoon to scoop food	
Sucks from a straw	

FEEDING – BY ABOUT 30 MONTHS	
Uses a fork to pick up food	
Uses a napkin to wipe face and hands	
Carries own lunch box or plate to table	
Opens own lunch box	
Opens Ziploc bags	
Unwraps partially opened food packaging	
Puts a straw into a juice box	
Peels a banana	
Takes off own bib	

FEEDING – BY ABOUT 48 MONTHS	
Uses the side of a fork to cut softer foods	
Uses a knife for spreading	
Uses a knife for cutting (softer foods)	
Keeps eating area reasonably clean while eating	
Unwraps most food packaging	
Opens milk or juice container	
Pours liquids into a cup or bowl (from a small pitcher or lunch thermos)	
Helps to prepare simple foods (spreading, stirring, using cookie cutters, holding a beater, measuring ingredients, pouring ingredients)	
Helps to set the table for meal s	
Takes dishes to the sink	
Wipes the table with a sponge or dish towel	

Fig. 8.10 (continued)

TOILETING – READINESS SKILLS – BY ABOUT 24 MONTHS	
Responds to reinforcement	
Follows simple directions	
Seems uncomfortable in soiled diapers	
Remains dry for 2 hours at a time	
Bowel movements are predictable and regular	
Pulls pants down	
Pulls pants up	
Can sit still for 2 minutes at a time	

TOILETING – BY ABOUT 36 MONTHS	
Has learned a word, sign or PECS for using the toilet (e.g., potty, pee, sign for toilet)	
Mands to use the toilet	
Unbuttons, unsnaps or unzips pants	
Sits on toilet	
Urinates on toilet	
Wipes after urinating (girls)	
Defecates on toilet	
Wipes after defecating (with assistance)	
Pulls underwear up	
Pulls pants up	
Zips, snaps or buttons pants (with some assistance)	
Flushes toilet	
Washes hands (with some assistance)	
Dries hands	

TOILETING – BY ABOUT 48 MONTHS	
Aims into toilet standing (boys)	
Wipes self (girls wipe from front to back)	
Zips front zippers	
Buttons front buttons	
Snaps front snaps	
Washes and dries hands - as part of the toileting routine	
Night-time trained (may still have accidents)	

Fig. 8.10 (continued)

(Q9) In the following case, what skills increased for Raja and what skills decreased for her that contributed to her overall quality of life? Why is it important to focus on both skill building and behavior reduction for individuals?

(Q10) The staff team in Raja's home continue taking data on the target behaviors and continue sending the data to the behavior analyst. As the behavior analyst continues to graph the data she notices that over the last three months, the data have been consistently level and stable. At what point should the staff stop collecting data? When can the behavior analyst terminate Raja's services? Have all the dimensions of applied behavior analysis been met?

Additional Web Links

Measuring Behavior: A Case Study Unit

https://iris.peabody.vanderbilt.edu/wp-content/uploads/pdf_case_studies/ics_measbeh.pdf

Behavioral Cusps

http://www.ncbi.nlm.nih.gov/pmc/articles/PMC1284293/pdf/11317984.pdf

References

Alnahdi, G. H. (2015). Single subject designs in special education: Advantages and limitations. *Journal of Research in Special Education Needs, 15*(4), 257–265.

Barlow, D. (2009). *Single case experimental designs: Strategies for studying behavior change.* Boston: Pearson.

Baer, D. M., Wolf, M. M., & Risley, T. R. (1968). Some current dimensions of applied behavior analysis. *Journal of Applied Behavior Analysis, 1*, 91–97.

Behavior Analyst Certification Board (2014). *Professional and ethical compliance code for behavior analysts.* Retrieved from http://bacb.com/wp-content/uploads/2016/01/160120-compliance-code-english.pdf

Bellini, S., & Pratt, C. (2011). From intuition to data: Using logic models to measure professional development outcomes for educators working with students on the autism spectrum. *Teacher Education and Special Education, 34*(1), 37–51.

Carman, J. (2007). Evaluation practice among community-based organizations: Research into the reality. *American Journal of Evaluation, 28*(1), 60–75.

Caring Homes Group. (2016). *Person-centred planning.* Retrieved from http://www.consensussupport.com/support/person-centred-plan-pcp/

Carr, E., Dunlap, G., Horner, R., Koegel, R., Turnbull, A., Sailor, W., et al. (2002). Positive behavior support: Evolution of an applied science. *Journal of Positive Behavior Interventions, 4*(1), 4–16.

Cooper, J., Heron, T., & Heward, W. (2007). *Applied behavior analysis* (2nd ed.). New Jersey: Pearson.

Crocker, A., Mercier, C., Lachappelle, Y., Brunet, A., Morin, D., & Roy, M. (2006). Prevalence and types of aggressive behavior among adults with intellectual disabilities. *Journal of Intellectual Disability Research, 50*(9), 652–661.

Educate Autism (2016). *Functional Behavior Assessment.* Retrieved from http://www.educateautism.com/functional-behaviour-assessment.html

Elsbree, A. (n.d.). *Secondary classroom management plan.* Retrieved from http://secondaryclassroommanagementplan.weebly.com/5-support.html

Gartlehner, G., Hansen, R. A., & Nissman, D. (2006). Criteria for distinguishing effectiveness from efficacy trials in systematic reviews. Rockville (MD): Agency for healthcare research and quality (US), April (Technical Reviews, No. 12.) Preface. Available from: https://www.ncbi.nlm.nih.gov/books/NBK44031/

Hogan, R. L. (2007). The historical development of program evaluation: Exploring the past and present. *Online Journal of Workforce Education and Development, 2*(4), 1–14.

Horner, R., Carr, E., Halle, J., McGee, G., Odom, S., & Wolery, M. (2005). The use of single subject research to identify evidence-based practice in special education. *Council for Exceptional Children, 71*(2), 165–179.

Hoskin, T. (n.d.). *Parametric and nonparametric: Demystifying the terms.* Retrieved from http://www.mayo.edu/mayo-edu-docs/center-for-translational-science-activities-documents/berd-5-6.pdf

Kaminski, J., Valle, L., Filene, J., & Boyle, C. (2008). A meta-analytic review of components associated with parent training program effectiveness. *Journal of Abnormal Child Psychology, 36*(4), 567–589.

Marchand, E., Stice, E., Rohde, P., & Becker, C. (2011). Moving from efficacy to effectiveness trials in prevention research. *Behavior Research and Therapy, 49*(1), 32–41.

Mayer, G. R., Sulzer-Azaroff, B., & Wallace, M. (2014). *Behavior analysis for lasting change* (3rd ed.). Sloan Publishing: Cornwall-on-Hudson, NY.

Ontario Centre of Excellence for Child and Youth Mental Health (2016). *Evaluation module: Planning evaluation.* Retrieved from http://www.excellenceforchildandyouth.ca/evaluation-module-1-planning-evaluation

Ryan, C. S. (2011). Applied behavior analysis: *Teaching procedures and staff training for children with autism.* Retrieved from https://www.researchgate.net publication/221915787_Applied_Behavior_Analysis_Teaching_Procedures_and_Staff_Training_For_Children_with_Autism

Sundberg, M. (n.d.). *Self-care checklist.* Retrieved from http://www.avbpress.com/updates-and-downloads.html

Sundberg, M. (2015). *ABA program evaluation form: Quick assessment.* Retrieved from http://www.avbpress.com/updates-and-downloads.html

Todd, A. W., Lewis-Palmer, T., Horner, R. H., Sugai, G., Thompson, N. K., & Phillips, D. (2012, February). *School-wide evaluation tool (SET): Implementation manual.* Retrieved from http://www.pbis.org/common/cms/files/pbisresources/SET_Manual_02282012.pdf

University of Calgary. (2005). Psychology & Science: Validity. Retrieved from http://pip.ucalgary.ca/psyc-312/introduction-to-research-methods/psychology-and-science/key_concepts_validity.html

Ward-Horner, J., & Sturmey, P. (2010). Component analysis using single-subject experimental designs: A review. *Journal of Applied Behavior Analysis, 43*(4), 685–704.

Wells, K. B. (1999). Treatment research at the crossroads: The scientific interface of clinical trials and effectiveness research. *American Journal of Psychiatry, 156*(1), 5–10.

Part V
Research and Ethics

Chapter 9
Preschool-to-School-Age Case Studies Constructed Around Research and Ethics

Abstract This chapter explores ethical considerations associated with the research and practice of applied behavior analysis (ABA). Through a series of case studies highlighting behavior difficulties experienced by preschool- and school-age children, learners are guided to consider standards of practice, areas of professional competence, and the three questions central to the study of ethics—What is the right thing to do? What is worth doing? And what does it mean to be a good behavior analyst? (Cooper et al. in applied behavior analysis. Pearson Prentice Hall, Upper Saddle River, NJ, 2007). Within the preschool- and school-age years, parental or guardian consent to participate in research or to receive ABA services is a central ethical consideration faced by behavior analysts. At the same time, behavior analysts must also consider the "assent" of the child in receipt of the behavior-change program, and the child's involvement in key decisions surrounding the behavior-change program he or she is receiving. This can be particularly complex when supporting children with developmental disabilities or cognitive impairments who may not be able to express their assent verbally or nonverbally. Throughout this chapter, the cases presented will highlight the similarities and differences between measurement of ABA practice and ABA research, and the ethical considerations associated with each. Further, learners will critically explore professional competencies required to conduct research and practice and consider the role of behavior analysts in advocating for the protection of those they are supporting. In this chapter, entitled "Preschool-to-School-Age Case Studies Constructed Around Research and Ethics," the challenges associated with ethical ABA practice are explored through five case scenarios in home, school, clinical, and community settings.

Keywords Preschool · School-age children · Professional competence · Ethical consideration · Ethics · Parental consent · Behavior-change program · Developmental disabilities · Cognitive impairments · Verbal · Nonverbal

© Springer International Publishing AG 2016　　　　　　　　　　　　　　311
K. Maich et al., *Applied Behavior Analysis*,
DOI 10.1007/978-3-319-44794-0_9

CASE: v-R1 Guest Author: Tricia van Rhijn

Stay, Play, and Talk with Me
Setting: Childcare   Age Group: Preschool
Guest Author, Tricia van Rhijn,
Assistant Professor, University of Guelph

LEARNING OBJECTIVE:

- To describe appropriate professional competence to conduct research in applied behavior analysis.

Professional and Ethical Compliance Code for Behavior Analysts:

- Conforming with Laws and Regulations (9.01),
- Characteristics of Responsible Research (9.02),
- Informed Consent (9.03),
- Acknowledging Contributions (9.08).

KEY TERMS:

- **Professional Competence**

  - Professional competence in applied behavior analysis is typically achieved through both academic training and professional experience. Academic training may include graduate-level coursework with a focus in ABA. Professional experience can include obtaining certification from the Behavior Analyst Certification Board, as well as supervised research and practice within an area of specialization; for example, an particular age group, a certain diagnoses, or specific types of challenging behaviors (BACB 2015).

- **Research Ethics Board**

- A research ethics board is responsible for determining the extent to which proposed research projects meet ethical standards and requirements. Research ethics boards are mandated to clear, reject, ask for modifications, or terminate research projects (Thomson 2012)

Stay, Play, and Talk with Me

As a new faculty member at a large university in a mid-sized city, Tamara was eager to take advantage of the opportunity to utilize the on-campus childcare center for the next phase of a research project which she had been working with a few trusted colleagues. The project focused on the *Stay, Play, and Talk* program, a manual-based, peer-mediated intervention.

A peer-mediated approach, Tamara wrote in her research notebook, involves teaching peers how to interact with the child with a disability, along with adult prompting in the application of these behaviors. Peer-mediated interventions, like Stay, Play, and Talk, have been shown to be one of the most researched, effective methods for increasing social interaction skills in children with social issues, characteristics of an autism spectrum disorder (ASD), or a diagnosis of an ASD (Kohler et al. 2007; Laushey and Heflin 2000; McConnell 2002).

Tamara's research team had focused the previous phases of the research on the children with identified or suspected ASD. Recognizing that social skills are an important developmental domain and the growth of these skills at the preschool age is an important area of research both for children with identified or suspected challenges as well as their typically developing peers. The next phase of the anticipated research would, excitedly, broaden the focus to include these typically developing peers. This childcare center had a strong focus on inclusion, because of this focus Tamara and her colleagues believed that it would be an excellent location to implement the Stay, Play, and Talk program within the centers daily programming. The research group would be interested in both the effectiveness of the program and its related child-based outcomes.

The director, supervisor, and staff at the childcare center were all very enthused about the program and its concurrent research project. Tamara began working on the first steps of the research project, the application to the university's **research ethics board** and planning out the numerous and specific details of running the project. The plan was to draw on the research team members' areas of **professional competence** and conduct a quasi-experimental, pretest/posttest design with a non-equivalent control group. Happily, all of the classrooms at the center were planning to participate with the exception of the three toddler rooms. *One of the preschool classes*, Tamara thought, *could act as a control group in which the Stay, Play, and Talk program would be implemented immediately following the conclusion of the research project. In the participating classrooms, parents and educators would be invited to complete pre- and posttest measures of social skills for all the children, both those with social-behavioral challenges as well as those typically developing individuals.*

She then planned out an additional component. Single-subject observational data would be collected for children diagnosed with ASD or those displaying traits of ASD. The project received ethics clearance that spring (in early April), training on the Stay, Play, and Talk program was carried out in mid-May, pretest measures were sent to the parents and educators, and the program was implemented within the classroom programming following the training. While carrying out the research project Tamara encountered two significant challenges. The first challenge was with implementation of the single-subject research component, and the second was with the research assistants working on the project with her and her colleagues.

Implementing the single-subject aspect of the research project proved to be challenging due to scheduling and cost. Carrying out the single-subject observations was a labor-intensive process, with student research assistants committed to observe the focal children at various times of day, in various activities (although primarily free play), beginning with baseline observations followed by observations over the five week course of the program implementation. Despite having daily schedules, the childcare center embraced an emergent curriculum and the flexibility that arose from this approach proved challenging when scheduling the student research assistants' observation times; there were conflicts when scheduled observation times did not match up with free play activities, which were the focus of the observations. In addition, the sheer number of observations that needed to be conducted with multiple classrooms, and some with more than one focal child to be observed, meant that the labor costs for the research assistants were excessively high, and the grant for the research was being stretched thin.

The research assistants working on the project were in their final term as undergraduate students. They both had interest and experience in early childhood education and had previously worked in various roles at the childcare center including practicum students, inclusion facilitators, and teaching assistants. The second challenge related to the research assistants because of their previous experience working at the childcare center. *Although their experience was ideal background for the research, it clearly was not a perfect fit*, reflected Tamara. The childcare center was purpose-built as a laboratory school and has observation booths available; but unfortunately, the observation booths were not available for all of the classrooms, only half of them! In order to be consistent in how the single-subject data were collected, the decision was made to have the research assistants conduct their observations from within the classrooms, rather than the observation booths. This way, they were better able to see and hear their focal child and their interactions with peers, but the downside to this was that the children knew the research assistants from their previous work and were happy to see them. The children did not understand that the research assistants could not play with them during their observation times; this caused confusion and frustration for the children and was a distraction for the research assistants. In addition, the research assistants' experiences in the center also meant that they knew the children and their capabilities very well. They were tempted to prompt the focal children to do engage in behaviors that they were not spontaneously demonstrating. The research assistants also knew what the study was about and found it challenging to conduct their observations in an unbiased manner.

"Good grief," mumbled Tamara at her computer screen while she wrote some additional notes while trying to develop her manuscript. "I had no idea this project was so full of problems that I would have to supervise and solve."

Ultimately the challenges were overcome by conducting frequent team meetings to respond to these issues as they arose. Recognizing that the research assistants were being challenged to be unbiased in their observations, Tamara submitted an ethics change request to allow video recording of the interactions of the focal child to allow for additional reliability checking by an additional observer without experience at the childcare center. Over time, and with support from the classroom educators, the children learned that when the research assistants had their clipboards, they were not to be disturbed. Scheduling challenges were worked out through communication and cooperation with the childcare center director, supervisor, and educators in each classroom. And the project was, according to everyone involved, a great success where all students learned and practiced new skills, and demonstrated use of them far beyond the boundaries of the walls of the childcare center and far past the months of the project itself.

The Response: Principles, Processes, Practices, and Reflections

Principles:

(Q1) Outline a process that Tamara may have used to recruit participants for this research project that meets the principle of free and informed consent (Reference Ethics Box 9.1, Behavior Analyst Certification Board, 2014).

Ethics Box 9.1

Professional and Ethical Compliance Code for Behavior Analysts

- 9.03 Informed Consent.
  Behavior analysts inform participants or their guardian or surrogate in understandable language about the nature of the research that they are free to participate, to decline to participate, or to withdraw from the research at any time without penalty; about significant factors that may influence their willingness to participate; and answer any other questions participants may have about the research.

(Q2) Should Tamara also include an "assent" process for the children participating? Why or why not? If so, what might the process look like (Reference Ethics Box 9.2, Behavior Analyst Certification Board, 2014)?

Ethics Box 9.2

Professional and Ethical Compliance Code for Behavior Analysts

- 1.05 Professional and Scientific Relationships.
  (b) When behavior analysts provide behavior-analytic services, they use language that is fully understandable to the recipient of those services while remaining conceptually systematic with the profession of behavior analysis. They provide appropriate information prior to service delivery about the nature of such services and appropriate information later about results and conclusions.

Processes:

(Q3) Since Tamara has applied to the research ethics board, are there other laws that she must abide by (Reference Ethics Box 9.3, Behavior Analyst Certification Board, 2014)? Why or why not?

Ethics Box 9.3

Professional and Ethical Compliance Code for Behavior Analysts

- 9.01 Conforming with Laws and Regulations.
  Behavior analysts plan and conduct research in a manner consistent with all applicable laws and regulations, as well as professional standards governing the conduct of research. Behavior analysts also comply with other applicable laws and regulations relating to mandated-reporting requirements.

(Q4) Tamara mentioned that she needs to resubmit an ethics change form to allow for videotaping of the children. Why does she need to complete this? What other considerations must be taken into account in the childcare center in regard to video taping (Reference Ethics Box 9.4, Behavior Analyst Certification Board, 2014)?

Ethics Box 9.4

Professional and Ethical Compliance Code for Behavior Analysts

- 9.02 Characteristics of Responsible Research.
  (a) Behavior analysts conduct research only after approval by an independent, formal research review board.

Practices:

(Q5) Tamara has thought a lot about the effects of having data collectors in the environment on the children's learning. How may this effect the intervention itself, and how could the researchers determine if their presence is having an effect on the intervention itself? Is this an ethical issue itself (Reference Ethics Box 9.5, Behavior Analyst Certification Board, 2014)?

Ethics Box 9.5

Professional and Ethical Compliance Code for Behavior Analysts

- 9.02 Characteristics of Responsible Research.
  (b) Behavior analysts conducting applied research conjointly with provision of clinical or human services must comply with requirements for both

intervention and research involvement by client-participants. When research and clinical needs conflict, behavior analysts prioritize the welfare of the client.
(l) Behavior analysts minimize interference with the participants or environment in which research is conducted.

(Q6) Outline a process for Tamara to train the research assistants in the study's procedures. How could she use Behavior Skill Training in this process? How might Tamara determine when the assistants are ready to begin work?
(Q7) What type of single-subject research design would you use in this case? What are any ethical concerns about using this approach?
(Q8) Looking at the Professional and Ethical Compliance Code for Behavior Analysts (BACB, 2014), guideline 9.08, Acknowledging Contributions, who will Tamara need to acknowledge or include in her research publication (Reference Ethics Box 9.6, Behavior Analyst Certification Board, 2014)?

Ethics Box 9.6

Professional and Ethical Compliance Code for Behavior Analysts

- 9.08 Acknowledging Contributions.
  Behavior analysts acknowledge the contributions of others to research by including them as co-authors or footnoting their contributions. Principal authorship and other publication credits accurately reflect the relative scientific or professional contributions of the individuals involved, regardless of their relative status. Minor contributions to the research or to the writing for publications are appropriately acknowledged, such as in a footnote or introductory statement.

(Q9) Which guidelines from the Professional and Ethical Compliance Code for Behavior Analysts (BACB 2014) highlights the importance of ensuring that data are accurate when there are multiple individuals collecting data?

Reflections:

(Q10) Does Tamara's employment at the university raise any ethical concerns pertaining to this research being conducted at the on-site childcare center (Reference Ethics Box 9.7, Behavior Analyst Certification Board, 2014)?

Ethics Box 9.7

> **Professional and Ethical Compliance Code for Behavior Analysts**
>
> - 9.02 Characteristics of Responsible Research.
>   (i) Behavior analysts minimize the effect of personal, financial, social, organizational, or political factors that might lead to misuse of their research.
>   (k) Behavior analysts avoid conflicts of interest when conducting research.

(Q11) Would Tamara's research assistants be able to ethically conduct their own single-subject design following the completion of this study (Reference Ethics Box 9.8, Behavior Analyst Certification Board, 2014)?

Ethics Box 9.8

> **Professional and Ethical Compliance Code for Behavior Analysts**
>
> - 9.02 Characteristics of Responsible Research.
>   (c) Behavior analysts conduct research competently and with due concern for the dignity and welfare of the participants.
>   (d) Behavior analysts plan their research so as to minimize the possibility that results will be misleading.
>   (e) Researchers and assistants are permitted to perform only those tasks for which they are appropriately trained and prepared. Behavior analysts are responsible for the ethical conduct of research conducted by assistants or by others under their supervision or oversight.
>   (f) If an ethical issue is unclear, behavior analysts seek to resolve the issue through consultation with independent, formal research review boards, peer consultations, or other proper mechanisms.
>   (g) Behavior analysts only conduct research independently after they have successfully conducted research under a supervisor in a defined relationship (e.g., thesis, dissertation, specific research project).
>   (h) Behavior analysts conducting research take necessary steps to maximize benefit and minimize risk to their clients, supervisees, research participants, students, and others with whom they work.
>   (i) Behavior analysts minimize the effect of personal, financial, social, organizational, or political factors that might lead to misuse of their research.

Additional Web Links

Teaching and Maintaining Ethical Behavior in a Professional Organization
http://www.ncbi.nlm.nih.gov/pmc/articles/PMC3592493/

Using private blog sites to collect interobserver agreement and treatment integrity data
http://psycnet.apa.org/journals/bdb/19/1/30.pdf&productCode=pa

Institutional Review Boards Frequently Asked Questions
http://www.fda.gov/RegulatoryInformation/Guidances/ucm126420.htm

CASE: v-R2

Show me the evidence
Setting: School   Age Group: School Age

LEARNING OBJECTIVE:

- To utilize knowledge of applied behavior analysis (ABA) standards of practice to guide evidence-informed decision-making.

Professional and Ethical Compliance Code for Behavior Analysts:

- Reliance on Scientific Knowledge (1.01),
- Responsibility (1.02),
- Maintaining Confidentiality (2.06),
- Maintaining Records (2.07),
- Documenting Professional Work and Research (2.10),
- Contracts, Fees, and Financial Arrangements (2.12),
- Behavior-Analytic Assessment (3.01),
- Environmental Conditions that Interfere with Success (4.07),
- Characteristics of Responsible Research (9.02),
- Timely Responding, Reporting, and Updating of Information Provided to the BACB (10.02),

KEY TERMS:

- **Ethics:**

  - Cooper et al. (2007) express that "ethics refers to three basic and fundamental questions: What is the right thing to do? What is worth doing? What does it mean to be a good behavior analyst?" (p. 660). Every day, these three questions guide every decision, interaction with colleagues, as well as clients, and the research and practice conducted by behavior analysts.

- **Embracing the Scientific Method:**

  - ABA is a science of understanding human behavior. As a science, scientific methods of inquiry such as objective measurement, data-based decision-making, and determining functional and replicable relations between an intervention technique (independent variable) and a behavior change (dependent variable) are adhered to and guide all research and practice within the discipline (Baer et al. 1968).

- **Right to Effective Behavioral Treatment:**

  - Behavior analysts have an obligation to provide only treatments and techniques that have been scientifically validated. In other words, only those interventions which have been demonstrated by research to be effective (Van Houten et al. 1988) based on their associations with improvements in pro-social behaviors, and/or a reduction in problem behaviors. These associations are typically documented in scientifically sound research studies published in peer-reviewed academic journals.

- **Standards of Practice for ABA:**
  - Standards of practice are written guidelines that outline expectations regarding conduct and service provision for practitioners within a field of practice (e.g., ABA). The Behavior Analysis Certification Board has written the "Professional and Ethical Compliance Code for Behavior Analysts" (Behavior Analysis Certification Board 2014) as the guiding standards of practice for behavior analysts. As of 2016, all Board Certification Behavior Analysts must comply with the expectations outlined in this standard.

Show Me The Evidence

As an employee of a community-based program in applied behavior analysis (ABA), Ivan had been working with Eva, a young not-quite-three-year-old child diagnosed with Autism Spectrum Disorder (ASD) for nearly six months. His program is partly privately funded, and as a result of this his program is less sought out by parents—not everyone can afford the fees—but it typically has no wait list for services. When Eva's parents approached Ivan's agency, he quickly began his assessment practices in careful consultation with her parents, shared the results, and made some solid goals to move forward with Eva's therapy. After working between 10 and 20 h a week for the past five months with Eva and her family using evidence-based practices in the field of ASD and ABA to help decrease challenging behavior, teach new skills, and prepare Eva for the preschool environment Ivan received a voice mail message that he was not expecting from her family.

Ivan listened to the voice mail message attentively and then listened again. "Chelation therapy? Dietary change? Seriously?" he spoke back to his cell phone. "What's this about?"

Ivan was in between community appointments with other clients when he had the chance to stop and check his phone and review his voice messages. He thought about how the last six months of service had been going with Eva and her family, the only concern he had, before receiving the phone call, was that Eva's parents seemed to be far less invested than anticipated with respect to the agreed-upon programs and protocols. For example, they forgot to fill out their data sheets last week, so Ivan was unable to graph evidence of any further gains in the ABA-base program.

He listened to the message for a third time. *Something is going on,* he thought. *But I don't get it. Eva has been doing so well; she is making great gains in her skills of everyday living, she has made significant leaps in her communication abilities. Her non-compliance and aggression have both decreased dramatically. So what's this about?* Finding it difficult to concentrate, he went to his next two appointments, trying to tuck this concern—a mystery, really—into the back of his mind, promising himself he would call the family as soon as his other responsibilities for the day were met.

Pulling into the parking lot outside his building, he quickly keyed in the entry code and went into his personal office to ensure that confidentiality was maintained in his impending conversation. *I will never get caught in that problem again*, he had promised himself many times, recalling when he had once been talking about clients at a restaurant with a colleague and had been inadvertently overheard. *I really understand the* **Standards of Practice in ABA**, *particularly in the areas of ethics and the importance of maintaining privacy. Hopefully, I can do both of those things and still help out these parents with whatever is going on right now.* Ivan had undertaken some additional continuing education credits in the last few years over that lapse in judgment and found that he really enjoyed the presentations and conversations around ethical principles, including the strong focus on **embracing the scientific method** the recommendation of scientifically validated interventions in his field of work.

He dialed his cell after carefully closing his door. "Hello?" Eva's mother answered after only a few rings.

"Hi." Ivan responded. "It's Ivan from *ABA Services Inc.* You left me a voicemail message earlier today and I am calling to follow up with you."

"Right!" she answered quickly. "Well, to summarize, Eva's father and I have been going to some talks and meetings with some other parents in the neighboring town. It's fun to get together with other parents who understand what we are going through, but also we have been learning about some new treatments that we want to try. I mentioned a few of them in your phone messages."

"Yes," Ivan responded in turn. "I was hoping to hear a little more."

"The thing we are really hoping to move forward with—and we were hoping you could help us—is that special diet. A lot of the other parents we have been talking to are using it and they all say that it has worked wonders for their children with autism. We have actually been trying it out some in the last few weeks. It is really hard right now to always give Eva the right foods, but I guess it will take up less of our time once we have bought all the supplies, and when we know where gluten-free, casein-free products are locally available." Eva's mother paused.

Oh boy, thought Ivan, *this isn't what I was expecting to hear. I thought they were going to ask me for information, not tell me that they are already implementing an un-validated treatment. True, it's not really an intrusive choice, but it's not one I can support. Both my boss and my credentialing agency would be highly unimpressed to hear me supporting this. I am probably going to be lucky if I keep my credentials if I don't handle this right. They have a* **right to effective behavioral treatment**, *not to the popular treatment trend of the time.*

"I think we should probably sit down and talk about this next time I am scheduled to come in ..." Ivan quickly thumbed through his planner and finished his sentence. "... the day after tomorrow."

As he reflected on his workday so far, Ivan further considered this issue, trying to set aside his own feelings, attitudes, and priorities. Is there really any harm in what these parents are doing? Maybe it would be better if I just "let" them do this diet alongside the things we are already doing—the ones we know work. Will that make them happy with me? What is the worst thing that could happen? I don't want to lose this client—or my job.

The Response: Principles, Processes, Practices, and Reflections

Principles:

(Q1) The Behavior Analysis Certification Board emphasizes that "Behavior Analysts rely on professionally derived knowledge based on science and behavior analysis when making scientific or professional judgments in human service provision, or when engaging in scholarly or professional endeavors" (BACB 2014, p. 4), but also "operate(s) in the best interest of clients" and uses "informed consent and respects the wishes of client" (BACB 2014, p. 6). Based on these statements, which two guidelines are potentially in conflict?

(Q2) What does it mean to provide "effective treatment" (Reference Ethics Box 9.9, Behavior Analyst Certification Board, 2014)?

Ethics Box 9.9

Professional and Ethical Compliance Code for Behavior Analysts

- 9.02 Characteristics of Responsible Research.
  (a) Clients have a right to e effective treatment (i.e., based on the research literature and adapted to the individual client). Behavior analysts always have the obligation to advocate for and educate the client about scientifically supported, most effective treatment procedures. Effective treatment procedures have been validated as having both long-term and short-term benefits to clients and society.
  (b) Behavior analysts have the responsibility to advocate for the appropriate amount and level of service provision and oversight required to meet the desired behavior-change program goals.
  (c) In those instances where more than one scientifically supported treatment has been established, additional factors may be considered in selecting interventions, including, but not limited to, efficiency and cost-effectiveness, risks and side effects of the interventions, client preference, and practitioner experience and training.
  (d) Behavior analysts review and appraise the effects of any treatments about which they are aware that might impact the goals of the behavior-change program, and their possible impact on the behavior-change program, to the extent possible.

Processes:

(Q3) Describe how you might guide a parent of a young child with a development disability through the process of selecting an intervention for their child. List the types of questions you would use to encourage parents to consider multiple approaches and scientific-based treatments?

(Q4) Ivan needs to do the billing for this family, as it is the end of the month. He is unsure what to do given what has just happened. List items he should have put in place before starting with the family that would assist in this situation and things that he may have to do now given this new turn of events, regarding billing (Reference Ethics Box 9.10, Behavior Analyst Certification Board, 2014).

Ethics Box 9.10

Professional and Ethical Compliance Code for Behavior Analysts

2.12 Contracts, Fees, and Financial Arrangements.

(a) Prior to the implementation of services, behavior analysts ensure that there is in place a signed contract outlining the responsibilities of all parties, the scope of behavior-analytic services to be provided, and behavior analysts' obligations under this Code.

(b) As early as is feasible in a professional or scientific relationship, behavior analysts reach an agreement with their clients specifying compensation and billing arrangements.

(c) Behavior analysts' fee practices are consistent with law and behavior analysts do not misrepresent their fees. If limitations to services can be anticipated because of limitations in funding, this is discussed with the client as early as is feasible.

(d) When funding circumstances change, the financial responsibilities and limits must be revisited with the client.

Practices:

(Q5) Ivan is worried about losing his client and the monetary implication that this may have, however, needs to abide by the Ethics Compliance Code (BACB 2014). What does Ivan need to be conscious of in this situation and describe the ethical path he should take (Reference Ethics Box 9.11, Behavior Analyst Certification Board, 2014)?

Ethics Box 9.11

Professional and Ethical Compliance Code for Behavior Analysts

1.01 Reliance on Scientific Knowledge
Behavior analysts rely on professionally derived knowledge based on science and behavior analysis when making scientific or professional judgments in human service provision, or when engaging in scholarly or professional endeavors.

1.02 Boundaries of Competence

(a) All behavior analysts provide services, teach, and conduct research only within the boundaries of their competence, defined as being commensurate with their education, training, and supervised experience.

(b) Behavior analysts provide services, teach, or conduct research in new areas (e.g., populations, techniques, behaviors) only after first undertaking appropriate study, training, supervision, and/or consultation from persons who are competent in those areas.

(Q6) Is the level of intrusiveness of the diet something that Ivan should be considering when weighing his options of whether he can support this approach or advocate for an evidence-based approach? Support with references.

(Q7) List all of the methods that Ivan completes to protect the privacy of his clients. What safeguards does he also have to have in place for their records and documentation? What would he do with the records if Eva is no longer a client (Reference Ethics Box 9.12, Behavior Analyst Certification Board, 2014)?

Ethics Box 9.12

Professional and Ethical Compliance Code for Behavior Analysts

2.06 Maintaining Confidentiality.

(a) Behavior analysts have a primary obligation and take reasonable precautions to protect the confidentiality of those with whom they work or consult, recognizing that confidentiality may be established by law, organizational rules, or professional or scientific relationships.

(e) Behavior analysts must not share or create situations likely to result in the sharing of any identifying information (written, photographic, or video) about current clients and supervisees within social media contexts.

2.07 Maintaining Records.

(a) Behavior analysts maintain appropriate confidentiality in creating, storing, accessing, transferring, and disposing of records under their control, whether these are written, automated, electronic, or in any other medium.

(b) Behavior analysts maintain and dispose of records in accordance with applicable laws, regulations, corporate policies, and organizational policies, and in a manner that permits compliance with the requirements of this Code.

2.10 Documenting Professional Work and Research.

(a) Behavior analysts appropriately document their professional work in order to facilitate provision of services later by them or by other professionals, to ensure accountability, and to meet other requirements of organizations or the law.

(b) Behavior analysts have a responsibility to create and maintain documentation in the kind of detail and quality that would be consistent with best practices and the law.

(Q8) Ivan mentions that Eva was doing very well in treatment, but also mentions that he has not been able to reliably graph the data because of the parents not following through with the intervention plan. List some of his next steps based on the guidelines in the Ethics Box 9.13 listed below (BACB, 2014)

Ethics Box 9.13

Professional and Ethical Compliance Code for Behavior Analysts

- 3.01 Behavior-Analytic Assessment.
  (b) Behavior analysts have an obligation to collect and graphically display data, using behavior-analytic conventions, in a manner that allows for decisions and recommendations for behavior-change program development.
  4.07 Environmental Conditions that Interfere with Implementation.
  (a) If environmental conditions prevent implementation of a behavior-change program, behavior analysts recommend that other professional assistance (e.g., assessment, consultation, or therapeutic intervention by other professionals) be sought.
  (b) If environmental conditions hinder implementation of the behavior-change program, behavior analysts seek to eliminate the environmental constraints, or identify in writing the obstacles to doing so.

Reflections:

(Q9) Do you agree that after Ivan was corrected for some of his ethical misconduct that he is able to continue to practice in the field? What would you be required to complete if Ivan broke these ethical principles again? Do you think that Ivan can continue to provide ABA services to Eva if he completes his due diligence and puts other parameters in place (Reference Ethics Box 9.14, Behavior Analyst Certification Board, 2014)?

Ethics Box 9.14

Professional and Ethical Compliance Code for Behavior Analysts

- 10.02 Timely responding, reporting, and updating of information provided to the BACB.
  (a) Behavior analysts must comply with all BACB deadlines including, but not limited to, ensuring that the BACB is notified within thirty (30) days of the date of any of the following grounds for sanctioning status:

A violation of this Code, or disciplinary investigation, action or sanction, ling of charges, conviction or plea of guilty or nolo contendere by a governmental agency, healthcare organization, third-party payer, or educational institution. Procedural note: Behavior analysts convicted of a felony directly related to behavior analysis practice and/or public health and safety shall be ineligible to apply for BACB registration, certification, or recertification for a period of three (3) years from the exhaustion of appeals, completion of parole or probation, or final release from confinement (if any), whichever is later (see also, 1.04d Integrity);

(b) Any public health- and safety-related fines or tickets where the behavior analyst is named on the ticket;

(c) A physical or mental condition that would impair the behavior analysts' ability to competently practice; and

(d) A change of name, address, or email contact.

Ethics Box 9.15

Professional and Ethical Compliance Code for Behavior Analysts

- 9.03 Informed Consent.
  Behavior analysts inform participants or their guardian or surrogate in understandable language about the nature of the research; that they are free to participate, to decline to participate, or to withdraw from the research at any time without penalty; about significant factors that may influence their willingness to participate; and answer any other questions participants may have about the research.

(Q10) Some feel that there is no harm in trying an invalidated treatment, provided that it deemed not very intrusive, may not pose any harm, and appears relatively safe. For example, some might say, "What harm is there in trying a new diet?" Or, "Taking some vitamin supplements seems harmless, since vitamins are good for you anyways." Do you agree? Why or why not?

Additional Web Links

Evidence-Based Practices for children and adolescents with Autism Spectrum Disorders: Review of the Literature and Practice Guide http://www. kidsmentalhealth.ca/documents/EBP_autism.pdf

Guidelines for Responsible Conduct for Behavior Analysts http://www.bacb. com/index.php?page=57

Introduction to Evidence-Informed Decision-Making http://www.cihr-irsc.gc.ca/
e/45245.html
Implementing Evidence-Informed Practice http://www.excellenceforchildand
youth.ca/sites/default/files/docs/implementation-toolkit.pdf

CASE: v-R3

Volunteered or Volun-*told*?
Setting: Childcare   Age Group: Preschool

LEARNING OBJECTIVE:

- To consider the ethical considerations surrounding the recruitment of research
  participants.

  Professional and Ethical Compliance Code for Behavior Analysts:

- Informed Consent (9.03),
- Using Confidential Information for Didactic or Instructive Purposes (9.04),
- Grant and Journal Reviews (9.06),
- Plagiarism (9.07).

KEY TERMS:

- **Research:**

  - Research typically refers to the process of scientific inquiry, or seeking an
    answer to a question in order to further scientific knowledge. This can be
    contrasted with evaluation, which refers to providing information for
    decision-making about a particular program and is often based on furthering
    policy and program interests.

- **Research Participants:**

  - A research participant is an individual that takes part in a research project.
    Research participants are the target of observations by researchers.
    Participating in a research project often begins with the potential participant
    providing free and informed consent, that is demonstrating that they have
    received information about the research study, they have the capacity to
    decide, their decision is voluntary and that they have been given enough
    information to make an informed decision about their participation (Bailey
    and Burch 2002).

Volunteered or Volun-*told*?

"Yes!" Darin Vineel crowed. Hovering over the inbox on his email account, he once again opened the most recent email that had just come through his system, alerting his various devices. *I am sure in the right place at the right time right now! Usually I don't get to read my emails properly until late at night, long after the busy-ness of the day has subsided. But I am glad to be here for this one!*

Congratulations! Your research grant proposal has been approved. Please open the attached document for more information. Because he could not quite believe it after months of waiting and wondering—not including the weeks it took him to prepare the grant application in the first place—he reopened and reread his "award letter."

Congratulations! Your grant proposal has been approved. Please open the attached document for more information. Your approved budget for your "Consulting Briefly with the Brief Consultation Model" research project has been reviewed, and you have been awarded $5000 for the next six months. These funds will be allocated to you as soon as you have received research ethics CLEARANCE and have supplied us with a certificate of clearance from the research ethics board. Best wishes in moving ahead with your project.

Still not quite believing this stroke of luck, he started to compose and internal email to the other staff of his behavior management team, asking them to attend a mandatory **research** meeting, next Thursday at 5:00 PM. *They need to know what is coming,* he thought. To be sure everyone attended (since he wanted everyone involved), he typed "MANDATORY MEETING!" in the subject line of his carefully prepared email and sent it to allstaff@behmgmt.com right away. He headed for home, but with this news still rolling around in his mind, he barely remembered the adrenaline-fueled trip. After dinner, he went into his home office and reviewed the proposal he had sent off months ago. *It is going to be so exciting for everyone,* he considered. *Rather than having a caseworker for years and years, sometimes with no significant progress, we are going to team up with families for short-term, goal-orientated interventions. Then, if the families still need more support, we can do it all over again!* He was sure of its success, after all he had read in the literature about its success in community settings, and even school environments. *I can't wait until next Thursday, when I get to tell everyone about the project they will be participating in for the next six months…At least!* he added in his head. *After all, we might like it and keep it. Even better: we might get some fantastic data!*

Eager for the project to move ahead, he downloaded his agency's research ethics forms and began to complete them, page by page. When he got to the subheading marked **RESEARCH PARTICIPANTS**, he cut-and-pasted a complex matrix that he had created in anticipation of this application. In this matrix, he matched up his staff with families, using "Therapist 1" and "Family A" and other pseudonyms. He explained in the application how he anticipated 100 % rate of participation from his staff, and his families who would be the recipients of this brief consultation model. *Who would ever want to turn this opportunity down!* Darin thought.

It only took a few days for a decision to be emailed back to him. *That was surprisingly fast*, he thought, very impressed with the speed of the ethics board. But when he read the email that night from ethics@behmgmt.com, he was surprised again, but this time it was a more disappointing surprise than he had experienced days earlier. Dear Darin, it began and continued:

We are unable to complete your ethics review for project 4241, and we are unable to clear it for you to move ahead and begin the data collection phase. Our primary concern is the lack of voluntary participation. Your expectation—and your supervisory role—in your agency may unduly coerce your staff members and your client family members into participation in this project. For example, you have noted that you plan to disseminate the recruitment posters for your research project, your letters of invitation, and consent forms yourself, which may cause potential participants to feel that they are required to take part. to be cleared, participation in this research must be entirely voluntary. When you have updated this section, please resubmit your work for a full review.

"I don't get it!" He spoke aloud in the empty room. "I keep hearing about how effective work depends on effective collaboration, positive relationships, and individualized attention. Shouldn't it be better if I meet with everyone and talk with each of them about this research in person? This change just goes against everything I have been taught about working with others in this field. What do I do?"

The Response: Principles, Processes, Practices, and Reflections

Principles:

(Q1) Do you agree with the response that the Research Ethics Board provided to Darin? Why or why not?

(Q2) Darin seems to be confusing voluntary participation with a collaborative approach to research. What distinguishes these concepts?

Processes:

(Q3) Outline a recruitment process that Darin could use that addresses the concerns expressed by the Research Ethics Board.

(Q4) How might Darin ensure that his potential participants are free to decline participation?

Practices:

(Q5) How might Darin ensure that participants are not only voluntarily participating in this research, but also that their decisions are based on informed consent?

(Q6) Describe what Guideline 9.04, *Using Confidential Information for Didactic or Instructive Purposes*, means in practice for Darin (Reference Ethics Box 9.16, Behavior Analyst Certification Board, 2014)?

Ethics Box 9.16

Professional and Ethical Compliance Code for Behavior Analysts

- 9.04 Using Confidential Information for Didactic or Instructive Purposes.
  (a) Behavior analysts do not disclose personally identifiable information concerning their individual or organizational clients, research participants, or other recipients of their services that they obtained during the course of their work, unless the person or organization has consented in writing or unless there is other legal authorization for doing so.
  (b) Behavior analysts disguise confidential information concerning participants, whenever possible, so that they are not individually identifiable to others and so that discussions do not cause harm to identifiable participants.

(Q7) How may decisions be biased based on the decision of Darin's grant review team and his Research Ethics board team if there were the same members (see Guideline 9.06)? What would you do if they were not members of the BACB (Reference Ethics Box 9.17, Behavior Analyst Certification Board, 2014)?

Ethics Box 9.17

Professional and Ethical Compliance Code for Behavior Analysts
9.06 Grant and Journal Reviews.
- Behavior analysts who serve on grant review panels or as manuscript reviewers avoid conducting any research described in grant proposals or manuscripts that they reviewed, except as replications fully crediting the prior researchers.

(Q8) In completing his Research Ethics Board application, Darin copy and pasted information from his grant. Is this considered plagiarism according to Guideline 9.07, Plagiarism (Reference Ethics Box 9.18, Behavior Analyst Certification Board, 2014)?

Ethics Box 9.18

Professional and Ethical Compliance Code for Behavior Analysts

- 9.07 Plagiarism.
  (a) Behavior analysts fully cite the work of others where appropriate.
  (b) Behavior analysts do not present portions or elements of another's work or data as their own.

Reflections:

(Q9) If you were a member of the Research Ethics Board reviewing Darin's project, what additional questions might you raise?

(Q10) How would you feel if you were a family being asked to participate in this research project given the current setup?

Additional Web Links
The TCPS 2 Tutorial Course on Research Ethics (CORE)
http://www.pre.ethics.gc.ca/eng/education/tutorial-didacticiel/
Plagiarism in Higher Education Research
http://www.ithenticate.com/plagiarism-detection
log/bid/87,315/Plagiarism-in-Higher-Education-Research#.V3aW2ldWu7Y
Voluntary Participation in Research
http://www.ncbi.nlm.nih.gov/pmc/articles/PMC4032563/

CASE: v-R4

Settle in—or Opt Out?
Setting: School   Age Group: School Age
LEARNING OBJECTIVE:

- To utilize ethical principles of research to advocate for the protection of a child with exceptionalities in a school setting.

Professional and Ethical Compliance Code for Behavior Analysts:

- Least Restrictive Procedures (4.09)
- Describing Behavior-Change Program Objectives (4.05)
- Describing Conditions for Behavior-Change Program Success (4.06)
- Environmental Conditions that Interfere with Implementation (4.07)

KEY TERMS:

- **Advocacy:**

  - Advocacy is a process in which an individual or a group works to influence decisions. Within the field of applied behavior analysis, for example, the "Association of Behavior Analysis International" works to support the growth of the science of behavior and the adoption of evidence-informed practice by conducting research, providing education, and disseminating best practices (ABAI 2012). Similarly, the Behavior Analyst Certification Board works to support high-quality behavioral practices and protect consumers of behavior analysis services by promoting and disseminating professional standards and increasing the availability of certified behavior analysts (BCBA 2014). *Autism Speaks* is example of an organization that is involved in advocacy, working to raise awareness to increase support for research and intervention for individuals with ASD. Individual behavior analysts may also act as advocates; for example, providing evidence to school personnel to support accommodations within a classroom for a child experiencing behavior difficulties. When combined, these activities work to influence decisions at organizational, community, and individual levels.

- **Capacity:**
  - An essential consideration for requesting research participation is whether the individuals being asked have the ability to understand the information provided to them and appreciate the consequences of their decision (e.g., able to weigh the risks and benefits of participation). For example, young children, individuals with developmental disabilities, or individuals with cognitive impairments may not have the capacity to make a decision on their own about their involvement in a research project (Canadian Institutes of Health Research 2010).

- **Conflict of Interest:**
  - Within a research project, a conflict of interest arises when activities place individuals at odds between the responsibilities of research and their organization's interests (Canadian Institutes of Health Research 2010).

- **Free and Informed Consent:**
  - Ethical principles, such as free and informed consent, work to ensure that individuals taking part in research activities are protected and treated respectfully. "Free" refers to consent to participate that is given voluntarily, without any influence or coercion, and that may be withdrawn at any time; and (2) "Informed" refers to ensuring that potential participants are provided with enough information about the project (e.g., study purpose, what is involved and expected of them, benefits, risks) to make a knowledgeable decision about participation (Canadian Institutes of Health Research 2010).

Settle In—Or Opt Out?

Demetrios and his family had moved to a large, urban center three years ago when Demetrios was six years old and entering grade one. That year after a lengthy process, most of the school year, he was diagnosed with an intellectual disability. Before moving to the urban area he and his family had been living in a beautiful, rural area where Demetrios enjoyed the freedom afforded to a child growing up in the country.

Once Demetrios entered formal school in his Kindergarten year, before the family's move, it became apparent that he struggled with basic academic tasks, socialization with his peers, and following the basic rules for behavior in a group environment. While his rural freedom had given him great joy in the outdoors and a great love for child-led exploration, it had left him bereft of same-age play partners. Demetrios was an only child with two devoted parents focusing on him, who made many efforts to find playmates and play dates for him, the distance between not only community activities and their home, but other neighbors with young children and their home, appeared to be a significant barrier to easy socialization. After all their efforts, when Demetrios's final report card at the end of Kindergarten still pointed to "persistent problems with peer-to-peer socialization," they started to make plans for a significant lifestyle change.

They chose their current community due to its proximity to two large hospitals, one connected to a university focused on training graduate students in clinical and developmental psychology. In the family's research, they found that the second hospital had an excellent reputation for adult mental health. The university attached to the hospital had a positive reputation for supporting the professional development of local schools, boards, and the educators within them. The university trained these professionals into developing a strong capacity for supporting students with exceptionalities within inclusive settings. A final draw to this specific community was a large, well-development children's developmental center that appeared to have excellent community support and, again, had the reputation for helping out with local families.

Demetrios's family chose a small home with a large yard nestled carefully within the boundaries of these service areas; in fact, they had limited their house search boundaries to the geographical area inside the area that was surrounded by these center-based services. With such a significant sacrifice, they felt assured that they were ready for what the future held. But they did not anticipate the downside that would work its way into their lives in a couple of years, specifically in Demetrios's grade four year.

Following the family's move and Demetrios's diagnosis of an intellectual disability, Demetrios—and his parents—settled into the community very well. With the diversity evident in their new they had no difficulty finding other parents who were in similar circumstances, they easily discovered a community of care for themselves and Demetrios, and they had no challenges finding a school community which supported full inclusion of all students in the neighborhood, which as a final bonus had plenty same-aged peers for Demetrios. Rather than facing a difficulty FINDING services, they were having difficulty DECLINING services. It seemed like every second day, a permission slip, an information letter, or an email arrived with requests for participation in special events, special services: even research projects from the university community! Their typical response was to "opt out" of most of these while they settled into their new homes and new lives, but as time moved on and Demetrios grew in size, age, and need, they selected a few opportunities for involvement here and there. However, they had strong concerns about their son becoming what they thought of as a "laboratory rat."

When grade four hit, the academic demands grew, peer socialization became even harder, and Demetrios really began to struggle in a way that he had not experienced before in his new school and inclusive classroom. A few incidents of aggression appeared at school but then these incidents gradually increased in strength, quantity, and intensity and became a daily concern. Demetrios's parents were called into school a first, second, and third time.

After the fourth call, they contacted an advocate at the local children's center and started working with an advocate to attend school meeting with them, as they were feeling overwhelmed with pressures from the school's special education staff. At both meetings two and three, the resource staff—whose role was to support the classroom teachers—strongly recommended including Demetrios in a clinical treatment center at the local university. While this would provide extra personnel and services for his classroom, it would also mean that Demetrios would be segregated in the university classroom and observed daily, and data about his behavior would be summarized. It would also mean that Demetrios would be included in a special, experimental intervention program that had proven results in decreasing aggression at school, and it would lead to more support for Demetrios's academic needs of the classroom. Although Demetrios's parents made it quite clear that they are uneasy about participating in segregated settings—and always have been—they felt a continuing pressure to do so.

On the fourth visit with the classroom teacher, the school administrators, the special education staff, Demetrios's parents, their advocate, and the researchers, problems came to a boiling point. Right before the meeting began, the advocate, whom the school personnel had not met, was waiting outside the staff washroom, and overheard the special education staff expressing their frustration with Demetrios's family in a less than positive way, and sharing ideas about how they might "convince them" to "get on board" and "just sign up and settle in already." The advocate became highly concerned about issues such as free and informed consent and conflict of interest, which undergird the ethics of inclusion and the parents and students rights to stay in the community setting. When she joined the meeting, she immediately raised her hand and said with a severe tone, "I have something urgent to add to our agenda, which I think should be the starting topic of our meeting here today."

The Response: Principles, Processes, Practices, and Reflections

Principles:

(Q1) List and describe at least three ethical issues present in Demetrios's case.
(Q2) Where the requirements of informed consent met? If so, please explain how they were met. If not, please explain why not?

Processes:

(Q3) If you were supporting Demetrios and his family, what informed consent process would you recommend for the school?
(Q4) Describe how Demetrios can be included in the consent process.

(Q5) Least Restrictive Procedures are important to try before moving to more restrictive procedures like a segregated setting. List what least restrictive procedures should have been applied first before moving Demetrios to a secluded setting (Reference Ethics Box 9.19, Behavior Analyst Certification Board, 2014).

Ethics Box 9.19

Professional and Ethical Compliance Code for Behavior Analysts

- 4.09 Least Restrictive Procedures.
  Behavior analysts review and appraise the restrictiveness of procedures and always recommend the least restrictive procedures likely to be effective.

Practices:

(Q5) If you were advocating on behalf of Demetrios and his family, how would you respond to the behavior of the school staff? List at least three steps.

(Q6) Given the case study, do you feel that the educators in the classroom have completed both of the Guidelines from the Professional and Ethical Compliance Code by the BACB: (a) Describe the Behavior Objectives (Guideline 4.05) and (b) Describe the Conditions for Program Success (Guideline 4.06 (Reference Ethics Box 9.20, Behavior Analyst Certification Board, 2014))?

Ethics Box 9.20

Professional and Ethical Compliance Code for Behavior Analysts

- 4.05 Describing Behavior-Change Program Objectives.
  Behavior analysts describe, in writing, the objectives of the behavior-change program to the client before attempting to implement the program. To the extent possible, a risk-benefit analysis should be conducted on the procedures to be implemented to reach the objective. The description of program objectives and the means by which they will be accomplished is an ongoing process throughout the duration of the client-practitioner relationship.
- 4.06 Describing Conditions for Behavior-Change Program Success.
  Behavior analysts describe to the client the environmental conditions that are necessary for the behavior-change program to be effective.

(Q8) List environmental conditions that may interfere with the behavior-change program (Guideline 4.07, Reference Ethics Box 9.21, Behavior Analyst Certification Board, 2014)?

Ethics Box 9.21

> **Professional and Ethical Compliance Code for Behavior Analysts**
>
> - 4.07 Environmental Conditions that Interfere with Implementation.
>   (a) If environmental conditions prevent implementation of a behavior-change program, behavior analysts recommend that other professional assistance (e.g., assessment, consultation, or therapeutic intervention by other professionals) be sought.
>   (b) If environmental conditions hinder implementation of the behavior-change program, behavior analysts seek to eliminate the environmental constraints, or identify in writing the obstacles to doing so.

Reflections:

(Q9) Why might it be important for Demetrios to be included in the informed consent process?

(Q10) What are the pros and cons of a segregated treatment setting versus his inclusive setting he is currently in?

Additional Web Links

Tri-Council Policy Statement: Ethical Conduct for Research Involving Humans

http://www.pre.ethics.gc.ca/archives/tcps-eptc/docs/TCPS%20October%202005_E.pdf

The consent process

http://www.pre.ethics.gc.ca/eng/policy-politique/initiatives/tcps2-eptc2/chapter3-chapitre3/

WHO informed consent form templates http://www.who.int/rpc/research_ethics/informed_consent/en/

CASE: v-R5

Ask for permission, or ask for forgiveness?
Setting: School   Age Group: School age

LEARNING OBJECTIVE:

- To distinguish between measurement of practice and research.

Professional and Ethical Compliance Code for Behavior Analysts:

- Rights and Prerogatives of Clients (2.05)
- Treatment/Intervention Efficacy (2.09)

- Ethical Violations by Others and Risk of Harm (7.02)
- Characteristics of Responsible Research (9.02)

KEY TERMS:

- **Ethical Review:**

  - An ethical review is when ethical principles governing research involving humans (e.g., respect for persons and concerns for welfare and justice) are used to evaluate an application for research. This review is typically conducted by an ethics review board, a group of individuals that meet to determine whether a research project meets ethical standards. Depending on the level of risk associated with a research project, an application might be reviewed by a full ethics board review (often projects involving greater risks), or delegated for review by only one or a few members of the research ethics board (often projects involving minimal levels of risk). The outcomes of an ethical review might involve clearance of research or requesting changes to ensure the protection of research participants (Canadian Institutes of Health Research 2010).

- **Intervention:**

  - In ABA, an intervention involves the application of the principles of behavior to change (increase or decrease) socially significant behaviors. These applications of the principles of behavior are called strategies or tactics and can take place in home, school, or community settings (Cooper et al. 2007).

- **Measurement of Practice:**

  - Measuring occurs when we assign numbers to objects or events. In applied behavior analysis, the effects of the application of behavioral principles on observable behaviors are measured through data collection (e.g., documenting observed behavior in response to behavior-change tactics), visualization (e.g., graphing of data points), and analysis (e.g., examining trends in the data over time). This differs from conducting an evaluation (e.g., determining, sometimes using research designs and methods, if a program being delivered is achieving the intended outcomes) or carrying out research (e.g., using research designs and methods to answer a scientific question) (Bloom et al. 2003).

Ask for Permission, or Ask for Forgiveness?

Ahmed was excited about his new plan. As a consultant hired by the school board, the main focus of his position was to act as an itinerant support for referrals generated by his "family" of 15 public schools in a busy, urban area. Inevitably, though, he found that he spent more time in a few of his schools. These three schools were informally labeled as "inner-city" schools and had many more needs when it came to challenging behaviors than his other schools did. Consequently, Ahmed got to know the staff quite well: the classroom teachers, the special education teachers, and even the school administration. Based on numerous conversations he had been engaged in through the school year, it seemed that there was an issue with not only specific, complex children identified with special needs and, simultaneously, problem behaviors, but also with general issues in classroom management such as noise levels, compliance, and task completion. This issue was seemingly pervasive across many classrooms in all of his family of schools, but was much more pronounced in these three inner-city schools.

His new plan was to focus on a proactive way to prevent—and decrease—these typically occurring problem behaviors. In order to help him consolidate his ideas, he started working through journal articles, in order to ensure the impact of this new, not-quite-yet planned, intervention in his three schools was effective. *This would make a fantastic research project,* he thought. *After all, if you are not collecting data, you are not doing ABA. And if we are collecting this data, we should be sure to publish and disseminate the results, so it can help other educators in similar situations.* That evening after work, he was so pumped about getting this on the go that he pulled out his laptop and dug right back into describing this hopefully upcoming intervention for ethics review and clearance. At the same time, he sent emails to the principals of these three schools, requesting time at each upcoming staff meeting to describe his plans, to request feedback from the involved teachers, and hopefully to elicit excitement about it!

The first two staff meeting presentations Ahmed had prepared slides and handouts filled with visuals, graphs, and descriptions from the literature of how other educators had decreased the incidence of problem behaviors in their own classroom environments with very doable strategies like greeting each student at the doorway every morning. However, he was met with a lot of resistance about the research project itself. Educators were willing to go forward with the intervention, but did not want to trouble of complying with the research ethics board.

At this third meeting, he stumbled over his words from beginning to end. The hot, angry glare from the grade one teacher completely discombobulated him. When she whispered time and time again to her colleagues seated next to her, he wondered what the conversations were, instead of focused on sharing his plans. Even though things were going along so poorly already, he was dreading the question-and-answer period he had planned for the last five minutes of time available to him.

"And why, exactly, would you call this *research*?" the grade one teacher asked, raising her hand as soon as she could. "Why would we do this ethics business instead of just focusing on *the children*? After all, we make changes to our pedagogy all the time. Just yesterday, for example, I decided that I would create an in-box for all the students' homework, pizza money, and permission forms, because I was tired of being handed things all the time, disrupting both teaching and learning. But I didn't have to ask our ethics board for *permission* to do this. It is just part of my professionalism as an educator. And I could take data on this if I wanted to do so. But it's just looking at measuring if this practice works for me and if it works for the students. I don't need to ask."

Ahmed froze a little, unsure of what to say next. He quickly scanned the room and noticed that even the principal was nodding agreement with this grade one teacher. He felt quite unsure and extremely uncomfortable, and did not know how to answer. They asked him to come and do the intervention and just not do formal research. Ahmed decided that it would be okay if they were willing to complete the research project with him. He just decided that he could not do formal research and would still be able to present the findings.

The Response: Principles, Processes, Practices, and Reflections

Principles:

(Q1) Research ethics are based on three principles: respect for person, concern for welfare, and justice. Describe each principle and outline how each might apply to Ahmed's situation.

(Q2) As "scientist-practitioners," behavior analysts are involved in measurement of practice and can become involved in conducting research. It would not be practical if an ethical review board process were required each time a behavior analyst was preparing to implement and measure the effects of an intervention. When does measurement of practice become research and require a review by an ethical review board?

(Q3) Define the differences between evaluation and research.

Processes:

(Q4) The Professional and Ethical Compliance Code for Behavior Analysts notes that "When research and clinical needs conflict, behavior analysts prioritize the welfare of the client" (BACB 2014, p. 18). How does this statement apply to Ahmed's dilemma?

(Q5) In some ways, Ahmed has followed the Guideline 2.09 for Treatment Efficacy/Intervention and in some ways he has not. List the ways he has followed this guideline and how he has dismissed it (Reference Ethics Box 9.22, Behavior Analyst Certification Board, 2014)?

Ethics Box 9.22

Professional and Ethical Compliance Code for Behavior Analysts

2.09 Treatment/Intervention Efficacy.

(a) Clients have a right to effective treatment (i.e., based on the research literature and adapted to the individual client). Behavior analysts always have the obligation to advocate for and educate the client about scientifically supported, most effective treatment procedures. Effective treatment procedures have been validated as having both long-term and short-term benefits to clients and society.

(b) Behavior analysts have the responsibility to advocate for the appropriate amount and level of service provision and oversight required to meet the defined behavior-change program goals.

(c) In those instances where more than one scientifically supported treatment has been established, additional factors may be considered in selecting interventions, including, but not limited to, efficiency and cost-effectiveness, risks and side effects of the interventions, client preference, and practitioner experience and training.

(d) Behavior analysts review and appraise the effects of any treatments about which they are aware that might impact the goals of the behavior-change program, and their possible impact on the behavior-change program, to the extent possible.

Practices:

(Q6) What guideline is Ahmed going against in his final course of action according to the BACB's *Professional and Ethical Compliance Code* (BACB, 2014)?

(Q7) Given the ethical decision-making model at the link below, determine what course of action you would take in the following case. Would it be the same as or different than Ahmeds?

http://www.ryerson.ca/content/dam/ethicsnetwork/downloads/model_G.pdf

(Q8) Since Ahmed will not publish the results and will only present them, does he now comply with the Guideline 9.01, Conforming with Laws and Regulations? In other words, if he does not get research ethics board approval, is he able to present this research (Reference Ethics Box 9.23, Behavior Analyst Certification Board, 2014)?

Ethics Box 9.23

Professional and Ethical Compliance Code for Behavior Analysts

2.05 Rights and Prerogatives of Clients.

(a) The rights of the client are paramount and behavior analysts support clients' legal rights and prerogatives.

(b) Clients and supervisees must be provided, on request, an accurate and current set of the behavior analyst's credentials.

(c) Permission for electronic recording of interviews and service delivery sessions is secured from clients and relevant staff in all relevant settings. Consent for different uses must be obtained specifically and separately.

(d) Clients and supervisees must be informed of their rights and about procedures to lodge complaints about professional practices of behavior analysts with the employer, appropriate authorities, and the BACB.

(e) Behavior analysts comply with any requirements for criminal background checks.

9.01 Conforming with Laws and Regulations

Behavior analysts plan and conduct research in a manner consistent with all applicable laws and regulations, as well as professional standards governing the conduct of research. Behavior analysts also comply with other applicable laws and regulations relating to mandated-reporting requirements.

Reflections:

(Q9) How might Ahmed's dual role as both a behavior analyst brought into support the staff and their students, and his desire to simultaneously be a researcher, be contributing to the difficulties he is experiencing with the school personnel? How might this dilemma be resolved?

(Q10) Would Ahmed's behavior be in compliance with the BACB? Would you be required to report his behavior (Reference Ethics Box 9.24, Behavior Analyst Certification Board, 2014)?

Ethics Box 9.24

Professional and Ethical Compliance Code for Behavior Analysts

7.02 Ethical Violations by Others and Risk of Harm.

(a) If behavior analysts believe there may be a legal or ethical violation, they first determine whether there is potential for harm, a possible legal violation, a mandatory-reporting condition, or an agency, organization, or regulatory requirement addressing the violation.

(b) If a client's legal rights are being violated, or if there is the potential for harm, behavior analysts must take the necessary action to protect the client, including, but not limited to, contacting relevant authorities, following organizational policies, consulting with appropriate professionals, and documenting their efforts to address the matter.

(c) If an informal resolution appears appropriate and would not violate any confidentiality rights, behavior analysts attempt to resolve the issue by bringing it to the attention of that individual and documenting their efforts to address the matter. If the matter is not resolved, behavior analysts report the matter to the appropriate authority (e.g., employer, supervisor, regulatory authority).

(d) If the matter meets the reporting requirements of the BACB, behavior analysts submit a formal complaint to the BACB (see also, 10.02 Timely Responding, Reporting, and Updating of Information Provided to the BACB).

Additional Web Links
Distinguishing Evaluation from Research
http://www.uniteforsight.org/evaluation-course/module10
Similarities and Differences Between Research and Evaluation
http://www.cihr-irsc.gc.ca/e/45336.html#a2.1

References

Baer, D., Wolf, M., & Risely, T. (1968). Some current dimensions of applied behavior analysis. *Journal of Applied Behavior Analysis, 1*(1), 91–97.

Bailey, J., & Burch, M. (2002). *Research methods in applied behavior analysis*. London: Sage Publications.

Behavior Analyst Certification Board. (2014). *Professional and ethical compliance code for behavior analysts*. Retrieved from http://www.bacb.com/Downloadfiles/BACB_Compliance_Code.pdf

Bloom, M., Fischer, J., & Orme, J. (2003). *Evaluating practice: Guidelines for the accountable professional* (4th ed.). Boston: Allyn & Bacon.

Canadian Institutes of Health Research, Natural Sciences and Engineering Research Council of Canada, and Social Sciences and Humanities Research Council of Canada. (2010, December). *Tri-council policy statement: Ethical conduct for research involving humans.*

Cooper, J., Heron, T., & Heward, W. (2007). *Applied behavior analysis* (2nd ed.). Upper Saddle River, N.J.: Pearson PrenticeHall.

Kohler, R. W., Greteman, C., Raschke, D., & Highnam, C. (2007). Using a buddy skills package to increase the social interactions between a preschool with autism and her peers. *Topics in Early Childhood Special Education, 27*(3), 155–163.

Laushey, K. M., & Heflin, L. J. (2000). Enhancing social skills of kindergarten children with autism through the training of multiple peers as tutors. *Journal of Autism and Developmental Disorders, 30*, 183–193.

McConnell, S. R. (2002). Interventions to facilitate social interaction for young children with autism: Review of available research and recommendations for educational intervention and future research. *Journal of Autism and Developmental Disorders, 32*(5), 351–372.

Thomson, C. J. H. (2012). Research ethics committees. In R. Chadwick (Eds.), Encyclopedia of Applied Ethics (Vol. 3, pp. 786–796). San Diego: Academic Press.

Van Houten, R., Axelrod, S., Bailey, J., Favel, J., Foxx, R., Iwata, B., et al. (1988). The right to effective behavioral treatment. *Journal of Applied Behavior Analysis, 21*(4), 381–384.

Chapter 10
Adolescence to Adulthood Case Studies Constructed Around Research and Ethics

Abstract In this chapter, ethical considerations surrounding research, program evaluation, and practice in applied behavior analysis (ABA) are explored through a series of case studies involving adolescents and adults in home, school, and community settings. When providing ABA services to adults, informed consent is a central ethical consideration faced by behavior analysts. This can be particularly complex with adults with developmental disabilities or cognitive impairments who may not have the capacity to make informed decisions. Throughout this chapter, learners are guided to identify and respond to violations of ethical standards while critically exploring issues such as breaches of confidentiality and conflicts of interest. Further, the cases presented will explore the difficult balance facing behavior analysts when charged with selecting the most evidence-based, yet least restrictive treatment available, including the ethical use of restraint. In this chapter, entitled "Adolescent to Adulthood Case Studies Constructed Around Research and Ethics," expectations of behavior analysts surrounding protecting the dignity, health, and safety of those they are supporting are explored through five case scenarios in home, school, work, and community settings.

Keywords Adolescents · Adults · Program evaluation · Practice · Ethics · Developmental disabilities · Cognitive impairments · Restraint · Informed decisions · Conflicts of interest

© Springer International Publishing AG 2016   343
K. Maich et al., *Applied Behavior Analysis*,
DOI 10.1007/978-3-319-44794-0_10

CASE: v-R6 Guest Author: John LaPorta

GUEST AUTHOR

John LaPorta, PhD, CEO Thames Valley Children's Centre
Include or Exclude?
Setting: Community   Age-Group: Adolescent

LEARNING OBJECTIVE:

- To evaluate the ethical considerations surrounding the adoption of least restrictive evidence-based interventions.

RESPONSIBLE CONDUCT FOR BEHAVIOR ANALYSTS LINKS:

- Integrity (1.04)

KEY TERMS:

- **Evidence-based Practice**

  – The American Psychological Association (2005) defines evidence-based practice as "the integration of the best available research with clinical expertise in the context of patient characteristics, culture, and preferences" (p. 5). Smith (2013), built on this definition, asserting that evidence-based practice in applied behavior analysis "entails more than the analysis of behavior. It requires synthesis of findings into a package that independent providers can adopt and that offers a thorough solution to problems presented by consumers" (p. 24).

- **Least Restrictive Alternative**

  – The Association for Behavior Analysis International (2011) defines the least restrictive treatment as "that treatment that affords the most favorable risk-to-benefit ratio, with specific consideration of probability of treatment success, anticipated duration of treatment, distress caused by procedures, and distress caused by the behavior itself" (p. 104). Before intrusive procedures such as seclusion or restraint are utilized, therefore, less intrusive or restrictive alternatives should be exhausted first (Vollmer et al. 2011).

Include or Exclude?

Derek, a 14-year-old teen with a confirmed diagnosis of Asperger's disorder, was just beginning high school and was determined to not be thought of as (in his words) "a goof" or "a geek." The first few days at school were, of course, trying for Derek—and his classmates—with all of the movement and noise as classes changed at unfamiliar times and in unfamiliar patterns. Right away, he became annoyed when he noticed some of the looks and remarks from his peers as they seemed to zoom right in on his anxiety-reducing mannerisms like rocking (hard) and humming loudly.

Along with his newfound plan to be "cool," Derek convinced his parents that getting himself back and forth from school on his own was a high school thing, so, obviously, he would do it. To get ready for this new adventure in independence, they mapped out a route and trialed it at times when the other neighborhood grade nine students would not likely be encountered. After a few days of walking the route, Derek eyed a shortcut that he quietly kept to himself. *Seems safe,* thought Derek the first time he came across this path. It was through a lightly wooded area and reduced his walk by 15 min each way.

As Derek was taking this shortcut after the third week of school, he was surprised to find a large dog lying on the path watching him, clearly tense and highly watchful. As he approached, the dog growled menacingly. Derek did not know what to do: His mind was flooded with fear and he felt frozen physically. The two of them (the dog and the teen) stayed motionless until the dog heard its owner calling and left immediately in the opposite direction. Derek breathed a huge sigh of relief and hurried home, avoiding this shortcut to school over the next few days.

Over the weekend, though, he obsessed over this issue of the dog blocking his path (*The dangerous cur,* he thought to himself) and his inability to act to protect himself or drive off the menacing creature. He resolved to try the shortcut again and, this time, act assertively toward the dog. *This would be like other kids would do and also, it would show my independence.*

The next school day while traveling through the wooded area, he rapidly noticed the dog's presence. This time, the dog scuttled right up to him, bit into his pant leg at the cuff and, growling, worked the material in his mouth, grinding it between his jaws. Again, Derek froze. He could not utter a word nor make any kind of gesture or action, and hot tears of helpless frustration filled his eyes. Again, boy and dog remained in their respective, tense states until the dog's owner thankfully called for him from the woods. On every instance after this occurrence when Derek tried to take the shortcut, the dog impeded his walk by aggressively dominating him into immobile submission.

Derek never told his parents because he desperately wanted to work this problem out for himself. However, they inadvertently found out about it one evening when, while walking home, the dog approached Derek and blocked his path. Derek was terrified. He stood very still tried to control his breathing until the dog's owner called for him. For some reason unknown to Derek, the call did not come. Derek's mind raced through many terrible possibilities as first dusk and then darkness settled. After nearly an hour, Derek thought *I can do this* and tried to quickly walk past the dog. As he did, the dog grasped Derek's hand in its mouth, hard enough to hold it firmly but without breaking the skin.

At the same time, his parents were also consumed with concern over Derek not having arrived from school at the agreed upon time. They set out to find him by covering the route they had mapped out with him earlier in the school year. While doing so, they came upon the entrance to the shortcut and hurried into it. With their flashlights, they illuminated the frightening scene of Derek's hand captured in the dog's mouth. His father strode up to the pair, eyed the dog, and simply said, "Bad dog! No!" in a firm, clear, deep voice. The dog released Derek's hand and lay down with a whine. In turn, Derek was embarrassed and ashamed at how easily his father had controlled the animal.

After returning home, Derek's parents wanted to call the local animal control agency and report the dog. Derek adamantly argued against this, expressing the desire to learn how to respond in this situation—*an important life skill,* he argued. His parents were in a quandary. They wanted to ensure their son's safety but they also wanted to assist him in his twin goals of growth and independence by providing the **least restrictive, evidence-based** intervention.

The Response: Principles, Processes, Practices, and Reflections

Principles

(Q1) Derek's parents believed they were adhering to the principal of "least restrictive alternative" when they allowed Derek to walk to and from school on his own. Where they correct? Why or why not?

(Q2) In what situation might a more restrictive option be more appropriate than a less restrictive alternative? Please provide an example. How might this apply to the case of Derek?

Processes

(Q3) In response to the incident between Derek and the dog, Derek's parents began walking him to school. How might Derek's parents begin to gradually fade their presence, while allowing him to gradually increase his independence?

(Q4) As Derek's parents move through the continuum of most to least intrusive supports for Derek, how might they determine when to fade each level of support?

Practices

(Q5) What evidence should Derek's parents seek to guide them through their decisions surrounding support for Derek?

(Q6) How might Derek's parents weigh the available evidence? How might you prioritize the types of evidence listed in Question#5? Please explain your decision.

(Q7) If you were a BCBA on this case, what ethical considerations would you need to consider (Reference Ethics Box 10.1, Behavior Analyst Certification Board, 2014)?

Ethics Box 10.1

Professional and Ethical Compliance Code for Behavior Analysts

1.04 Integrity.

(a) Behavior analysts are truthful and honest and arrange the environment to promote truthful and honest behavior in others.

(b) Behavior analysts do not implement contingencies that would cause others to engage in fraudulent, illegal, or unethical conduct.

(c) Behavior analysts follow through on obligations and contractual and professional commitments with high-quality work and refrain from making professional commitments they cannot keep.

(d) Behavior analysts' behavior conforms to the legal and ethical codes of the social and professional community of which they are members. (See also, 10.02a Timely Responding, Reporting, and Updating of Information Provided to the BACB).

(e) If behavior analysts' ethical responsibilities conflict with law or any policy of an organization with which they are affiliated, behavior analysts make known their commitment to this Code and take steps to resolve the conflict in a responsible manner in accordance with law.

Reflections

(Q8) When determining the least restrictive alternative available for Derek, what ethical dilemmas will his parents have to consider?

(Q9) How might Derek's parents address each ethical dilemma listed in Question#7?

(Q10) Looking at your own values and beliefs, aside from the ethics codes, what would be your instinct to do in this case if you were consulting?

Additional Web Links
Evidence-Based Guidelines to Reduce the Need for Least Restrictive Practices in the Disability Sector

https://www.psychology.org.au/Assets/Files/Restrictive-Practices-Guidelines-for-Psychologists.pdf

Balancing the right to habilitation with the right to personal liberties: the rights of people with developmental disabilities to eat too many doughnuts and take a nap.

http://www.ncbi.nlm.nih.gov/pmc/articles/PMC1286212/

CASE: v-R7

MALCOLM'S IN THE MIDDLE

Setting: Community   Age-Group: Adolescence

LEARNING OBJECTIVE:

* To identify and address violations of ethical standards.

RESPONSIBLE CONDUCT FOR BEHAVIOR ANALYSTS LINKS:

* Disclosures (2.08)
* Considerations Regarding Punishment Procedures (4.08)

- Least Restrictive Procedures (4.09)
- Providing Feedback to Supervisees (5.06)
- Being Familiar with This Code (10.06)
- Discouraging Misrepresentation by Noncertified Individuals. (10.07)

KEY TERMS:

- **Breach of Confidentiality**

  - In research, a breach of confidentiality occurs when a researcher shares information about a research subject without first obtaining that subject's free and informed consent. A breach of confidentiality can also occur when a third party (e.g., other researchers looking to replicate a study) attempts to gain access to research records (Tri-Council Policy Statement 2014).

- **Confidentiality**

  - In research, confidentiality refers to the obligation of an individual or organization to safeguard information, for example, protecting information from unauthorized access, use, or disclosure (TCPS-2, 2014). An important consideration within confidentiality is security, or the steps taken to protect information. This includes physical considerations such as locked filing cabinets, administrative policies such as organizational rules about who can access information, and technical safeguards such as computer passwords, firewalls, anti-virus software, and encryption (Tri-Council Policy Statement 2014).

- **Physically Restraining**

  - Restraint can be defined as "physically holding or securing the individual, either (a) for a brief period of time to interrupt and intervene with severe problem behavior or (b) for an extended period of time using mechanical devices to prevent otherwise uncontrollable problem behavior (e.g., self-injurious behavior) that has the potential to produce serious injury" (Vollmer et al. 2011, p. 104).

- **Protection of dignity**

  - A guiding principle of all research is respect for human dignity. This can include bodily, psychological, and cultural protections (Tri-Council Policy Statement 2014).

Malcolm's in the Middle

Malcolm not-too-gently put down the last recycling bin from cleaning after the summer's first weekend sports program, and stood up slowly, his hand automatically searching the pockets on his cargo shorts for his car keys. *Not there*, he mumbled to himself, exhausted by only 9:00 PM after a rousing, rowdy weekend playing recreational sports and games with a group of adolescents with develop-mental disabilities. *What was I thinking?* He further wondered, *thinking* ahead to the remaining seven weeks before college returned to session. *I had no idea that taking on this program leadership role would be quite so physically tiring. But I also had no idea that it would be quite so much fun.*

Giving up searching, he pulled open the heavy steel doors back to the inside of the recreation center and made his way back through the gym to the staff room, his footfalls echoing in the strangely quiet gym: a contrast to the rest of the weekend. Figuring that he left his keys either on the staff room table or his locker, he reached out to pull that door open next, pausing to smell the delicious wafts of pizza-scented air that he had just purchased for his staff, which only added to his positive mood. *They worked so hard this weekend*, he thought. *They sure deserve a treat.* But the laughter and conversation he overheard stopped him in his tracks, his hand frozen on the doorknob.

"No way!" crowed one voice. "You have got to be kidding! That is so hilarious. And she didn't notice it until when? How did you stop yourself from laughing?" Malcolm continued listening and quickly realized they were referring to a fifteen-year-old girl who had come to the program not only with her skirt tucked into the back of her underwear, but also with a nonstatic dryer sheet stuck to her clothing.

"This place is the best!" another voice emphasized. "I had no idea this was going to be so much fun." *Not exactly the kind of fun I was thinking about just now*, Malcolm grimaced, finally pushing his way back into the staffroom with great reservations.

His group of five staff jumped up guiltily from their seats, where they had been crowded around a laptop, its screen facing Malcolm. On the screen he could see a photograph of that very girl posted on a social media website, and the sentences accompanying it were certainly not flattering. Although he only had a brief glimpse before its owner quickly shut the cover, he knew enough to know that this situation was very, very wrong. Malcolm quickly moved from elation from a job well done to growing feeling of revulsion. *"What is going on here?"* He managed to eke out hoarsely.

An hour later, the true story of the weekend had emerged. *I guess I should have expected this from an inexperienced staff, but I thought these things were just basic common sense that anyone would know*, he reflected, while listening. And the stories just went from bad to worse. Phrases he had learned in his leadership and health and safety training came back to him—**confidentiality, breach of confidentiality, protection of dignity**—scrolling through his mind at a horrifyingly fast pace. At one point, an incident was explained where one of his staff members (the same one using social media to mock the camp attendee with the unfortunate wardrobe malfunction) referred to **physically restraining** one of the youth in a very off-hand manner. When Malcolm rather vehemently questioned him, the staff member shot back, "It wasn't a big deal. This one kid was pulling food of this other kid's lunch and tossing it into the garbage can, so I just held his arm behind his back for a second. That's all it took. It wasn't fair on the first kid. Plus, it wasn't like I had time to run around and ask permission for something like that. Anyhow, I know what these things are like—what happens at camp stays at camp, right?"

Malcolm, unsure what to do next, sat down heavily, his formerly elated mood now completely replaced with growing anxiety. His staff members quietly crept around the room packing up their belongings and heading out the door to home, one by one, with their former chatter and laughter noticeably absent. As they were leaving, he heard one of them call himself a behavior analyst, a BCaBA. He was sure that this student was still in university and hadn't graduated. *What now?* He thought, unable yet to speak again. He wasn't even sure what the BACB Professional and Ethical Compliance Code said about this. Feeling significantly uncomfortable, he wondered how he would get through the next seven weeks. *How do I balance the significant needs of these vulnerable kids with building understanding, skills, and ethical behavior in my staff?* The next seven weeks were now looming long in front of him, and his physical exhaustion was replaced with a feeling of great trepidation as he thought about what to do next.

The Response: Principles, Processes, Practices, and Reflections

Principles

(Q1) Look up possible sources for confidentiality legislation for your jurisdiction. What principles are you bound by for confidentiality and breaches of confidentiality? (Q2) For different professionals, limits to confidentiality exist (e.g., when to report harm to self or others to authorities), including for behavior analysts. For your jurisdiction and role, what are the limits to confidentiality and when it can or must be broken (Reference Ethics Box 10.2, Behavior Analyst Certification Board, 2014)?

Ethics Box 10.2

Professional and Ethical Compliance Code for Behavior Analysts

2.08 Disclosures.

- Behavior analysts never disclose confidential information without the consent of the client, except as mandated by law, or where permitted by law for a valid purpose, such as (1) to provide needed professional services to the client, (2) to obtain appropriate professional consultations, (3) to protect the client or others from harm, or (4) to obtain payment for services, in which instance disclosure is limited to the minimum that is necessary to achieve the purpose. Behavior analysts recognize that parameters of consent for disclosure should be acquired at the outset of any defined relationship and is an ongoing procedure throughout the duration of the professional relationship.

Processes

(Q3) What information or proof does Malcolm need to report to governing bodies or his recreation center regarding the behavior of the staff? (Q4) List all of the potential ethical concerns that Malcolm must address with the staff. Which concerns would you address first? Why?

Practices

(Q5) What situations in the scenario would require Malcolm to break confidentiality about what occurred? Who would Malcolm be likely to report to, in his circumstances?

(Q6) The *Professional and Ethical Compliance Code for Behavior Analysts* state that Malcolm is responsible to address ethical violations by colleagues as per guideline 7.02. Does the breeching of confidentiality that occurred supersede this principle of talking to colleagues? What would you do first (Reference Ethics Box 10.3, Behavior Analyst Certification Board, 2014)?

Ethics Box 10.3

Professional and Ethical Compliance Code for Behavior Analysts

7.02 Ethical Violations by Others and Risk of Harm.

(a) If behavior analysts believe there may be a legal or ethical violation, they first determine whether there is potential for harm, a possible legal violation, a mandatory-reporting condition, or an agency, organization, or regulatory requirement addressing the violation.

(b) If a client's legal rights are being violated, or if there is the potential for harm, behavior analysts must take the necessary action to protect the client, including, but not limited to, contacting relevant authorities, following organizational policies, and consulting with appropriate professionals, and documenting their efforts to address the matter.

(c) If an informal resolution appears appropriate, and would not violate any confidentiality rights, behavior analysts attempt to resolve the issue by bringing it to the attention of that individual and documenting their efforts to address the matter. If the matter is not resolved, behavior analysts report the matter to the appropriate authority (e.g., employer, supervisor, regulatory authority).

(d) If the matter meets the reporting requirements of the BACB, behavior analysts submit a formal complaint to the BACB. (See also, 10.02 Timely Responding, Reporting, and Updating of Information Provided to the BACB)

(Q7) The use of restraints has been very controversial and thus has to be implemented with caution and appropriate design. Design a procedure for the implementation of restraints that has multiple steps before restraint would be used and abides by guidelines (4.08) Considerations Regarding Punishments Procedures and (4.09) Least Restrictive Procedures (Reference Ethics Box 10.4, Behavior Analyst Certification Board, 2014).

http://www.dhs.vic.gov.au/__data/assets/pdf_file/0005/845348/Toolkit-section-4-Useful-assessment-tools-and-forms-0913.pdf (pp. 20–21).

Ethics Box 10.4

Professional and Ethical Compliance Code for Behavior Analysts

4.08 Considerations Regarding Punishment Procedures.

(a) Behavior analysts recommend reinforcement rather than punishment whenever possible.

(b) If punishment procedures are necessary, behavior analysts always include reinforcement procedures for alternative behavior in the behavior-change program.

(c) Before implementing punishment-based procedures, behavior analysts ensure that appropriate steps have been taken to implement reinforcement-based procedures unless the severity or dangerousness of the behavior necessitates immediate use of aversive procedures.

(d) Behavior analysts ensure that aversive procedures are accompanied by an increased level of training, supervision, and oversight. Behavior analysts must evaluate the effectiveness of aversive procedures in a timely manner and modify the behavior-change program if it is ineffective. Behavior analysts always include a plan to discontinue the use of aversive procedures when no longer needed.

4.09 Least Restrictive Procedures.

Behavior analysts review and appraise the restrictiveness of procedures and always recommend the least restrictive procedures likely to be effective.

Reflections

(Q8) What proactive strategies could Malcolm implement to prevent some of these situations from occurring in the future?

(Q9) Given the state of technology in workplaces today, what other ethical concerns could occur and may need to be addressed in these situations?

(Q10) How would you have reacted in the moment to the situation as a supervisor given the BACB's suggestions for feedback to supervisees? What do you do when a staff claimed they were a BCaBA, and you are quite sure they were not (Reference Ethics Box 10.5, Behavior Analyst Certification Board, 2014)?

Ethics Box 10.5

Professional and Ethical Compliance Code for Behavior Analysts

5.06 Providing Feedback to Supervisees.

(a) Behavior analysts design feedback and reinforcement systems in a way that improves supervisee's performance.

(b) Behavior analysts provide documented, timely feedback regarding the performance of a supervisee on an ongoing basis. (See also, 10.05 Compliance with BACB Supervision and Coursework Standards)

10.06 Being Familiar with This Code.

Behavior analysts have an obligation to be familiar with this Code, other applicable ethics codes, including, but not limited to, licensure requirements for ethical conduct, and their application to behavior analysts' work. Lack of awareness or misunderstanding of a conduct standard is not itself a defense to a charge of unethical conduct.

10.07 Discouraging Misrepresentation by Noncertified Individuals.

Behavior analysts report noncertified (and, if applicable, nonregistered) practitioners to the appropriate state licensing board and to the BACB if the practitioners are misrepresenting BACB certification or registration status.

Additional Web Links
Notice of Alleged Violation—BACB
http://bacb.com/notice/
Ethics in Social Media
https://appliedbehavioralstrategies.wordpress.com/2016/04/26/ethics-in-social-media-2/
To Report or Not to Report
https://appliedbehavioralstrategies.wordpress.com/2013/05/14/to-report-or-not-to-report/

CASE: v-R8

Skilled Practice or Practice Skills?
Setting: Clinic   Age-Group: Adult

LEARNING OBJECTIVE:

- To recognize the boundaries of competence and professional practice.

RESPONSIBLE CONDUCT FOR BEHAVIOR ANALYSTS LINKS:

- Boundaries of Competence (1.02)
- Maintaining Competence through Professional Development (1.03)
- Multiple Relationships and Conflicts of Interest (1.06)
- Accepting Clients (2.01)
- Referrals and Fees (2.14)
- Avoiding False or Deceptive Statements (8.1)
- Intellectual Property (8.02)
- Statement by Others (8.03)
- Media Presentations and Media-Based Services (8.04)
- Testimonials and Advertising (8.05)
- In-Person Solicitation (8.06)

KEY TERMS:

- **Autism Spectrum Disorder**

  - Autism Spectrum Disorder (ASD) is characterized by persistent deficits in social communication and social interaction, restricted and repetitive patterns of behavior, interests, or activities. These symptoms must be present in the early developmental period and result in clinically significant impairment in social, occupational, and/or other areas of functioning. These symptoms may or may not have accompanying intellectual and language impairments (APA 2013; Baio 2014).

- **Down syndrome**

  - Down syndrome is a genetic disorder caused when an individual has an extra copy of chromosome 21. Common physical characteristics include low muscle tone, small stature, and an upward slant to the eyes (NDSS 2015). Down syndrome is a developmental disability, meaning that an individual has deficits in intellectual and adaptive functioning that occur, or are noticed, during the developmental period (during childhood or adolescence). Approximately 1 in 691 babies in the USA are born with Down syndrome (NDSS 2015).

- **Private Practice**

  - The field of behavior analysis continues to grow. The number of practitioners receiving certification as BCBAs is steadily increasing, resulting in many practitioners establishing their own private practices (Dorsey et al. 2009). A private practice is when practitioners choose to be self-employed, open their own businesses to deliver services. In the context of ABA, this might involve an individual that has received their BCBA certification opening up their own business to deliver behavior-analytic services to children, youth, and/or adults.

- **Supervised Practice**

  - The purpose of supervised practice is to ensure the delivery of high-quality behavior-analytic services. This process typically involves a "supervisor" (often a BCBA or Board-Certified Behavior Analyst—Doctoral) observing and providing feedback to a "supervisee" (often a practitioner delivering behavior-analytic services) regarding the extent to which their practice meets standards (BACB 2014).

Skilled Practice or Practice Skills?

"Annnnnnd, enter!" Amelia crowed, stretching her arms and cracking her knuckles in victory, after sending her form off into cyberspace. She took a sip of ice water, followed it up with a hearty, "Ahhhh!" and got to her feet. She picked up the piece of paper her printer sent right onto her carpet, and reviewed it, smiling. She scanned the logo for her business application for her new **private practice** as a behavior consultant specializing in applied behavior analysis (ABA) and reread the business she had created: "Quality Behavioral Consulting." With pleasure, she inserted it into a large brown envelope along with her payment and other required information to have an official business account number. *That's it, then!* she thought, satisfied that this long process was finally coming to an end.

Amelia, a fairly new behavior analyst, had been working in the field of ABA supporting individuals with **Autism Spectrum Disorders** (ASD) for about the past five years, first as a student receiving **supervised practice**, and then as a certified professional. She had never worked for a hospital, school, or a large, state-funded program, but had been quite satisfied working under the guidance and supervision of a more experienced behavior analyst who had been running a fairly small enterprise in a small geographic area that did not require much driving within the work day. However, she found the drive at the beginning and at the end of the day a little tiring after these five years and thought about finding something a little closer to home. With her graduate degree in ABA now completed, and her certification as a Board-Certified Behavior Analyst in place, she thought perhaps she was ready to do things a little more on her own terms.

On one of her long trips home about a month ago, she had noticed a sign in the window of one of the community agencies in town that supported small, local business enterprises. She pulled over and took a photograph of the sign with her cell phone to read over later, but its title "Start Your Own Business: Grants Available" really got her *thinking* deeply about making a change. In the weeks since her revelation—both personal and professional—she started the process to do just that, start her own behavior therapy business, ending with the moment of sending that very special brown envelope by registered mail. Then came the more challenging and unexpectedly difficult task of writing a resignation letter to her supervisor, who had been responsible for the development of not only her professional skills, but her professional confidence and competence in providing ABA services for children with ASD and their families. At this point, she was very excited and very ready to take these next steps, but also a little nervous as she imagined her professional future stretching out far ahead of her.

She turned back to her computer and signed into her brand-new email address: amelia@qualitybehaviorconsulting.com. After all her preparations for this series of exciting moments, she was once again thrilled to see that she had new email, including a referral for her business. She was aware that her kind and understanding now former boss—but also a friend and colleague—would be sending her referrals for her home town if they came up, but she was not expecting it to happen so quickly. She quickly scanned the text of the email and read it again more carefully. *Hmmmmm*, she thought as she read it once again, *I am not sure about this.*

Dear Amelia, it read. *I have been given your name as a possibility for behavior consultation from a friend of mine who has a child with ASD. She says you have been doing a really good job. To give you a brief idea of our need here at home, I have a daughter who has **Down Syndrome**. She isn't diagnosed with ASD, though a few professionals have told me she is showing signs of this as well. She is a delightful six-year-old who is the joy of our lives. But she is also struggling with what her teacher calls "bad behavior" and we are seeing this at home, too. It has been getting pretty hard for us and we think that we need some help. We are wondering if you would meet with us and think about working with us.*

Well, she thought, tapping the keys of her computer as she considered this request. *Behavior is behavior and problem behavior is problem behavior. It doesn't matter if the child has ASD, Down Syndrome, or if the child has no diagnosis at all. Right? The skills I have learned and the experiences I have had will be effective across the board. And in any case, it's really important for me to get things started and to learn more along the way so that my business will be successful. So, it's a YES.* Her decision made, she clicked "reply" and started to compose her first professional email in her own business as her own boss, making her own decisions.

Ethics Box 10.6

> **Professional and Ethical Compliance Code for Behavior Analysts**
>
> 2.01 Accepting Clients.
> Behavior analysts accept as clients only those individuals or entities whose requested services are commensurate with the behavior analysts' education, training, experience, available resources, and organizational policies. In lieu of these conditions, behavior analysts must function under the supervision of or in consultation with a behavior analyst whose credentials permit performing such services.

The Response: Principles, Processes, Practices, and Reflections

Principles

(Q1) In many situations, the statement that ABA works for all behavior is somewhat true, as research has been published with its techniques for many different populations. What do you see, however, as the primary concern with Amelia taking on a client with Down syndrome (Reference Ethics Box 10.7, Behavior Analyst Certification Board, 2014)?

Ethics Box 10.7

Professional and Ethical Compliance Code for Behavior Analysts

1.02 Boundaries of Competence.

(a) All behavior analysts provide services, teach, and conduct research only within the boundaries of their competence, defined as being commensurate with their education, training, and supervised experience.

(b) Behavior analysts provide services, teach, or conduct research in new areas (e.g., populations, techniques, behaviors) only after first undertaking appropriate study, training, supervision, and/or consultation from persons who are competent in those areas.

(Q2) What research has been published in ABA that demonstrates its effectiveness for individuals with Down syndrome? Find and summarize one or two examples.

Processes

(Q3) List 10 differences that need to be addressed when working with the two different populations in this case study (between individuals with ASD and Down syndrome). Why is it important that Amelia be aware of these differences?

(Q4) Read the following article on cultural competence:

http://www.apa.org/gradpsych/2010/09/culturally-competent.aspx

How might this apply to Amelia's case?

Practices

(Q5) Before accepting the client, what could Amelia do to increase her competency in order to work with the client who has been referred?

(Q6) Indicate how the guideline (1.06) *Multiple Relationships and Conflicts of Interest* (Reference Ethics Box 10.8, Behavior Analyst Certification Board, 2014) may apply in this situation. Is there anything about which Amelia needs to be particularly conscientious?

Ethics Box 10.8

Professional and Ethical Compliance Code for Behavior Analysts

1.06 Multiple Relationships and Conflicts of Interest.

(a) Due to the potentially harmful effects of multiple relationships, behavior analysts avoid multiple relationships.

(b) Behavior analysts must always be sensitive to the potentially harmful effects of multiple relationships. If behavior analysts and that, due to unforeseen factors, a multiple relationship has arisen, they seek to resolve it.

(c) Behavior analysts recognize and inform clients and supervisees about the potential harmful effects of multiple relationships.

(d) Behavior analysts do not accept any gifts from or give any gifts to clients because this constitutes a multiple relationship.

(Q7) In her new business, we can imagine that in the future, Amelia receives many requests from families with children with Down syndrome. Design a retraining program that would ensure that Amelia is competent in delivering services to this population and indicate how would she maintain this (Reference Ethics Box 10.9, Behavior Analyst Certification Board, 2014).

Ethics Box 10.9

Professional and Ethical Compliance Code for Behavior Analysts

1.03 Maintaining Competence through Professional Development.
Behavior analysts maintain knowledge of current scientific and professional information in their areas of practice and undertake ongoing efforts to maintain competence in the skills they use by reading the appropriate literature, attending conferences and conventions, participating in workshops, obtaining additional coursework, and/or obtaining and maintaining appropriate professional credentials.

(Q8) Look at the following checklist (p. 63) to determine if Amelia is competent to practice in this area. What items from the list do you feel are the most critical for her to have obtained or continue to obtain going forward both with individuals with ASD and Down syndrome?
https://books.google.ca/books?id=dWiTAgAAQBAJ&pg=PA60&lpg=&dq=how+to+become+competent+applied+behavior+analysis&source=bl&ots=UOhhu2mY xT&sig=ZMyuruBL0e-2TYeS8ykF_w0mLgI&hl=en&sa=X&ved=0CFcQ6AEw CWoVChMI5t31j5SdyAIVxouSCh1pNAEj#v=onepage&q=how%20to%20beco me%20competent%20applied%20behavior%20analysis&f=false

Reflections

(Q9) What are other ethical concerns that are common mistakes that new behavior therapists starting their own business may face? What considerations should they take in terms of Public Statements (Guideline 8.0, Reference Ethics Box 10.10, Behavior Analyst Certification Board, 2014)?

Ethics Box 10.10

Professional and Ethical Compliance Code for Behavior Analysts

- 8.0 Public Statements.
  Behavior analysts comply with this Code in public statements relating to their professional services, products, or publications, or to the profession of behavior analysis. Public statements include, but are not limited to, paid or unpaid advertising, brochures, printed matter, directory listings, personal resumes or curriculum vitae, interviews or comments for use in media, statements in legal proceedings, lectures and public presentations, social media, and published materials.

8.01 Avoiding False or Deceptive Statements.

(a) Behavior analysts do not make public statements that are false, deceptive, misleading, exaggerated, or fraudulent, either because of what they state, convey, or suggest or because of what they omit, concerning their research, practice, or other work activities or those of persons or organizations with which they are affiliated. Behavior analysts claim as credentials for their behavior-analytic work, only degrees that were primarily or exclusively behavior analytic in content.

(b) Behavior analysts do not implement nonbehavior-analytic interventions. Nonbehavior-analytic services may only be provided within the context of nonbehavior-analytic education, formal training, and credentialing. Such services must be clearly distinguished from their behavior-analytic practices and BACB certification by using the following disclaimer: "These interventions are not behavior analytic in nature and are not covered by my BACB credential." e-disclaimer should be placed alongside the names and descriptions of all nonbehavior-analytic interventions.

(c) Behavior analysts do not advertise nonbehavior-analytic services as being behavior analytic.

(d) Behavior analysts do not identify nonbehavior-analytic services as behavior-analytic services on bills, invoices, or requests for reimbursement.

(e) Behavior analysts do not implement nonbehavior-analytic services under behavior-analytic service authorizations.

8.02 Intellectual Property.

(a) Behavior analysts obtain permission to use trademarked or copyrighted materials as required by law. This includes providing citations, including trademark or copyright symbols on materials that recognize the intellectual property of others.

(b) Behavior analysts give appropriate credit to authors when delivering lectures, workshops, or other presentations.

8.03 Statements by Others.

(a) Behavior analysts who engage others to create or place public statements that promote their professional practice, products, or activities retain professional responsibility for such statements.

(b) Behavior analysts make reasonable efforts to prevent others whom they do not oversee (e.g., employers, publishers, sponsors, organizational clients, and representatives of the print or broadcast media) from making deceptive statements concerning behavior analysts' practices or professional or scientific activities.

(c) If behavior analysts learn of deceptive statements about their work made by others, behavior analysts correct such statements.

(d) A paid advertisement relating to behavior analysts' activities must be identified as such, unless it is apparent from the context.

8.04 Media Presentations and Media-Based Services.

(a) Behavior analysts using electronic media (e.g., video, e-learning, social media, electronic transmission of information) obtain and maintain knowledge regarding the security and limitations of electronic media in order to adhere to this Code.

(b) Behavior analysts making public statements or delivering presentations using electronic media do not disclose personally identifiable information concerning their clients, supervisees, students, research participants, or other recipients of their services that they obtained during the course of their work, unless written consent has been obtained.

(c) Behavior analysts delivering presentations using electronic media disguise confidential information concerning participants, whenever possible, so that they are not individually identifiable to others and so that discussions do not cause harm to identifiable participants.

(d) When behavior analysts provide public statements, advice, or comments by means of public lectures, demonstrations, radio or television programs, electronic media, articles, mailed material, or other media, they take reasonable precautions to ensure that (1) the statements are based on appropriate behavior-analytic literature and practice, (2) the statements are otherwise consistent with this Code, and (3) the advice or comment does not create an agreement for service with the recipient.

8.05 Testimonials and Advertising.

Behavior analysts do not solicit or use testimonials about behavior-analytic services from current clients for publication on their Web pages or in any other electronic or print material. Testimonials from former clients must identify whether they were solicited or unsolicited, include an accurate statement of the relationship between the behavior analyst and the author of the testimonial, and comply with all applicable laws about claims made in the testimonial.

Behavior analysts may advertise by describing the kinds and types of evidence-based services they provide, the qualifications of their staff, and objective outcome data they have accrued or published, in accordance with applicable laws.

8.06 In-Person Solicitation.

Behavior analysts do not engage, directly or through agents, in uninvited in-person solicitation of business from actual or potential users of services who, because of their particular circumstances, are vulnerable to undue influence. Organizational behavior management or performance management services may be marketed to corporate entities regardless of their projected financial position.

(Q10) In wanting to thank her former boss for the referral, Amelia was thinking of sending him a gift card to a coffee shop that they used to go to together. Do you feel this would be appropriate (Reference Ethics Box 10.11, Behavior Analyst Certification Board, 2014)?

Ethics Box 10.11

> **Professional and Ethical Compliance Code for Behavior Analysts**
>
> 2.14 Referrals and Fees.
> Behavior analysts must not receive or provide money, gifts, or other enticements for any professional referrals. Referrals should include multiple options and be made based on objective determination of the client need and subsequent alignment with the repertoire of the referee. When providing or receiving a referral, the extent of any relationship between the two parties is disclosed to the client.

Additional Web Links
Standards of Practice for Behavior Analysts in Ontario
http://www.ontaba.org/pdf/Standards.pdf
The Case for Licensure of Applied Behavior Analysts
http://www.ncbi.nlm.nih.gov/pmc/articles/PMC2854065/

CASE: v-R9

What's Wrong with a Little Deception?
Setting: Community   Age-Group: Adult

LEARNING OBJECTIVE:

- To recognize conflicts of interest and the importance of disclosure of treatment objectives and interventions.

RESPONSIBLE CONDUCT FOR BEHAVIOR ANALYSTS LINKS:

- Multiple Relationships and Conflicts of Interest (1.06)
- Exploitative Relationships (1.07)
- Debriefing (9.05)
- Promoting and Ethical Culture (7.01)

KEY TERMS:

- **Organizational Behavior Management**

  - Organizational Behavior Management is a subdiscipline of applied behavior analysis. It utilizes the principles of ABA to produce behavior change among employee performance within organizations. Specific emphasis is placed on the identification and modification of environmental variables that might affect observable employee behavior (Williams and Grossett 2011).

- **Conflict of interest**

  - A conflict of interest can arise when an individual in a position of authority has competing professional or personal interests (Gast 2010).

What's Wrong with a Little Deception?

Dr. Ken Bedard, a BCBA-D and supervisor of workplace productivity at (of all things) a vinyl factory, was contemplating just that—workplace productivity—as he watched the factory floor through the observation window of the atrium just adjacent to the factory's large and complex maze of administrative offices. *Sometimes it feels like such an enigma*, he contemplated, *but other times, it seems like the interventions I try around here meet with easy success, just like behavioral science tells me it should. Never, in a million years, would I have believed that my behavior studies and my clinical background would lead me to this place*, he thought, still in awe of his surroundings. Below, he could see what an untrained eye would perceive as an efficient and effective organization of workers and products on the floor. He followed the flow of work, gazing from the raw materials—mostly heavy rolls and piles of multicolored vinyl—to the huge industrial sewing machines, to the packed boxes of gloves, covers for electronic equipment and BBQs, and varied pieces of sporting equipment, ready to ship out into retail outlets. Behind, he thought about the many administrators he had met, organizing, controlling, and leading all with all of the larger departments like finance, to the smaller niche subdivisions like multilingual packaging, and the hard-to-categorize sectors like the creative marketing folks, easy to spot in the hallways with their easy laughter, casual clothes, and their heightened sense of fun. Although he has training in **organizational behavior management**, *measuring their productivity has been a particular challenge*, he recalled from his last struggle at graphing productivity change from the first to second business quarter of this fiscal year. *Whenever I asked questions*, he remembered, *they answered with comments like, "It's a creative process," "It can't be pinned down," and "We need room to fly."* He wasn't even sure what this last one really meant.

The next morning at work found Ken reading a series of articles around—*what else?*—workplace productivity. As part of his regular morning search for literature in his field, he had logged into the behavior databases and found reference to a new series on schedules of reinforcement and workplace productivity in factory settings. Basically, they focused on how employees responded to these different schedules of reinforcement, providing a framework for easy implementation in other similar settings. *How did I miss this?* He wondered, carefully downloading and filing each article in this very exciting series that had been published about five years ago. *I am so going to suggest we do something like this.*

He sent the vice president of the company—his immediate supervisor—a quick text scheduling an afternoon meeting for the next day and settled back down to reading, scrolling, highlighting, and making notes.

During the meeting, Ken and the VP had no trouble making the mutual decision to target the creative folks with their new plan. To collect some baseline data of time on task and time off task as well as "output units" (the number of completed advertising projects), they decided to install the same software that was presented in the literature series that Ken had printed and brought into the meeting. "We can have our tech team install it for us," suggested the VP, making a note on his to-do list. "I mean, we are always installing new programs and doing upgrades on everyone's systems. Nobody will think anything of it, least of all these creative types."

"Super," responded Dr. Bedard, standing up from his seated position in the conference area near his boss's desk. "Then the data will come directly to me in a daily summary. Like I have shown you before, I will graph each of these variables daily, and when we see a stable plan, we can start to implement our first reinforcement condition."

"Right," said the VP. More impatiently now, he gestured for Ken to sit back down while checking the time on his cell phone. "But we need to decide now what that will be so we can move ahead right away, as soon as we are ready. After all, we can just do it. It's not like we need anyone else's permission to get it going. I really want to have some results for next month's staff meeting. After that dismal second quarter, they are going to really grab on to any good news about better productivity. And if this goes well, I should be able to increase your contract with us."

Sitting back down, Ken quickly contemplated both the potential **conflict of interest** he is now facing, as well as the options they had discussed, and followed up with, "Well, how about when the data are stable, we do your first idea: Giving each of the creativity team members who finish a large project a ticket for lottery draw to win a gift certificate for free monthly admission to the new arts center downtown. If we don't see any success with that, we can try something more immediate, like a smaller prize given right away for our small or large projects, rather than waiting for a draw. They talk a lot about art supplies. Maybe something like that?"

"Great," said the VP, standing himself this time, rapping his knuckles on the top of his briefcase and preparing to head off. "Obviously, you have got this, and you have my full support."

A little astounded at the easy success of his suggested initiative, Ken returned to his office to start putting plans in place. Feeling slightly hesitant, he recognized that even though he had support for this project, a little concern about deception was nagging at him, from coursework of years ago in research ethics. But my professors cannot have meant for something like this, Ken quieted those nagging concerns. This isn't real research; it's just for us. And besides, sometime a little bit of deception is necessary. After all, we all know that if someone knows they are being "watched," in any way, their behavior is going to be different that it would otherwise be, and all of our data would be meaningless."

The Response: Principles, Processes, Practices, and Reflections

Principles

(Q1) Describe when a research ethics board would need to be consulted and when it would not. Would this situation with Ken require ethics clearance to apply a system that employees were not aware of to measure productivity (Reference Ethics Box 10.12, Behavior Analyst Certification Board, 2014)?
(Q2) Describe Ken's conflict of interest.

Ethics Box 10.12

> **Professional and Ethical Compliance Code for Behavior Analysts**
>
> 1.06 Multiple Relationships and Conflicts of Interest.
> (a) Due to the potentially harmful effects of multiple relationships, behavior analysts avoid multiple relationships.
> (b) Behavior analysts must always be sensitive to the potentially harmful effects of multiple relationships. If behavior analysts and that, due to unforeseen factors, a multiple relationship has arisen, they seek to resolve it.
> (c) Behavior analysts recognize and inform clients and supervisees about the potential harmful effects of multiple relationships.
> (d) Behavior analysts do not accept any gifts from or give any gifts to clients because this constitutes a multiple relationship.

Processes

(Q3) What are the ethical dilemmas with having a productivity tracking device on each employee's computer without individual consent?

(Q4) What would be the benefits and downfalls of having individuals aware of the productivity tracking device on their computer?

Practices

(Q5) If Ken were to have his project cleared by a research ethics board, what safeguards would need to be in place for him to put productivity tracking software on employee's computers without their knowledge? What would need to occur after the intervention (Reference Ethics Box 10.13, Behavior Analyst Certification Board, 2014)?

Ethics Box 10.13

> **Professional and Ethical Compliance Code for Behavior Analysts**
>
> 9.05 Debriefing.
> Behavior analysts inform the participant that debriefing will occur at the conclusion of the participant's involvement in the research.

(Q6) Why did Ken want to wait until the productivity information was stable before implementing the reinforcement condition? What would be another research design Ken could have used?

(Q7) How are multiple relationships different than exploitive relationships? Do you think that this situation could potentially be called an exploitive relationship (Reference Ethics Box 10.14, Behavior Analyst Certification Board, 2014)?

Ethics Box 10.14

Professional and Ethical Compliance Code for Behavior Analysts

1.07 Exploitative Relationships.

(a) Behavior analysts do not exploit persons over whom they have supervisory, evaluative, or other authority such as students, supervisees, employees, research participants, and clients.

(b) Behavior analysts do not engage in sexual relationships with clients, students, or supervisees, because such relationships easily impair judgment or become exploitative.

(c) Behavior analysts refrain from any sexual relationships with clients, students, or supervisees, for at least two years a er the date the professional relationship has formally ended.

(d) Behavior analysts do not barter for services, unless a written agreement is in place for the barter that is (1) requested by the client or supervisee; (2) customary to the area where services are provided; and (3) fair and commensurate with the value of behavior-analytic services provided.

Reflections

(**Q8**) What would you have done differently in this situation if your boss approached you and asked you to complete this work on employees' computers without their knowledge? What safeguards would you have put in place to avoid some of the situations Ken has faced?

(**Q9**) Given the conflict of interest that Ken is embroiled in, what course of action do you think he should take?

(**Q10**) How does the role of deception affect the workplace (Reference Ethics Box 10.15, Behavior Analyst Certification Board, 2014)?

Ethics Box 10.15

Professional and Ethical Compliance Code for Behavior Analysts

7.01 Promoting and Ethical Culture.
Behavior analysts promote an ethical culture in their work environments and make others aware of this Code.

Additional Web Links
What is OBM?
http://www.obmnetwork.com/what_is_obm
Applying Behavioral Analysis in Organizations: Organizational Behavior Management
https://www.researchgate.net/publication/232529712_Applying_Behavior_Analysis_in_Organizations_Organizational_Behavior_Management
Research Ethics: Deception
http://psc.dss.ucdavis.edu/sommerb/sommerdemo/ethics/deception.htm

CASE: v-R10

Include or Exclude?
Setting: Community   **Age-Group: Senior**

LEARNING OBJECTIVE:

- To identify and address ethical considerations associated with program evaluation.

RESPONSIBLE CONDUCT FOR BEHAVIOR ANALYSTS LINKS:

- Behavior Analysts as Supervisors (5.0)
- Supervisory Competence (5.01)
- Supervisory Volume (5.02)
- Supervisory Delegation (5.03)
- Designing Effective Supervision and Training (5.04)
- Communication of Supervision Conditions (5.05)
- Providing Feedback to Supervisees (5.06)
- Evaluating the Effects of Supervision (5.07)
- Behavior Analysts' Ethical Responsibility to the Profession of Behavior Analysis (6.0)
- Affirming Principles (6.01)
- Disseminating Behavior Analysis (6.02)
- Accuracy and Use of Data (9.09)

KEY TERMS:

- **Multidisciplinary Program Evaluation Team**

  - A multidisciplinary program evaluation team is a group of professionals from differing disciplines (e.g., psychology, speech and language pathology, physical therapy, occupational therapy, nursing, medicine) who work together as a team to support the evaluation of a program (Moore et al. 2012).

- **Stakeholders**

  - Stakeholders are those individuals or groups that are affected by an organizations decisions, policies, and outcomes. Stakeholders may include an individual receiving intervention, his or her family, the staff delivering the intervention, and the organization delivering the intervention program (Needham et al. 2011).

Include or Exclude?

After many meetings, careful budgeting, and layers of approval, a local day program for seniors finally decided to "green light" a program evaluation. Although the intention of the evaluation was formally described and transcribed in the paperwork as leading to improved programming for clients of the program, the undercurrent of conversation—and the body language of the staff—clearly indicated that it would also lead to increased (or decreased) levels of funding from their supporting charitable agency. The BCBA acting supervisor of the program, budget now in hand, led the process of hiring an external consultant to complete the internal program evaluation, along with a **multidisciplinary program evaluation team** chaired by himself. *Since I am acting as a BCBA and an administrator, I will hire a person who is working towards their credentials as the consultant on this case to make it "worth their while."*

After a careful planning process and an even more carefully planned hiring process, a behavior consultant (Delores Vanderveen) was chosen as a best fit for examining patterns of individual behavior changes in the clients of the day program. She had also began her course work for the BACB requirements to become a BCBA, so could start to accrue her hours. Along with the program **stakeholders**, she began to formally develop evaluation plans for what she was informed was an "implementation evaluation," so she began her work with that term. She found that an implementation evaluation can be defined as one which is "needed if a new program is being implemented or if data indicate the goals of an existing program are not being met," and that it can also help elucidate inform about strengths, challenges, resources, quality, and more (Mertens and Wilson 2012, p. 275). Pretty excited with the prospects about digging deeply into her program evaluation literature once more, she continued to read and make notes throughout the day. Some of her points were from her literature review, including more than one dense textbook from the fields of program evaluation and behavior analysis, as well as her consultations with her multidisciplinary program evaluation team members (and the project chair) who appeared to be heavily invested in a successful evaluation, including these handwritten notes in her project journal:

- *I need to gather data on outcome measures. For example, I must combine some sort of pretest and posttest measure with observational behavioral data.*
- *I need to also spend time gathering output measures. So this could include descriptive data such as the number of clients served on average per month, the number of programs attended (e.g., arts-and-crafts classes).*
- *I need to not only collect these data, but also analyze it, and write up a formal report.*
- *Although I will take the lead on all of this, I need to work closely through each step with the involved agency, its team, the chair, and the important stakeholders.*
- *The final report will be written with all team members as collaborative coauthors, though, again, I will be taking the lead.*
- *Consensus is important and valued here!*

Fast-forwarding six months ahead that flew by like five minutes, Delores stood beside the conference table quite proudly. Carefully stapled copies of her report watermarked diagonally with "DRAFT" on every page were distributed and reviewed, and she put down the remote control for her slide presentation with a flourish. "Well, what do you think?" she asked, surprised by the wall of silence around her, the obvious glances between staff members, and the raised brows of more than one. The BCBA acting supervisor starred in awe as he realized that each week when he signed her papers, he had not really investigated her behavior approach. In working with as many students as he had at the time, he forgot to check over her methodology, as it was not necessarily going to be the best approach for this population, and in fact would not capture the effects of the intervention.

The chair of the program evaluation stood slowly and spoke tentatively. "Delores, first I think it's important to thank you for all the hard work you have put into this. I know that you have been very careful about meeting with everyone and communicating by email, as well, at every phase of this program evaluation. As you know, I have been off for the last few weeks on a long-planned vacation, so I am afraid that I have missed some essential information. I am sure everyone else has some input, but I would like to talk to you about some of the graphs that related to program participation. They really don't show very good results and, in fact, make our program look rather badly run or badly managed, or both. I feel like this is not the kind of information that we want to share with our stakeholders. It's really going to hurt our opportunities moving forward. Can't we just leave these off and focus on the positives?" Delores answers, "Sure, I am sure that should be no problem, as it was just the graphs, and I wasn't really sure how to do them!"

The BCBA acting supervisor stared in disbelief in the situation he found himself in—with multiple ethical dilemmas in his hands.

The Response: Principles, Processes, Practices, and Reflections

Principles

(Q1) List all of the ethical dilemmas that are at play in this scenario.

(Q2) In what manner would a pre-test and posttest group design measure inform a study of this nature? Is this traditional single-subject research design? Why or why not?

Processes

(Q3) When presenting research studies, not all data can always be included due to space restrictions. What are methods that researchers can use in order to be ethical while not presenting all of their research (Reference Ethics Box 10.16, Behavior Analyst Certification Board, 2014)?

Ethics Box 10.16

Professional and Ethical Compliance Code for Behavior Analysts

9.09 Accuracy and Use of Data.

(a) Behavior analysts do not fabricate data or falsify results in their publications. If behavior analysts discover errors in their published data, they take steps to correct such errors in a correction, retraction, erratum, or other appropriate publication means.

(b) Behavior analysts do not omit findings that might alter interpretations of their work.

(c) Behavior analysts do not publish, as original data, data that have been previously published. This does not preclude republishing data when they are accompanied by proper acknowledgment.

(d) After research results are published, behavior analysts do not withhold the data on which their conclusions are based from other competent professionals who seek to verify the substantive claims through reanalysis and who intend to use such data only for that purpose, provided that the confidentiality of the participants can be protected and unless legal rights concerning proprietary data preclude their release.

(Q4) The BACB supervisor finds himself in a scenario where his supervisee did not understand the methodology used and the single-subject research design. He also finds himself in a difficult situation, as he took too many students on and didn't supervise her as much as he should have. What are his next steps in correcting this (Reference Ethics Box 10.17, Behavior Analyst Certification Board, 2014)?

Ethics Box 10.17

Professional and Ethical Compliance Code for Behavior Analysts

5.0 Behavior Analysts as Supervisors.

When behavior analysts are functioning as supervisors, they must take full responsibility for all facets of this undertaking. (See also, 1.06 Multiple Relationships and Conflict of Interest, 1.07 Exploitative Relationships, 2.05 Rights and Prerogatives of Clients, 2.06 Maintaining Confidentiality, 2.15 Interrupting or Discontinuing Services, 8.04 Media Presentations and Media-Based Services, 9.02 Characteristics of Responsible Research, 10.05 Compliance with BACB Supervision and Coursework Standards.)

5.01 Supervisory Competence.

Behavior analysts supervise only within their areas of defined competence.

5.02 Supervisory Volume.

Behavior analysts take on only a volume of supervisory activity that is commensurate with their ability to be effective.

5.03 Supervisory Delegation.

(a) Behavior analysts delegate to their supervisees only those responsibilities that such persons can reasonably be expected to perform competently, ethically, and safely.

(b) If the supervisee does not have the skills necessary to perform competently, ethically, and safely, behavior analysts provide conditions for the acquisition of those skills.

5.04 Designing Effective Supervision and Training.

Behavior analysts ensure that supervision and trainings are behavior analytic in content, effectively and ethically designed, and meet the requirements for licensure, certification, or other defined goals.

5.05 Communication of Supervision Conditions.

Behavior analysts provide a clear written description of the purpose, requirements, evaluation criteria, conditions, and terms of supervision prior to the onset of the supervision.

5.06 Providing Feedback to Supervisees.

(a) Behavior analysts design feedback and reinforcement systems in a way that improves supervisee's performance.

(b) Behavior analysts provide documented, timely feedback regarding the performance of a supervisee on an ongoing basis. (See also, 10.05 Compliance with BACB Supervision and Coursework Standards)

5.07 Evaluating the Effects of Supervision.

Behavior analysts design systems for obtaining ongoing evaluation of their own supervision activities.

Practices

(Q5) Suppose Delores finds herself in an ethical dilemma with two conflicting ethical principles: protecting the confidentiality of the research participants but also potentially withholding data from her research results. In this situation, which ethical principle(s) would you follow and how would you proceed?

(Q6) As a result of the agency supervisors' actions, what is his responsibility to the profession of ABA (Reference Ethics Box 10.18, Behavior Analyst Certification Board, 2014)?

Ethics Box 10.18

Professional and Ethical Compliance Code for Behavior Analysts

6.0 Behavior Analysts' Ethical Responsibility to the Profession of Behavior Analysis.

Behavior analysts have an obligation to the science of behavior and profession of behavior analysis.

6.01 Affirming Principles.

(a) Above all other professional training, behavior analysts uphold and advance the values, ethics, and principles of the profession of behavior analysis.

(b) Behavior analysts have an obligation to participate in behavior-analytic professional and scientific organizations or activities.

6.02 Disseminating Behavior Analysis.

Behavior analysts promote behavior analysis by making information about it available to the public through presentations, discussions, and other media.

(Q7) How could Delores discuss some of the negative aspects of the program evaluation in a respective and constructive way?

Reflections

(Q9) How could the agency supervisor respond to her boss's question at the presentation, so to not embarrass him but inform him of the ethical and research guidelines?
(Q10) What safeguards and assistance would the ethics committees provide Delores in this situation?

Additional Web Links
Requirements for Supervisors of Experience for those Pursuing Certification
http://bacb.com/supervision-requirements/
Clinical Supervision and Professional Development of the Substance Abuse Counselor: Information You Need to Know
http://www.ncbi.nlm.nih.gov/books/NBK64848/

References

American Psychological Association. (2005). *Policy statement on evidence-based practice in psychology*. Retrieved from http://www.apa.org/practice/guidelines/evidence-based-statement.aspx

Baio, J. (2014). Prevalence of autism spectrum disorder among children aged 8 years. *Centre for Disease Control and Prevention Surveillance Summaries, 63*(2), 1–24.

Behavior Analyst Certification Board (2014). *Professional and ethical compliance code for behavior analysts*. Retrieved from http://bacb.com/wp-content/uploads/2016/01/160120-compliance-code-english.pdf

Tri-Council Policy Statement (TCPS): Ethical Conduct for Research Involving Humans, December 2014. Retrieved from http://www.pre.ethics.gc.ca/pdf/eng/tcps2-2014/TCPS_2_FINAL_Web.pdf

Dorsey, M., Weinberg, M., Zane, T., & Guidi, M. (2009). The case for licensure of applied behavior analysts. *Behavior Analysis in Practice, 2*(1), 53–58.

Gast, D. (2010). *Single subject research methodology in behavioral sciences*. New York: Routledge.

Mertens, D. M., & Wilson, A. T. (2012). *Program evaluation theory and practice: A comprehensive guide*. New York: Guilford Press.

Moore, A., Patterson, C., White, J., House, S., Riva, J., Nair, K., et al. (2012). Interprofessional and integrated care of the elderly in a family health team. *Canadian Family Physician, 58*(8), 436–441.

Needham, D., Davidson, J., Cohen, H., et al. (2011). Improving long-term care outcomes after discharge from intensive care unit: Report from a stakeholders conference. *Critical Care Medicine, 40*(2), 502–509.

Smith, T. (2013). What is evidence-based behavior analysis? *The Behavior Analyst, 36*(1), 7–33.

Vollmer, T., Hagopian, L., Bailey, J., Dorsey, M., Hanley, G., Lennox, D., et al. (2011). The Association for Behavior Analysis International position statement on restraint and seclusion. *The Behavior Analyst, 34*(1), 103–110.

Williams, D., & Grossett, D. (2011). Reduction of restraint of people with intellectual disabilities: An organizational behavior management (OBM) approach. *Research in Developmental Disabilities, 32*(6), 2336–2339.

Ethics Index

Case Study Reference to the Professional and Ethical Compliance Code

1.0	**Responsible Conduct of Behavior Analysts**	
1.01	Reliance on Scientific Knowledge	v-R2
1.02	Boundaries of Competence	ii-P6, v-R2, v-R8
1.03	Maintaining Competence Through Professional Development	v-R8
1.04	Integrity	i-A2, v-R6
1.05	Professional and Scientific Relationships	i-A3, ii-P6, v-R1
1.06	Multiple Relationships and Conflicts of Interest	v-R8, v-R9
1.07	Exploitative Relationships	v-R9
2.0	**Behavior Analysts' Responsibility to Clients**	i-A6
2.01	Accepting Clients	v-R8
2.02	Responsibility	i-A5
2.03	Consultation	i-A5, iii-I5
2.04	Third-Party Involvement in Services	i-A4, ii-P2, ii-P10, iv-E5
2.05	Rights and Prerogatives of Clients	v-R5
2.06	Maintaining Confidentiality	v-R2
2.07	Maintaining Records	v-R2
2.08	Disclosures	v-R7
2.09	Treatment/Intervention Efficacy	i-A2, i-A6 (twice), v-R5
2.10	Documenting Professional Work and Research	v-R2
2.11	Records and Data	iii-I2
2.12	Contracts, Fees, and Financial Arrangements	v-R2
2.13	Accuracy in Billing Reports	
2.14	Referrals and Fees	v-R8
2.15	Interrupting or Discontinuing Services	iv-E6

(continued)

(continued)

3.0	**Assessing Behavior**	
3.01	Behavior-Analytic Assessment	i-A6, iii-I4, v-R2
3.02	Medical Consultation	ii-P10, iv-E5
3.03	Behavior-Analytic Assessment Consent	iv-E1
3.04	Explaining Assessment Results	i-A5
3.05	Consent-Client Records	i-A5
4.0	**Behavior Analysts and the Behavior-Change Program**	
4.01	Conceptual Consistency	
4.02	Involving Clients in Planning and Consent	i-A6, iv-E7
4.03	Individualized Behavior-Change Programs	iii-I9, iv-E1, iv-E5
4.04	Approving Behavior-Change Programs	iv-E1, iv-E4
4.05	Describing Behavior-Change Program Objectives	v-R4
4.06	Describing Conditions for Behavior-Change Program Success	ii-P8, iv-E5, v-R4
4.07	Environmental Conditions that Interfere with Implementation	iii-I1, iv-E4, v-R2, v-R4, v-R6
4.08	Considerations Regarding Punishment Procedures	ii-p3, ii-p9, iii-I3, iii-I7, v-R7
4.09	Least Restrictive Procedures	iii-I3, v-R4, v-R7
4.10	Avoiding Harmful Reinforcers	iv-E10
4.11	Discontinuing Behavior-Change Programs and Behavior-Analytic Services	iv-E6
5.0	**Behavior Analysts as Supervisors**	v-R10
5.01	Supervisory Competence	v-R10
5.02	Supervisory Volume	v-R10
5.03	Supervisory Delegation	v-R10
5.04	Designing Effective Supervision and Training	v-R10
5.05	Communication of Supervision Conditions	v-R10
5.06	Providing Feedback to Supervisees	v-R7, v-R10
5.07	Evaluating the Effects of Supervision	v-R10
6.0	**Behavior Analysts' Ethical Responsibility to the Profession of Behavior Analysts**	v-R10
6.01	Affirming Principles	v-R10
6.02	Disseminating Behavior Analysis	v-R10
7.0	**Behavior Analysts' Ethical Responsibility to Colleagues**	
7.01	Promoting an Ethical Culture	v-R9
7.02	Ethical Violations by Others and Risk of Harm	v-R5, v-R7
8.0	**Public Statements**	v-R8
8.01	Avoiding False or Deceptive Statements	v-R8
8.02	Intellectual Property	v-R8
8.03	Statements by Others	v-R8

(continued)

(continued)

8.04	Media Presentations and Media-Based Services	v-R8
8.05	Testimonials and Advertising	v-R8
8.06	In-Person Solicitation	v-R8
9.0	**Behavior Analysts and Research**	
9.01	Conforming with Laws and Regulations	v-R1, v-R5
9.02	Characteristics of Responsible Research	v-R1, v-R2
9.03	Informed Consent	v-R1, v-R2
9.04	Using Confidential Information for Didactic or Instructive Purposes	v-R3
9.05	Debriefing	
9.06	Grant and Journal Reviews	v-R3
9.07	Plagiarism	v-R3
9.08	Acknowledging Contributions	v-R1
9.09	Accuracy and Use of Data	v-R10
10.0	**Behavior Analysts' Ethical Responsibility to the BACB**	
10.01	Truthful and Accurate Information Provided to the BACB	
10.02	Timely Responding, Reporting, and Updating Information Provided to the BACB	v-R2
10.03	Confidentiality and the BACB Intellectual Property	
10.04	Examination Honestly and Irregularities	
10.05	Compliance with the BACB Supervision and Casework Standards	
10.06	Being Familiar with This Code	v-R7
10.07	Discouraging Misrepresentation by Non-Certified Individuals	v-R7

Behavior Analyst Certification Board. (2014). Professional and ethical compliance code for behavior analysts. Retrieved from http://bacb.com/wp-content/uploads/2016/03/160321-compliance-code-english.pdf

BACB 4th Edition Task List Index

Case Study Reference to the BACB 4th Edition Task List

Task List	Definition	Case Study
A-01	Measure frequency (i.e., count).	i-A2, i-A7, iii-I1, iii-I2, iii-I3, iii-I6, iii-I8
A-02	Measure rate (i.e., count per unit time).	i-A2, iii-I8
A-03	Measure duration.	i-A7, iii-I1, iii-I3, iii-I8
A-04	Measure latency.	i-A2, iii-I8
A-05	Measure interresponse time (IRT).	i-A2, i-A7
A-06	Measure percent of occurrence.	i-A6, iii-I6, iv-E1, iv-E10
A-07	Measure trials to criterion.	iii-I6
A-08	Assess and interpret interobserver agreement.	iii-I6
A-09	Evaluate the accuracy and reliability of measurement procedures.	iii-I6, iii-I8, iv-E3, iv-E8, iv-E10
A-10	Design, plot, and interpret data using equal-interval graphs.	i-A6, iii-I6
A-11	Design, plot, and interpret data using a cumulative record to display data.	iv-E6
A-12	Design and implement continuous measurement procedures (e.g., event recording).	i-A2, ii-P2, iii-I1, iii-I6, iii-I8
A-13	Design and implement discontinuous measurement procedures (e.g., partial & whole interval, momentary time sampling).	ii-P6, iii-I4, iii-I8
A-14	Design and implement choice measures.	i-A7, ii-P4, iii-I9, iv-E10
B-01	Use the dimensions of applied behavior analysis (Baer, Wolf, & Risley, 1968) to evaluate whether interventions are behavior analytic in nature.	i-A3, ii-P1, iv-E2, iv-E10

(continued)

© Springer International Publishing AG 2016
K. Maich et al., *Applied Behavior Analysis*,
DOI 10.1007/978-3-319-44794-0

(continued)

B-02	Review and interpret articles from the behavior-analytic literature.	i-A9, iii-I3, iv-E1, iv-E3, iv-E7, iv-E9
B-03	Systematically arrange independent variables to demonstrate their effects on dependent variables.	iii-I10, iv-E1, iv-E2, iv-E4, iv-E7, iv-E8
B-04	Use withdrawal/reversal designs.	iii-I10, iv-E4
B-05	Use alternating treatments (i.e., multielement) designs.	iv-E4
B-06	Use changing criterion designs.	iii-I4, iv-E4
B-07	Use multiple baseline designs.	iv-E4
B-08	Use multiple probe designs.	iv-E5
B-09	Use combinations of design elements.	iv-E5
B-10	Conduct a component analysis to determine the effective components of an intervention package.	i-A9, iv-E5
B-11	Conduct a parametric analysis to determine the effective values of an independent variable.	iv-E7
C-01	State and plan for the possible unwanted effects of reinforcement.	ii-P2, ii-P7
C-02	State and plan for the possible unwanted effects of punishment.	i-A8, ii-P2, iii-I7
C-03	State and plan for the possible unwanted effects of extinction.	i-A8, ii-P2, ii-P4, iii-I4
D-01	Use positive and negative reinforcement.	i-A9, ii-P4, iii-I3, iii-I4
D-02	Use appropriate parameters and schedules of reinforcement.	i-A6, i-A9, i-A10, iii-I3, iii-I4, iii-I6
D-03	Use prompts and prompt fading.	i-A10, iii-I1, iii-I4, iii-I8, iv-E1
D-04	Use modeling and imitation training.	iii-I, iii-I5
D-05	Use shaping.	iii-I3, iii-I5
D-06	Use chaining.	iii-I5
D-07	Conduct task analyses.	i-A10, iii-I3, iii-I8
D-08	Use discrete-trial and free-operant arrangements.	iii-I1, iv-E1
D-09	Use the verbal operants as a basis for language assessment.	iii-I1, iii-I5, iii-I10, iv-E1
D-10	Use echoic training.	
D-11	Use mand training.	i-A5
D-12	Use tact training.	
D-13	Use intraverbal training.	i-A5, iii-I5
D-14	Use listener training.	iii-I1, iii-I9, iii-I10, iv-E1
D-15	Identify punishers.	i-A2, i-A5, ii-P8, iii-I7
D-16	Use positive and negative punishment.	ii-P3, iii-I7

(continued)

(continued)

D-17	Use appropriate parameters and schedules of punishment.	ii-P3, iii-I7
D-18	Use extinction.	i-A8, iii-I4, iii-I7
D-19	Use combinations of reinforcement with punishment and extinction.	ii-P8, ii-P9, iii-I7
D-20	Use response-independent (time-based) schedules of reinforcement (i.e., noncontingent reinforcement).	iii-I8, iii-I9
D-21	Use differential reinforcement (e.g., DRO, DRA, DRI, DRL, DRH).	iii-I3, iii-I4, iii-I5, iii-I6, iii-I10, iv-E3, iv-E10
E-01	Use interventions based on manipulation of antecedents, such as motivating operations and discriminative stimuli.	iii-I9
E-02	Use discrimination training procedures.	iii-I9, iii-I10
E-03	Use instructions and rules.	i-A10, iii-I5
E-04	Use contingency contracting (i.e., behavioral contracts).	i-A5
E-05	Use independent, interdependent, and dependent group contingencies.	
E-06	Use stimulus equivalence procedures.	iii-I10
E-07	Plan for behavioral contrast effects.	i-A10, iii-I9
E-08	Use the matching law and recognize factors influencing choice.	i-A7, i-A10
E-09	Arrange high-probability request sequences.	i-A7, i-A10, ii-P4, iii-I8
E-10	Use the Premack principle.	i-A10, ii-P4, iii-I8
E-11	Use pairing procedures to establish new conditioned reinforcers and punishers.	i-A7, i-A10
E-12	Use errorless learning procedures.	iii-I2
E-13	Use matching-to-sample procedures.	
F-01	Use self-management strategies.	i-A10, ii-P4, ii-P8, iii-I8, iv-E3
F-02	Use token economies and other conditioned reinforcement systems.	iii-I4, iv-E7
F-03	Use Direct Instruction.	iii-I4
F-04	Use precision teaching.	iv-E9
F-05	Use personalized systems of instruction (PSI).	
F-06	Use incidental teaching.	ii-P7, iv-E6
F-07	Use functional communication training.	i-A2, ii-P4, iii-I10
F-08	Use augmentative communication systems.	ii-P4, iii-I10
G-01	Review records and available data at the outset of the case.	i-A1, i-A3, i-A5, ii-P1, ii-P2, ii-P7, ii-P8, ii-P9, ii-P10

(continued)

(continued)

G-02	Consider biological/medical variables that may be affecting the client.	i-A1, i-A3, ii-P1, ii-P10, iv-E5, iv-E10
G-03	Conduct a preliminary assessment of the client in order to identify the referral problem.	i-A1, i-A2, i-A4, ii-P1, ii-P2, ii-P3, ii-P7, ii-P8, ii-P9, ii-P10, iii-I5
G-04	Explain behavioral concepts using nontechnical language.	i-A2, i-A3, ii-P1, ii-P2, ii-P6, iii-I2, iii-I5
G-05	Describe and explain behavior, including private events, in behavior-analytic (nonmentalistic) terms.	i-A3, ii-P1, ii-P2, ii-P6
G-06	Provide behavior-analytic services in collaboration with others who support and/or provide services to one's clients.	i-A2, i-A3, i-A4, ii-P1, ii-P2, ii-P3, ii-P6, ii-P7, ii-P8, ii-P9, ii-P10, iii-I2, iii-I5, iv-E2, iv-E5
G-07	Practice within one's limits of professional competence in applied behavior analysis, and obtain consultation, supervision, and training, or make referrals as necessary.	ii-P1, ii-P6, ii-P10
G-08	Identify and make environmental changes that reduce the need for behavior analysis services.	i-A4, ii-P1, ii-P8, ii-P10
H-01	Select a measurement system to obtain representative data given the dimensions of the behavior and the logistics of observing and recording.	i-A2, i-A4, i-A5, i-A7, ii-P2, ii-P6, ii-P7, ii-P8, ii-P10, iii-I2, iii-I4, iv-E7, iv-E10
H-02	Select a schedule of observation and recording periods.	i-A2, i-A5, i-A7, ii-P2, ii-P6, ii-P7, ii-P10, iii-I2, iii-I4
H-03	Select a data display that effectively communicates relevant quantitative relations.	i-A2, ii-P6, ii-P7, ii-P10, iii-I2, iii-I4, iii-I5, iii-I6, iv-E7
H-04	Evaluate changes in level, trend, and variability.	i-A6, ii-P10, iii-I2, iii-I4, iii-I5, iii-I6, iv-E1
H-05	Evaluate temporal relations between observed variables (within & between sessions, time series).	ii-P6, iii-I2, iii-I5, iii-I10, iv-E1
I-01	Define behavior in observable and measurable terms.	i-A1, i-A2, i-A8, ii-P6, iii-I4
I-02	Define environmental variables in observable and measurable terms.	i-A1, i-A6, ii-P6
I-03	Design and implement individualized behavioral assessment procedures.	i-A1, i-A2, i-A6, i-A8, ii-P4, ii-P6, iv-E10
I-04	Design and implement the full range of functional assessment procedures.	i-A3, i-A9, ii-P4, iii-I1, iii-I10
I-05	Organize, analyze, and interpret observed data.	i-A6, i-A8, iii-I1, iv-E10

(continued)

(continued)

I-06	Make recommendations regarding behaviors that must be established, maintained, increased, or decreased.	i-A4, ii-P2, ii-P3, ii-P4, iii-I1, iv-E10
I-07	Design and conduct preference assessments to identify putative reinforcers.	ii-P2, ii-P9, iii-I8
J-01	State intervention goals in observable and measurable terms.	iii-I1, iii-I6
J-02	Identify potential interventions based on assessment results and the best available scientific evidence.	ii-P5, iii-I1, iii-I5, iii-I6
J-03	Select intervention strategies based on task analysis.	i-A10
J-04	Select intervention strategies based on client preferences.	ii-P5, iii-I6
J-05	Select intervention strategies based on the client's current repertoires.	ii-P5, iii-I10
J-06	Select intervention strategies based on supporting environments.	ii-P5, iii-I9
J-07	Select intervention strategies based on environmental and resource constraints.	ii-P1, ii-P5, iii-I9
J-08	Select intervention strategies based on the social validity of the intervention.	ii-P5, iii-I9, iii-I10
J-09	Identify and address practical and ethical considerations when using experimental designs to demonstrate treatment effectiveness.	iv-E2, iv-E3
J-10	When a behavior is to be decreased, select an acceptable alternative behavior to be established or increased.	iii-I6, iii-I10
J-11	Program for stimulus and response generalization.	iii-I5, iii-I10, iv-E5
J-12	Program for maintenance.	ii-P5, iii-I10
J-13	Select behavioral cusps as goals for intervention when appropriate.	iii-I10, iv-E10
J-14	Arrange instructional procedures to promote generative learning (i.e., derived relations).	ii-P7, iii-I1, iii-I5
J-15	Base decision-making on data displayed in various formats.	iii-I10
K-01	Provide for ongoing documentation of behavioral services.	iii-I9
K-02	Identify the contingencies governing the behavior of those responsible for carrying out behavior-change procedures and design interventions accordingly.	i-A8, ii-P2, iii-I9, iv-E2, iv-E6

(continued)

(continued)

K-03	Design and use competency-based training for persons who are responsible for carrying out behavioral assessment and behavior-change procedures.	i-A8, ii-P2, iii-I6, iii-I7, iv-E3
K-04	Design and use effective performance monitoring and reinforcement systems.	ii-P2, iii-I6
K-05	Design and use systems for monitoring procedural integrity.	i-A8, ii-P2, iii-I6, iii-I7, iii-I9
K-06	Provide supervision for behavior-change agents.	i-A8, ii-P2, iii-I6, iii-I7, iii-I9, iv-E2, iv-E6, iv-E7
K-07	Evaluate the effectiveness of the behavioral program.	iii-I6, iii-I7, iv-E6, iv-E7, iv-E8
K-08	Establish support for behavior-analytic services from direct and indirect consumers.	
K-09	Secure the support of others to maintain the client's behavioral repertoires in their natural environments.	ii-P2, iii-I9, iv-E2
K-10	Arrange for the orderly termination of services when they are no longer required.	iv-E6, iv-E10

Behavior Analyst Certification Board. (2012). Fourth edition task list. Retrieved from http://bacb. com/wpcontent/uploads/2016/03/160101-BCBA-BCaBA-task-list-fourth-edition-english.pdf

Copyright Acknowledgements

Chapter 1

Bicard, S. C., Bicard, D. F., & the IRIS Center (2012). *Measuring behavior.* Retrieved on from: http://iris.peabody.vanderbilt.edu/wp-content/uploads/pdf_case_ studies/ics_measbeh.pdf. Used with Permission of Vanderbilt Peabody College, Claremont Graduate University.

Chapter 3

Doher, P. (n.d.). *Three term contingency.* Retrieved from: http://abaapplied behavioranalysis.weebly.com/three-term-contingency.html. Used with permission of the author.

Chapter 4

Gulick, R. F., & Kitchen, T. P. (2007). *Effective instruction for children with autism: An applied behavior analytic approach.* The Dr. Gertrude A. Barber National Institute: Erie, PA. Used by permission of the publisher.

Chapter 5

Davis, A. (n.d.). *4 Functions of Behaviour.* Retrieved from: http://in1.ccio.co/sB/ w2/OC/c0c8d6261e5bcbe325bc445c85518241.jpg. Used by permission of Geneva Centre for Autism.

Chapter 6

Maryland State Department of Education. (n.d.). *Discipline of Students with Disabilities.* Retrieved from: http://www.marylandpublicschools.org/NR/rdonlyres/5F4F5041-02EE-4F3A-B495-5E4B3C850D3E/22801/DisciplineofStudentswithDisabilities_ September2009.pdf. Used by permission of the author.

Pyramid Educational Consultants. (2012). *PECS Phases.* Retrieved from: http://1. bp.blogspot.com/-M5TuLSDMlm8/UeW2mXgKIkI/AAAAAAAADPY/WYJ_ nYQQmGo/s1600/Poster+layout-PECS+Phases+copy.jpg. Used by permission of the author.

Chapter 7
Sundberg, M. L. (2008).*Verbal Behavior Milestones Assessment and Placement Program (VB-MAPP)*. Concord, CA: AVB Press. Used by permission of the publisher.

Chapter 8
Sundberg, M. (n.d.). *Self-care Checklist*. Retrieved from: http://www.avbpress.com/updates-and-downloads.html. Used by permission of AVB Press.

Index

Note: Page numbers followed by b, f, and t refer to boxes, figures, and tables, respectively

A
AB design, 238–240, 244
ABLLS-R, 47
Acceptance and commitment therapy, 46, 49
Accuracy of data, 364–365b
Accuracy of measurement, 59f
Adolescence
  behavior assessment, 46–76
  case studies
    evaluation-centered, 267–284, 294–306
    implementation-based, 192–204
    planning-focused, 119–151
  research and ethics, 343–353
Adulthood
  behavior assessment, 77–82
  case studies
    evaluation-centered, 267–305
    implementation-based, 204–225
    planning-focused, 126–151
  research and ethics, 343–365
Advertising, 360d
Advocacy, 331
Affirming principles, 370b
Alternating treatment design, 252, 254, 256t
Antecedent-behavior-consequence
  (ABC) chart, 7, 12–14, 16t, 158, 161
  data documentation chart, 109t
  for direct observational data, 32t
  sample observation form, 8t
Antecedent behavior consequence template, 74t
Antecedent stimulus, 211, 213
Applied Behavior Analysis (ABA)
  adolescence, 46–76
  adulthood, 76–81
  preschool children, 4–26, 158–169, 175–187
  school-age children, 26–41, 169–176
Assessment

adolescence, 46–76
adulthood, 76–81
preschool children, 4–26
results, explaining, 40b
school-age children, 26–41
Attention deficit/hyperactivity disorder
  (AD/HD), 61, 62–63
Augmentative and alternate communication
  (AAC) system, 90t
Autism spectrum disorder (ASD), 121, 313, 354, 355
Avoidance contingency, 67, 70

B
Baseline phase, 228, 229
Behavior, 93, 94
  analysis, disseminating, 366b
  consequences to, 135t
  consultation, 4, 7
  data, 236
  function questionnaire, 296f
  functions of, 21, 31, 160f
  intervention plan, 74f
  measurement procedures, 60f
  objective into teaching steps, breaking, 233f
  reduction tactics, 189
Behavior analysts
  as supervisors, 365b
  ethical responsibility to profession, 366b
  professional and ethical compliance code
    for (*see* Behavior analysts, professional and ethical compliance code for)
  responsibility to clients, 53b
Behavior analysts, professional and ethical compliance code for
  accepting clients, 352b
  accuracy and use of data, 364–365b
  advertising, 356b
  affirming principles, 366b

Behavior analysts, professional and ethical
    compliance code for (*cont.*)
  assessment results, explaining, 40*b*
  behavior-analytic assessment, 54*b*, 179*b*,
      321*b*
    consent, 234*b*
  behavior-analytic services, discontinuing,
      272*b*
  behavior-change programs (*see*
      Behavior-change programs)
  competence, boundaries of, 125*b*, 320*b*,
      353*b*
  confidential information for didactic or
      instructive purposes, using, 325–326*b*
  conforming with laws and regulations,
      312*b*, 337*b*
  consent-client records, 40*b*
  consultation, 40*b*, 186*b*
  contracts, fees, and financial arrangements,
      319*b*
  contributions, acknowledging, 313*b*
  debriefing, 360*b*
  designing effective supervision and
      training, 365–366*b*
  disclosures, 346*b*
  disseminating behavior analysis, 366*b*
  environmental conditions, implementation
      of, 160*b*, 253*b*, 332*b*
  ethical violations by others and risk of
      harm, 337*b*, 347*b*
  exploitative relationships, 361*b*
  false or deceptive statements, avoiding,
      355*b*
  feedback to supervisees, providing,
      348–349*b*, 366*b*
  grant and journal reviews, 330*b*
  harmful reinforcers, avoiding, 297*b*
  informed consent, 315*b*, 326*b*, 332*b*
  in-person solicitation, 360*b*
  integrity, 18*b*, 346, 347*b*
  intellectual property, 359*b*
  interrupting or discontinuing services, 274*b*
  involving clients in planning and consent,
      54*b*, 237*b*, 283*b*
  least restrictive procedures, 173*b*, 335*b*,
      346, 352*b*
  maintaining
    competence through professional
        development, 358*b*
    confidentiality, 324*b*
  media presentations and media-based
      services, 359, 364*b*

  medical consultation, 150*b*, 264*b*
  misrepresentation by noncertified
      individuals, discouraging, 353*b*
  multiple relationships and conflicts of
      interest, 357*b*, 360*b*
  plagiarism, 330*b*
  professional and scientific relationships,
      25*b*, 125*b*, 315*b*
  promoting and ethical culture, 365*b*
  public statements, 358*b*
  punishment procedures, 104*b*, 144*b*, 173*b*,
      203*b*, 352*b*
  records and data, 169*b*
  referrals and fees, 361*b*
  reliance on scientific knowledge, 323, 324*b*
  responsibility, 41*b*
  responsible research, characteristics of, 316,
      318*b*
  right to effective behavioral treatment, 364*b*
  rights and prerogatives of clients, 340*b*
  statements by others, 359*b*
  supervision effects, evaluation of, 370*b*
  supervisory delegation, 369*b*
  supervisory volume, 369*b*
  testimonials, 360*b*
  third-party involvement in services, 34*b*,
      95–96*b*, 150*b*, 262, 263*b*
  treatment/intervention efficacy, 18*b*,
      53–54*b*, 339, 340*b*
Behavior-analytic assessment, 54*b*, 180*b*, 325*b*
    consent, 237*b*
Behavior-analytic services, discontinuing, 275*b*
Behavior assessment
  adolescence, 46–76
  adulthood, 76–81
  methods, 80*f*
  preschool children, 4–26
  school-age children, 26–41
Behavior-change programs, 162*b*, 164, 172,
      173*b*, 178, 180*b*, 236*b*
  approving, 236*b*, 256*b*
  discontinuing, 274*b*
  individualized, 215*b*, 264*b*
  objectives, describing, 335*b*
  success, conditions for, 139*b*, 265*b*, 339*b*
Behavioral dimensions, 41*f*
  recording systems, 139*f*
Behavioral interview, 4–5, 7
Behaviorism, 99, 101
Best practices, 85
Biological factors, 146, 151
Bio-psycho-social model, 132, 134

Board Certified Behavior Analyst (BCBA),
    112–114, 121, 142–144
Breach of confidentiality, 348, 349

C

Capacity, 332
Caregivers, 155
Chaining, 181–182, 184
Changing criterion design, 250, 252, 254*t*, 256*f*
Choice board, 105, 107, 108*f*, 109*t*
Classroom management, 26–27, 29, 31*f*
Clients
    accepting, 352*b*
    behavior analysts' responsibility to, 53*b*
    involving, in planning and consent, 54*b*,
        234*b*, 281*b*
    rights and prerogatives of, 336*b*
Cognitive impairments, 189, 328, 339
Communication, functional, 12, 14
Comorbid diagnosis. *See* Dual diagnosis
Competence
    boundaries of, 125*b*, 320*b*, 353*b*
    professional, 308, 309
    through professional development,
        maintaining, 354*b*
Component analysis, 274, 276
Comprehensive treatment models (CTMs). *See*
    Intervention package
Confidential information for didactic or
    instructive purposes, using, 325–326*b*
Confidentiality, 344, 345
    maintaining, 320*b*
Conflict resolution, 185*t*
Conflicts of interest, 328, 353*b*, 357, 359
Conforming with laws and regulations, 312*b*,
    337*b*
Consent-client records, 40*b*
Consequence, 99, 101
Construct validity, 289*t*
Consultation, 40*b*, 186*b*
    behavior, 4, 7
    medical, 149*b*, 262*b*
Contingency
    avoidance, 67, 70
    escape, 68, 70
    three-term, 102*f*
Contracts, 319*b*
Contributions, acknowledging, 313*b*
Conversation skills, 185*t*
Cooperative play, 171*t*
Core vocabulary approach to teaching
    language, 90*t*
Culture, 140, 143

    ethical, 361*b*
Cumulative record, 266, 268, 270*f*, 271*f*

D

Data-based decision-making, 157
Data path, 176
Data quality, 234*f*
Debriefing, 364*b*
Deficits, 127, 128
Dependent variable, 245, 247
Developmental disabilities, 218, 332, 354
Developmental pediatrician, 86, 88
Developmentally appropriate, 5, 6
Differential reinforcement, 170–171, 172
    of Alternate Behavior (DRA), 103*f*, 195,
        197, 297
    of Incompatible Behavior (DRI), 103*f*, 195,
        197
    of Low Rates of Responding (DRL), 103*f*,
        197
    of Other Behavior (DRO), 103*f*, 178, 179,
        181, 193, 195–197, 289
Differentiated instruction, 36, 38
Direct assessment of individuals, 30*t*
Direct measurement of behavior, 294, 295
Direct replication, 288, 290
Disclosures, 350*b*
Discrimination training, 217, 219
Discriminative stimulus (SD), 211, 213
Disseminating behavior analysis, 370*b*
Down syndrome, 354, 356
Dual diagnosis, 132
Duration, 159, 161

E

Effectiveness of behavioral interventions, 268,
    269, 290*t*
Efficacy of behavioral interventions, 268, 269,
    290*t*
Embracing scientific method, 319, 321
Empiricism, 164
Employment, 141, 143
Engagement, 281, 297
Environment, 120, 122
Environment–behavior relationship, 45
Environmental conditions, implementation of,
    162*b*, 255*b*, 335*b*
Equal-interval graphs, 46, 49
Escape contingency, 68, 70
Establishing operation, 68, 70
Ethical consideration, 327–331
Ethical culture, 365*b*
Ethical guidelines, 191

Ethical review, 337
Ethical violations by others, 341b, 351b
Ethics, 319
Evaluation-centered case studies
    adolescence, 267–283, 293–306
    adulthood, 267–306
    preschool children, 229–265
    school-age children, 229–265
Event recording, 55, 58
    devices and created strategies for, 60t
Evidence-based practice, 344, 346
Experiential factors, 62, 63, 67, 70
Experimental Analysis of Behavior (EAB), 99, 101
Experimental designs, 238, 240, 245, 252, 254, 268, 276, 278
Exploitative relationships, 365b
External validity, 288, 290, 291t
Extinction, 62, 63, 65f

F
False or deceptive statements, avoiding, 359b
Family conference, 147, 148
Feedback to supervisees, providing, 352–353b, 370b
Fees, 323b, 361b
Financial arrangements, 323b
First/then board, 105, 107
Focused intervention packages, 241f
Free consent, 332
Frequency, 159, 161
Friendship skills, 186t
Full inclusion, 36, 38
Function-based definition of behavior, 159
Functional assessment, 161
    interview, 116f
    procedures, 75f
    summary statement/hypothesis, 209t
Functional behavior assessment
    conditions for, 76f
    correlation versus causation within, 279f
Functional communication, 12, 14
    phases of, 223f
Functional communication training (FCT), 217, 219, 221f
Functional perspective, 147, 149
Functional relation, 93, 95
Functionally equivalent, 111, 113
Functions of behavior, 21, 31, 162f

G
Gait, 56, 57
Gender identity, 121

Generalization, 183, 185
    types of, 262f
Goal
    long-term, 90t
    short-term, 90t
Grant reviews, 330b
Graph, 176, 178, 179f
    behavioral data, displays of, 46–47, 49, 51–52t, 53f, 229
Group homes, 127, 128

H
Habilitation, 27
Harmful reinforcers, avoiding, 297b
High-probability request sequence, 205, 206

I
Imitation, 183, 185
Implementation, 280–281
Implementation-based case studies
    adolescence, 191–203
    adulthood, 204–224
    preschool children, 158–169, 175–188
    school-age children, 169–175
Incidental teaching, 271f
Inclusive classroom, 36, 37
Independent living, 127, 288
Independent variable, 245, 247
Indirect assessment of individuals, 30t
Indirect measurement of behavior, 294, 295
Individualized behavior-change programs, 215b, 265b. See also Behavior-change programs
Informed consent, 315b, 326b, 332
    checklist, 33t
Informed decisions, 343
In-person solicitation, 360b
Integrity, 18b, 346–347b
    procedural, 64, 66t
Intellectual disability, 294
Intellectual property, 359b
Intensity, 159, 161
Intensive behavioral intervention (IBI), 11, 12
    transition to full-time school setting, timeline for, 23f
Interdisciplinary team, 86–87, 88
Internal validity, 289t
Interobserver agreement (IOA), 193, 195, 196, 197t, 296
Interrupting or discontinuing services, 274b
Intervention, 86–88, 93, 95, 96f, 97f, 111, 337
    condition, 233
    phases of, 230

planning, 85
programs, 119
Intervention package, 68, 70, 241f
Intraverbal training, 183, 185
Interverbals, 36
Interviews, 111, 113
    functional assessment, 116f
"I want ..." board, 106, 107, 109

J
Journal reviews, 330b

K
Knowledge, 25, 62, 164

L
Language delay, 93
Learning, 58
    disability, 68, 69, 71, 76
Least restrictive procedures, 173b, 335b, 346,
    352b
Least-to-most prompt hierarchy, 230, 233
Level, 238, 240
Life span, 68, 119
Living, 46
Logic model, 284, 285
Long-term goal, 90t

M
Maintenance, 111, 113
Mand, 36
Mastery criteria for behavior assessment, 66t
Measurement, 246, 255, 275, 276, 284, 292t
    of practice, 337
Media-based services, 359–360b
Media presentations, 359–360b
Mediator model of behavior intervention, 62,
    63, 93, 95, 96f, 97f, 157, 237, 249, 251f
Medical causes, 147, 147f, 148
Medical consultation, 150b, 265b
Misrepresentation by noncertified individuals,
    discouraging, 353b
Multidisciplinary program evaluation team,
    366, 367
Multidisciplinary teams, 86, 218
Multiple baseline design, 252, 254, 256t
Multiple relationships, 357b, 364b
Multiple treatment designs, types of, 242–243t

N
Natural environment teaching (NET), 111, 113
Negative punishment, 98t, 135t

Negative reinforcement, 68, 70, 135t
Noncertified individuals, discouraging, 353b
Nonexperimental designs, 229
Nonverbal behavior, 311

O
Objective measurement systems, 191
Observations, 112, 113
Occupational therapists (OT), 19, 21, 88, 89,
    219
Operationalizing, 121, 122
Organizational behavior management, 361, 362
Outcome measures, 286
Output measures, 282, 286
Overcorrection, 199, 200
    procedures, 202f
    restitutional, 199, 200, 202f

P
Parametric analysis, 276, 278
Paraprofessionals, 27, 28, 121, 197t
Parental consent, 311
Parents, 157, 166–167, 171–172, 175
Peer(s)
    comparison chart, for interval recording,
        168t
    pushing behavior, during afterschool care,
        168f
    relationships, 49, 56, 57, 64, 70
Person-centered planning, considerations in
    utilizing, 281f
Physically restraining, 348, 349
Physicians, 85
Picture exchange communication system,
    phases of, 109f, 220f
Plagiarism, 330b
Planning-focused case studies
    adolescence, 119–151
    adulthood, 126–151
    preschool children, 86–105, 110–117,
        119–126
    school-age children, 105–110
Positive behavior support (PBS), 275, 277
    evaluation questionnaire, 282t
Positive punishment, 98t, 135t
Positive reinforcement, 135t, 159, 170, 176
Practice
    best, 85
    evidence-based, 344, 346
    measurement of, 337
    skills, 355–361
    standards of, 320, 321

Premack principle, 205, 207
Preschool children
    behavior assessment, 4–26
    case studies
        evaluation-centered, 229–266
        implementation-based, 158–169,
            175–188
        planning-focused, 86–105, 110–117,
            119–126
    research and ethics, 308–314, 323–327
Private practice, 354, 355
Problematic behaviors, 160, 175, 275, 276
Procedural adherence, 62, 213
Procedural drift, 199, 201
Procedural identity checks, 191
Procedural integrity, 64
    checklist, 66t
Professional competence, 312, 313
Professional development, maintaining
    competence through, 358b
Professional relationships, 25b, 125b, 315b
Program evaluation, 268, 269, 366–367, 368
    form, quick assessment, 301t
Progressive discipline, 141
Prompt(s/ing), 205, 365b
    response, 137–138t
    stimulus, 136–137t
    verbal, 12
Property destruction behavior, 299t
Protection of dignity, 348, 349
Psychological Assessment Screen for Adults
    with Developmental Disabilities
    (PAS-ADD), 295
Psychological factors, 119, 132
Psychologists, 85
Public statements, 358b
Punishment, 38, 100, 102, 172, 184
    difficulties with, 98t
    negative, 98t, 135t
    positive, 98t, 135t
    procedures, 104b, 144b, 173b, 203b, 352b
Pyramid model for school-wide positive
    behavior, 280f

Q
Quality of life, 5, 41
Questionnaires, 112, 113
Questions about Behavior Function (QABF)
    questionnaire, 295

R
Rapport, 87, 88
Rating matrix, 50t
Receptive identification, 231f

Receptive language, 230
    training, issues and solutions during, 236t
Records, 169 b
Reinforcement, 11, 16, 17, 62
    negative, 68, 70, 135t, 170, 176
    positive, 135t, 170, 176
    procedures, types of, 103f
    schedules of, 50f, 193
Reinforcer, 193
    survey, 205, 206
Relationships
    environment–behavior, 45
    exploitative, 365b
    functional, 93, 95
    multiple, 357b, 364b
    peer, 49, 57, 64, 71
    professional, 25b, 125b, 315b
    scientific, 25b, 125b, 315b
Relevance of behavior rule, 27, 29
Reliability of measurement, 55, 59, 59f
Reliance on scientific knowledge, 323–324b
Repeatability, 164, 166
Replacement behaviors, 111, 161
Replication, 288
    systematic, 288, 290
Reporting, 325–326b
Research, 327, 328
    ethics board, 312, 313
    participants, 327, 328
Resistance, 112, 113
Response interruption and redirection (RIRD)
    program, 297, 298
Response prompts, 137–138t
Responsibility, 41b
Responsible research, characteristics of,
    316–318b, 318b
Restitutional overcorrection, 199, 201, 203f
Restraint, 348, 349
Reversal/withdrawal treatment design, 238,
    240, 256t
Rewards, 141, 143
Rights and prerogatives of clients, 340b
Right to effective behavioral treatment (RBT),
    319–320, 317, 358b
Risk of harm, 341b, 351b

S
Safe space, 148, 149
Scatterplot, 259, 260
School
    challenging behavior at, 124t
    children (*see* School-age children)
School-age children
    behavior assessment, 26–41

case studies
    evaluation-centered, 229–265
    implementation-based, 169–176
    planning-focused, 105–110
  research and ethics, 319–326, 331–341
Science, 164
Scientific merit rating scale (SMRS), 292*t*
Scientific relationships, 25*b*, 125*b*, 315*b*
Self-care checklists, 302–305*f*
Self-injurious behavior, 259, 264*f*
Self-management, 77, 79
Self-monitoring, 77, 79, 247
Seniors, 191, 277, 278
  research and ethics, 366–371
Shaping, 171, 172
Short-term goal, 90*t*
Sign language, 20, 21
Skill acquisition template, 174–175*t*
Skill-deficit approach versus strength-based
    approach, 129*t*
Skill development, 47, 49, 191
Skilled practice, 355–361
Social activities, 267
Social factors, 119
Social significance, 5, 7, 22*f*, 259
  checklist for determining, 15*t*
Social skills, 56, 57, 58, 128
  teaching, data collection in, 279*t*
Special education teachers, 85
Speech and language pathologists (SLP), 19,
    21, 89
Stakeholders, 366, 367
Standards of Practice for ABA, 320, 321
Statements by others, 359*b*
Stimulus
  antecedent, 211, 213
  control, 211, 213, 215*f*
  delta, 214*f*
  discriminative, 211, 214
  equivalence, 217, 219, 222*f*, 224*t*
  prompts, 136–137*t*
Strength-based approach, 129*t*
  case examples using, 130*t*
  versus skill-deficit approach, 129*t*
Strengths checklist, 24*f*
Structure, 100
Successive approximations, 171
Supervised practice, 354, 355
Supervisees, providing feedback, 352–353*b*,
    370*b*
Supervision
  effective, designing, 370–371*b*

effects, evaluation of, 370*b*
Supervisors, behavior analysts as, 369*b*
Supervisory delegation, 369*b*
Supervisory volume, 369*b*
Systematic replication, 288, 290

T
Tact, 218, 219
Target behavior, 5
Teachers, 157, 178, 185
Teaching targets, 231, 233, 232–233*f*
Technology, 157
Temporal extent, 164, 166
Temporal locus, 165, 166
Terminal behavior, 171
Terms of reference, developing, 89*t*
Testimonials, 360*b*
Text-to-speech, 132, 133
Third-party involvement in services, 34*b*, 96*b*,
    151*b*, 263*b*
Three-term contingency, 102*f*
Timely response, 325–326*b*
Time-out, 11, 18*t*, 159
Token economy, cycle of, 181*f*
Topography-based definition of behavior, 159
Transition planning, 126, 128, 129
Treatment drift, 247, 249*f*
Treatment fidelity, 245, 247
  assessment grid, 250*t*
  checklist, 249*f*
Treatment/intervention efficacy, 18*b*, 54*b*,
    339–340*b*
Trend, 236, 237
Triadic mediator model of interaction, 251*f*
Typically developing, 5, 6

U
Unstructured time, 121, 122
Updating of information provided to BACB,
    325–326*b*
Use of data, 368–369*b*

V
Validity
  construct, 291*t*
  internal, 291*t*
  external, 288, 290, 291*t*
  of measurement, 56, 59, 59*f*
Variability, 239, 240
VB-MAPP, 47, 256, 257*f*
Verbal behavior, 183, 184, 311
  approach to teaching language, 90*t*

Verbal operants, 159, 161, 187*f*
Verbal prompt, 12
Visual analysis, 177
    of graphed data, difficulties with, 272*f*
Visual schedule, 77, 78, 107
    implementation of, 208*f*

W
Wechsler Individual Assessment Test-II
    (WIAT-II), 74

Wechsler Intelligence Scale for Children
    (WISC-V), 73
Word prediction, 132, 133

X
X-axis, 177

Y
Y-axis, 177

9 783319 447926